Early praise for
Emerging Adulthood
A Psychodynamic Approach to the New Developmental Phase of the 21st Century

"In the closing chapters of their 2014 book, *Normal Child and Adolescent Development: A Psychodynamic Primer*, Karen J. Gilmore, M.D., and Pamela Meersand, Ph.D., make a clear distinction between development of late adolescents from ages 17 to 21 and that of emerging adults during the "Odyssey years" from 21 to 30. In this new book, the authors challenge contemporary characterizations of emerging adulthood as one phase spanning the years 18 to 30 and provide further cogent arguments for differentiating two segments, each with its own tasks, achievements, and attitudes. They carefully articulate aspects of experimentation and exploration during the late adolescent/early emerging adult years in the late teens and early 20s, when adult realities still seem far off in the future, in contrast to late emerging adulthood, when choices about that future become imperative. This work stands out for its integration of multiple perspectives, its illuminating vignettes that show many paths toward adulthood followed not only by college students but also by other emerging adults, and its focus on the mental health vulnerabilities and needs of this cohort. Throughout, the authors convey the value of psychoanalytic and psychodynamic principles and insights for understanding and treating young people who are headed for an adulthood that is itself undergoing transformations."

Denia G. Barrett, M.S.W., Co-Editor-in-Chief, Psychoanalytic Study of the Child; Past President, Association for Child Psychoanalysis; and Faculty, Chicago Psychoanalytic Institute

"First and foremost, the psychoanalytic model of the mind is a developmental one. From its beginnings, psychoanalysts have emphasized that current-day mental function and dysfunction are rooted in and affected by developmental and maturational experiences. One of the most prominent supports for psychoanalysis as an evidence-based science and therapy is, in fact, its long history of developmental research. This history is the context for this new and very important book by Karen J. Gilmore, M.D., and Pamela Meersand, Ph.D. It joins their other books on child and adolescent development and on the importance of play as an essential vehicle for bringing psychoanalysis into the twenty-first century.

In this book, they bring Arnett's concept of emerging adulthood into the psychoanalytic fold, enriching both. Doing so deepens Arnett's intriguing thinking by integrating a psychodynamic, intrapsychic perspective into an otherwise more phenomenological, sociocultural emphasis. Their integration also strengthens a weak link in psychoanalytic developmental thinking—that stage traditionally called *late adolescence*. This amorphous period of the life cycle, lying between adolescence proper and adulthood, has been an ambiguous area for psychoanalysis with its ever-expanding age range and its vaguely articulated characteristics.

In particular, they emphasize the huge sociocultural shifts in Western society during this century. These shifts have profoundly altered the anticipation of and planning for the future in those who graduate high school. As they say, this generation has taken to heart the mantra that there is no hurry to decide what one will be or do when one grows up. This newfound attitude delays traditional markers of adulthood like marriage and career longer and longer. Gilmore and Meersand note that these markers are no longer even seen as signifiers of adulthood by those in the emerging adulthood field.

To date, there has not been a comprehensive review of the research on this new developmental concept or attempt to consider its clinical ramifications. This volume accomplishes these tasks impressively. In addition, it uses the challenges to traditional developmental thinking posed by the concept of emerging adulthood to reconsider and reorganize our psychoanalytic developmental theory of the mind. Hence, it is a must-read for all psychodynamically oriented clinicians and students in allied fields."

Alan Sugarman, Ph.D., Training and Supervising Child, Adolescent, and Adult Psychoanalyst, San Diego Psychoanalytic Center; and Former and Founding Head of the Department of Psychoanalytic Education, American Psychoanalytic Association

EMERGING ADULTHOOD

A Psychodynamic Approach to the
New Developmental Phase of the 21st Century

EMERGING ADULTHOOD

A Psychodynamic Approach to the
New Developmental Phase of the 21st Century

Karen J. Gilmore, M.D.
Pamela Meersand, Ph.D.

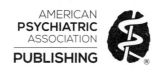

AMERICAN
PSYCHIATRIC
ASSOCIATION
PUBLISHING

Copyright © 2024 American Psychiatric Association Publishing
ALL RIGHTS RESERVED
First Edition
Manufactured in the United States of America on acid-free paper
27 26 25 24 23   5 4 3 2 1

American Psychiatric Association Publishing
800 Maine Avenue SW, Suite 900
Washington, DC 20024-2812
www.appi.org

Library of Congress Cataloging-in-Publication Data
Names: Gilmore, Karen J., 1948- author. | Meersand, Pamela, 1956- author. | American Psychiatric Association Publishing, issuing body.
Title: Emerging adulthood : a psychodynamic approach to the new developmental phase of the 21st century / Karen J. Gilmore, M.D., Pamela Meersand, Ph.D.
Description: First edition. | Washington, DC : American Psychiatric Association Publishing, 2023. | Includes bibliographical references and index.
Identifiers: LCCN 2023010706 (print) | LCCN 2023010707 (ebook) | ISBN 9781615374199 (paperback ; alk. paper) | ISBN 9781615374205 (ebook)
Subjects: MESH: Psychology, Adolescent | Adolescent Behavior | Adolescent Development | Young Adult--psychology
Classification: LCC RJ503 (print) | LCC RJ503 (ebook) | NLM WS 462 | DDC 616.8900835--dc23/eng/20230714
LC record available at https://lccn.loc.gov/2023010706
LC ebook record available at https://lccn.loc.gov/2023010707

British Library Cataloguing in Publication Data
A CIP record is available from the British Library.

Contents

PART I

Introduction

PART II

Phases of Emerging Adolescence

PART III

Developmental Tasks and the Role of the Peer Group in Emerging Adulthood

PART IV

Mental Health in Emerging Adulthood

Video Access: www.appi.org/GilmoreEmerging

About the Authors

Karen J. Gilmore, M.D., is Clinical Professor of Psychiatry in the Department of Psychiatry at Columbia University College of Physicians and Surgeons and Training and Supervising Analyst at Columbia University Center for Psychoanalytic Training and Research in New York, New York.

Pamela Meersand, Ph.D., is Associate Clinical Professor of Medical Psychology in the Department of Psychiatry at Columbia University College of Physicians and Surgeons and Director of the Child Division at Columbia University Center for Psychoanalytic Training and Research in New York, New York.

Disclosure of Interests

The authors affirm that they have no competing interests or affiliations that present or could appear to present a conflict of interest with regard to the content and publication of this book.

Preface

The idea of emerging adulthood as a new developmental phase was proposed by Jeffrey Arnett, Ph.D., in an article titled "Emerging Adulthood: A Theory of Development From the Late Teens Through the Twenties" (Arnett 2000). This proposal and the research that soon followed have had a remarkable effect on contemporary views about the years preceding adulthood, how these are traversed, and what kind of development happens. Although the recognition of *something* of developmental significance between late adolescence and adulthood has been present in the literature for about half a century—termed *youth*, the *transition to adulthood*, *late adolescence*, *young adulthood*, and the like—the full emergence of a phase with its own tasks and challenges awaited the radical technological, informational, and communicational changes of twenty-first-century Western society. Despite controversy and detractors (see Côté 2014; Kloep and Hendry 2011; Swanson 2016; Twenge 2013), the presence of this entity—that is, a cohort with recognizable features, not quite adult and no longer adolescent—is increasingly acknowledged by many neighboring disciplines: research psychology, developmental psychology, sociology, psychoanalysis, psychiatry, pediatrics, and adolescent psychiatry. Similarly, its bidirectional interfaces with cultural transformations are widely recognized. Given the vast number of research papers devoted to the new concept of emerging adulthood (more than 1.5 million in a recent library search during May 2023), our mission in this book is to create a psychodynamic synthesis of the accumulated research on emerging adults in juxtaposition with a deeper exploration of emerging adulthood as a developmental phase.

This paradigm shift in conceptualizing the arc of human development occurred midstream in our consecutive roles directing the Child and Adolescent Psychoanalysis program at the Columbia University Center for Psychoanalytic Training and Research, where we taught a year-long course on human development. Although we have always considered the immediate post–high school years to be properly understood as late adolescence, a subphase of adolescence with its own developmental tasks and trajectory, Arnett's new conceptualization ultimately incorporated age 18 years through the third decade in its entirety. To us, this conflated the contemporary but nonetheless recognizable late adolescent journey with elements extending deep into the 20s. Although it could be argued that this extension is just the same process attenuated, to us the extension signals the real change in the process, because it suggests that the tasks of late adolescence, historically understood as individuation and resolution of the identity crisis, not only are unresolved but also remain fluid for a decade-long evolution as young people gradually become engaged in the rest of their lives. As a consequence, our preference is to see the emerging adult time frame as meaningfully partitioned into two segments: early emerging adulthood (late adolescence) and late emerging adulthood.

The most important change is this decade of something new between the end of compulsory schooling and adulthood, accompanied by its own developmental challenges, emerging ego capacities, alterations in mental life, and sensibilities. The traditional progression of late adolescence to adulthood has expanded into more than a decade of experimentation, a space in which young people on the brink of adulthood explore identity and commitments as they enter into real life—a real life that is markedly different from the past and likely to continue its relentless transformations into the future. Although we disagree with Arnett's elimination of late adolescence as a unique developmental entity, which we discuss in detail in Chapter 3 ("Late Adolescence: The First Phase of Emerging Adulthood"), we concur that emerging adulthood (which, despite its early wobbly parameters, typically comprises most of the third decade of life) should be considered a developmental entity in its own right. It is not merely a prolongation or an extension of the adolescent process but rather a new chapter in role exploration and identity formation that has distinct experiential qualities. Furthermore, despite its lack of biological markers, it is typically accompanied by a sharp subjective sense of onset and of closure.

In addition, the idea of emerging adulthood has proved illuminating in the clinic; our experience with people in this age group resonates with many of the ideas that evolved from Arnett's theory. It stimulated us to reformulate the way we conceptualize the years approaching adulthood in teaching and writing. Beginning with a chapter in our earlier book *Normal Child and Adolescent Development* (Gilmore and Meersand 2014), we explored this period, felicitously termed *the Odyssey years* by David Brooks; this was followed by papers and presentations by ourselves and other psychoanalytic thinkers (Gilmore 2019; Knight and Miller 2017; Miller 2017; Schechter et al. 2018; Shulman 2017). The massive research literature is nonetheless challenging to tackle. We present this book as an attempt to integrate psychiatric, psychological, sociological, psychoanalytic, and research findings about the typical development of emerging adults for trainees and experienced clinicians in psychoanalysis, psychiatry, and psychology. We hope that this admittedly ambitious synthesis provides a foundation for ongoing developmental insights into this age group and for a growing understanding of the active interface of twenty-first-century cultural changes and the process and meaning of achieving adulthood in today's world.

To our way of thinking, developmental considerations are insufficiently integrated into clinical thinking, especially as they relate to patients past mid-adolescence. The recognition and delineation of the developmental phase of emerging adulthood in the twenty-first century highlight—even insist on—the importance of developmental factors for understanding a cohort whose more dramatic problems and behaviors tend to dominate assessments. Attention is directed mostly to their problems (including borderline personality disorder, risky behaviors, suicidality, and other dramatic manifestations of psychopathology) or to behaviors incomprehensible to the current adult generation (such as nonbinary approaches to gender and sexuality, the obsession with new media, and the tendency to engage in peer groups of their own making). Evidence of psychopathology is the usual focus, eclipsing the developmental challenges of stabilizing identity in a rapidly transforming society, sustaining a moral compass, and discovering personal meaning in a globalized world. Today, the power and status of the parent generation are not the typical sources of inspiration: emerging adults do not idealize and aspire to the model of venerated adults whose accomplishments rest on tradition and the canon; rather, their heroes are wildly successful and/or creative peers. Even more alien to the parent generation is the reality that an individual's true maturational status, resiliency, and social adaptation are continuously challenged by a rapidly changing culture, which makes flexibility, adaptability, and vision key capacities for traversing adulthood.

In Chapter 1, "A Brief Review of Developmental Theory," we offer a selective review of the many theories of development that have been proposed historically and are still in use, review our basic approach to human development as described in our book *Normal Child and Adolescent Development* (Gilmore and Meersand 2014), and apply and elaborate that approach to illuminate this stage. Certainly, every aspect of developmental progression is affected by the insertion of this extended period when adult commitments are postponed in favor of exploration, experimentation, and the freedom to *not commit*. Therefore, it is inevitable that late adolescence bears its impact; this is equally the case regarding the concept of adulthood, especially as adulthood has been unchanged for almost a century and is in need of examination (Hunter 2009). In this regard, the notion of "established adulthood" (Mehta et al. 2020) is a beginning, but it fails to encompass the effect on mental life of a global culture, a world where emulation of the prior generation is markedly diminished relative to the importance of peers, where achievements achieve affirmation via social media, and where invention occurs in a mediated environment. Chapter 2, "Development in the Period Between Adolescence and Adulthood," is an introduction to a developmental perspective on the new phase; we review Arnett's criteria that, with a single exception, have limited developmental import and examine the problems with his original theory that have affected subsequent research and resisted efforts to deepen its basic premises. We then look at the lively interface between contemporary culture and human development. We highlight what happens to identity formation and sense of self as a significant member of the global culture in addition to the effect of the vastly augmented role of the peer group.

The part consisting of Chapter 3 and Chapter 4 ("What Is Distinct About the Second Part of Emerging Adulthood?") is dedicated to detailed descriptions of the developmental process leading to adulthood and the progression of developmental tasks. In Chapter 3, we discuss today's late adolescence as the first phase of emerging adulthood, highlighting the ego capacities, developmental tasks and challenges, and changing relationships of the group ages 18 to 23. We describe the ways in which the unique aspects of this phase, in which the young adult embarks on a period of increasing autonomy and beginning identity exploration, and its social context distinguish it from both earlier adolescence and later emerging adulthood.

In Chapter 4, we examine what we consider the new developmental phase proper, extending from ages 24 to 30. In this lengthy interval, social changes interface with individual development and shape its contours. Today's young people are evolving in the midst of a kaleidoscope of changes in contemporary society, including technological advances, global communication, social media, the disappearance of privacy, artificial intelligence, and other twenty-first-century phenomena.

In Chapter 5, "Identity in Emerging Adulthood," we examine the concept of identity, its crucial function in personality, and the process by which young individuals begin to experiment within different domains of self-expression and self-definition. We review contemporary research on the identity exploration process, on major identity domains such as gender, and on problems of identity consolidation. For our segment on racial/ethnic identity, we sought consultation with Dr. William Cross, a renowned scholar on the subject of race and development.

In Chapter 6, "Youth Culture," we explore a phenomenon that began after World War II and flowered in the twenty-first century. It consists of the spontaneous formation of peer groups that evolve from shared interests and lifestyle. In some ways, participation in a youth culture provides the guide rails for the future, taking over the role of college campuses, parental advice, and broader community identifiers in the process of identity formation.

In Chapter 7, "Psychopathology and Emerging Adulthood," we discuss the socioemotional challenges and psychiatric conditions that tend to arise during the late teens and 20s. Our developmental and psychodynamic framework examines psychopathology within the context of the emerging adult's unique personal history, attachments, and biologically based vulnerabilities as well as the pressures and demands of emerging adult life. We cover an array of mental health conditions, including anxiety and depression, suicidality, alcohol and substance use, eating disorders, and problems of identity.

In Chapter 8, "Therapeutic Modalities in the Treatment of Emerging Adults," we outline the array of mental health interventions available for this age group and consider their relative success in engaging a population in an unprecedented developmental period distinguished by rapid flux and transformation and by resistance to traditional categories and definitive statements about identity and indeed favoring no commitments and the freedom to choose in all aspects of identity formation. In contrast to some previous youth generations' cultivated mistrust of adults, the obstacle in communication today seems to originate in the adult generation's profound, but nonetheless sincere, lack of comprehension of the pathways and identities, the rate of change, and the dissolution of conventional hierarchies and boundaries that the emerging adult generation presents; the adult mental health professional frequently mistakes these for psychopathology.

Chapter 9, "Conclusion," is our summary and conclusion, in which we observe that some familiar descriptors of maturation reflect processes at work in the late emerging adult. However, this is not a maturation that would suit any epoch in history; it is a kind of maturation that favors flexibility and readiness to change course. Given the degree to which the tasks of emerging adulthood poach a decade from adulthood, it can only mean that these are capacities that foster adaptation to the extraordinary evolutionary, social, and technological advances in today's world.

References

Arnett JJ: Emerging adulthood: a theory of development from the late teens through the twenties. Am Psychol 55(5):469–480, 2000 10842426

Côté JE: The dangerous myth of emerging adulthood: an evidence-based critique of a flawed developmental theory. Appl Dev Sci 18(4):177–188, 2014

Gilmore K: Is emerging adulthood a new developmental phase? J Am Psychoanal Assoc 67:625–653, 2019

Gilmore KJ, Meersand P: Normal Child and Adolescent Development: A Psychodynamic Primer. Arlington, VA, American Psychiatric Publishing, 2014

Hunter JD: Wither adulthood? The Hedgehog Review, Spring 2009. Available at: https://hedgehogreview.com/issues/youth-culture/articles/wither-adulthood. Accessed November 17, 2022.

Kloep M, Hendry LB: A systemic approach to transitions to adulthood, in Debating Emerging Adulthood: Stage or Process? Edited by Arnett JJ, Kloep M, Hendry LB, et al. New York, Oxford University Press, 2011, pp 53–76

Knight R, Miller JM: Emerging adulthood: a developmental phase: an introduction to the section. Psychoanal Study Child 70:5–7, 2017

Mehta CM, Arnett JJ, Palmer CG, et al: Established adulthood: a new conception of ages 30 to 45. Am Psychol 75(4):431–444, 2020 32378940

Miller JM: Young or emerging adulthood: a psychoanalytic view. Psychoanal Study Child 70(1):8–21, 2017

Schechter M, Herbstman B, Ronningstam E, et al: Emerging adults, identity development, and suicidality: implications for psychoanalytic psychotherapy. Psychoanal Study Child 71(1):20–39, 2018

Shulman S: The emerging adulthood years: finding one's way in career and intimate love relationships. Psychoanal Study Child 70:40–62, 2017

Swanson JA: Trends in literature about emerging adulthood: review of empirical studies. Emerg Adult 4:391–402, 2016

Twenge JM: Overwhelming evidence for generation me: a reply to Arnett. Emerg Adulthood 1:21–26, 2013

Acknowledgments

The copyrighted lyrics used in Chapter 6 were reprinted with permission as follows:

CHANGES
Words and Music by DAVID BOWIE
© 1973 (Renewed) TINTORETTO MUSIC and BMG RIGHTS MANAGEMENT (US) LLC
All Rights for TINTORETTO MUSIC Administered by WARNER-TAMERLANE MUSIC.
All Rights Reserved
Used by Permission of ALFRED MUSIC

Changes
Words and Music by David Bowie
Copyright© 1971 EMI Music Publishing Ltd., Tintoretto Music and BMG Rights Management (UK) Limited
Copyright Renewed
All Rights on behalf of EMI Music Publishing Ltd. Administered by Sony Music Publishing (US) LLC, 424 Church Street, Suite 1200, Nashville, TN 37219
All Rights on behalf of Tintoretto Music Administered by Warner-Tamerlane Publishing Corp.
All Rights on behalf of BMG Rights Management (UK) Ltd. Administered by BMG Rights Management (US) LLC
International Copyright Secured   All Rights Reserved
Reprinted by Permission of Hal Leonard Europe Ltd.

The Bigger Picture
Words and Music by Dominique Jones, Noah Pettigrew and Rai'Shaun Williams
Copyright© 2020 UNIVERSAL MUSIC CORP., QUALITY CONTROL QC PRO, WOLF PACK GLOBAL MUSIC PUBLISHING,

THE BIGGER PICTURE

Video Guide

**The companion videos can be viewed online at
www.appi.org/GilmoreEmerging**

Callouts in the text identify the videos by name, as shown in the following example:

 Video #: Video Title

The videos are streamed via the internet and can be viewed online by navigating to **www.appi.org/GilmoreEmerging** and using the embedded video player. The videos are optimized for most current operating systems, including mobile operating systems.

This video series comprises eight brief clips, drawn from our individual interviews with emerging adults between ages 20 and 30 years. Each young person was asked open-ended questions designed to elicit how they think and feel about themselves within major areas of life, including family, friendships, romantic connections, work, values, and interests. We hoped to learn how this small group of open and articulate emerging adults are negotiating interpersonal and societal challenges, linking their current with their younger selves, and envisioning their future lives. Responses to one or two more pointed queries, such as how the coronavirus SARS-CoV-2 disease (COVID-19) pandemic affected or interrupted daily life, are included in some of the video segments. In their own unique ways, all eight of the interviewees show the trends of the emerging adulthood developmental period: they are interested in self-development, there is a sense that things are not yet settled, the future is seen as offering possibilities, they explore various aspects of identity, and they conceptualize themselves as on the way to but not yet quite within adulthood proper.

When viewed in tandem with the book, these short videos provide a tangible and highly individualized depiction of the broader concepts addressed more abstractly within the text; in particular, they highlight the complicated, multifaceted, and gradual process of identity development, in which emerging adults explore and synthesize domains of self-definition (beliefs and values, sense of family and community, interests and goals, gender and sexuality). The young people in the videos describe their unique journeys from childhood and adolescence toward adulthood, weaving new experiences, family relationships, personal history and culture, peer influences, and mentors with their evolving self-concepts. These eight emerging adults represent a small but diverse group with a range of racial/ethnic identities, family attachments, personal obstacles, and ambitions for the future. We hope that the video dimension of this volume engages the reader/viewer in a multimodal learning experience that vividly conveys the richness and complexity of the emerging adulthood years.

How to Use the Book and Videos Together

The reader should use the **boldface video prompts** embedded in the text of Chapters 3 through 6 as signals for viewing the associated clips online by navigating to www.appi.org/GilmoreEmerging and using the embedded video player.

The following section contains further details about each individual video clip.

Video Descriptions

The eight video clips depict different aspects of the emerging adulthood experience, illustrated through the lens of each individual's unique family background, current occupations and relationships, and visions for their future. In each video, the young person looks backward and creates short autobiographical narratives that represent meaningful links between past and present; in addition, current situations (work, recreation, relationships) are described, and hopes and worries for the future are also referenced.

Chapter 3: Late Adolescence: The First Phase of Emerging Adulthood

- **Video 1: Adjusting to life without parental oversight (20-year-old student) (14:55)**

- **Video 2: Finding a place in the gaming world (20-year-old gamer) (22:16)**

Video 1, **"Adjusting to life without parental oversight,"** depicts a 20-year-old college student who is negotiating a range of identity domains while staying closely connected to family. They have to grapple with the tasks of managing newfound freedoms without the familiar parental support and supervision. Enrolled in a 4-year university program, their lifelong interests in creative arts, and more recent explorations into self and gender, create inner tension when they are considered in light of traditional-minded Asian parents who strongly favor more conventional professions. They anticipate a need to integrate their chosen career path, in the arts, with some pragmatic concerns, such as earning a living. In addition, we hear about the effect of the COVID-19 pandemic, which restricted the college social experience.

Video 2, **"Finding a place in the gaming world,"** illustrates a different trajectory taken by a 20-year-old gamer who left community college after a year and began to fulfill an intense, lifelong interest in gaming. After he joined a video gaming organization, which provided a platform for competitive playing and access to a large group of like-minded individuals who saw gaming as a way of life, he discovered a community in which he found friendship and mentorship, the opportunity to pursue philosophical and historical interests, and a potential pathway toward financial independence. He has other strong bonds, such as those to his girlfriend and to his mother, whom he sees as having sacrificed a great deal for his welfare and development.

Chapter 4: What Is Distinct About the Second Part of Emerging Adulthood?

- **Video 3: Creating a professional identity during emerging adulthood (25-year-old young architect) (16:07)**
- **Video 4: Late emerging adult and a creative path forward (26-year-old graduate student) (19:02)**

In Video 3, **"Creating a professional identity during emerging adulthood,"** a 25-year-old architect reflects on a demanding and specific career pathway, which overstructured his college experience and may have prematurely foreclosed his identity exploration, and looks back on the ways in which it shaped choices and opportunities in his late teens and 20s. He is beginning to look forward in a serious way, wondering if his professional role will support the kind of future he envisions, ultimately with a partner and children. In addition, he discusses the importance of his family and of their culture and the influence of his immigrant experience as a child, moving from Venezuela to the United States and then to Costa Rica. He also describes the role of a slightly older mentor, who shares some of his professional and personal experiences and who has provided guidance and support. The architect's drive, his commitment, his success in his career, and his mature relationship heighten the impression that he moved into adulthood too quickly, albeit successfully, perhaps to manage the geographic instability of his earlier years and to set an independent course.

Video 4, **"Late emerging adult and a creative path forward,"** features a 26-year-old graduate student who is studying creative writing and working toward a master of fine arts degree. He reflects on the academic and personal experiences that led him to pursue writing. During the pandemic, he had an identity crisis and battled ruminations, self-doubt, uncertainty, and low mood for a year while preparing his application to programs in creative writing. Much of this state (which had clear depressive overtones) resolved with his admission to an excellent program. He is conscious of his friends' and parents' attitudes toward this potentially ambiguous course of study and aware that it offers a less definite and pragmatic direction than a previous choice (journalism), which he ultimately jettisoned. In addition, he grapples with the consequences of pursuing graduate school and deferring a full-time job, which has created financial dependence on his family and thereby limited his independence.

Chapter 5: Identity in Emerging Adulthood

- **Video 5: Integrating the identity process with a chronic medical condition (29-year-old recruiting and human resources manager) (26:25)**
- **Video 6: Late emerging adult grapples with responsibilities while exploring different roles (27-year-old multimedia artist) (13:11)**

In Video 5, **"Integrating the identity process with a chronic medical condition,"** a 29-year-old recruiting and human resources manager reflects on the effect of a lifelong disability that impedes mobility and causes chronic pain on her evolving sense of self, social experience, and decisions made during her emerging adulthood decade. She recounts how these physical challenges have shaped her visions for the future and her ability to pursue freely her passions and dreams, imposing a need for reality-based considerations. At the same time, her unique struggles have contributed to her own capacity for empathy and understanding and have guided her selection of a life partner toward an individual who is similarly sensitive, serious, and compassionate.

Video 6, **"Late emerging adult grapples with responsibilities while exploring different roles,"** describes how a 27-year-old multimedia artist and dog walker weaves her many creative interests and talents into a lifestyle that takes into account her need to support herself financially. She describes the childhood experiences that she considers formative, such as adjusting to the language and culture of grade school in the United States, at age 6 years, after leaving St. Lucia. She attended college for a time while living at home with her mother, but the pressures of having to study and earn money simultaneously were too burdensome. Her attitude toward her future is optimistic and open; she feels confident that her pattern of working while exploring multiple fields will ultimately yield a good life.

Chapter 6: Youth Culture

- **Video 7: Passion for an athletic activity becomes a life's work (30-year-old parkour expert) (20:13)**
- **Video 8: The "in-between" experience of emerging adulthood (26-year-old former raver) (25:27)**

Video 7, **"Passion for an athletic activity becomes a life's work,"** depicts a 30-year-old parkour expert who has converted a personal passion into a professional and social life. He describes how, as a young college student, he first became enamored of parkour, gradually finding friends, a welcoming and inclusive community, and ultimately a way to earn a living via teaching and coaching. For him, parkour encompasses multiple identity domains: health and wellness, philosophy, social connection, and professional ambitiousness.

Video 8, **"The 'in-between' experience of emerging adulthood,"** features a 26-year-old former raver and ambitious pharmaceutical sales representative who describes integrating various identities, including serious career ambitions, the traditional Jewish values of her family, and her own immersion in "the dating scene" and "the music scene." She enjoys participating in her youth culture by weekend partying but uses her judgment to stay safe. Looking back, she discusses how her initial college choices, which included a major in chemistry, gave way to a realization that she would not be happy in a research field and wanted to gravitate toward a professional path with more interpersonal interactions.

PART I
Introduction

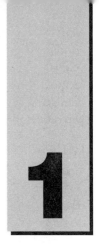

A Brief Review of Developmental Theory

Developmental Theories

Arnett's (2000) theory of emerging adult development joins a host of pre-existing developmental theories that differ by virtue of their comprehensiveness and identification of mechanisms that may operate over the entire trajectory of a life or apply to only one period. Adolescence has famously garnered a host of phase-specific theories since the turn of the twentieth century, including offerings by Anna Freud, Daniel Offer, Peter Blos, Moses Laufer, and others. In contrast, adulthood has received less attention and little theorizing, despite the obvious fact that it is a phase of considerable interest. Arnett's phase of emerging adulthood, positioned between these two phases, has appropriated a substantial segment between ages 18 and 29, borrowing from both the prior late adolescent and the following adult periods. Interestingly, the theory, its description, and its mechanisms have remained relatively unchanged since Arnett's first publication, generating controversy and debate but not refinement or elaboration, despite the massive outpouring of research.

What Is Development?

Development is a common word with general as well as context-specific applications, ranging from the conventional to the highly technical and spanning a wide range of disciplines, from economics to the study of human development. The multiplicity of uses, the many levels of abstraction, and the complexity among the different sectors using the concept are extraordinary. Despite the vast adaptability of the term, there is a shared recognition that it invokes a *change*, an event of significance, typically embedded in a process: some shift has happened that takes things to a new level of organization, size, complexity, or other indicator of difference from what was before. And although the implication is often progressive and positive, that aspect is certainly not universal.

Most disciplines that include such a process incorporate a theory or theories, whether named as such or not, to explain movements within their subject of interest: economists' theories, historians' theories, and scientists' theories all concern themselves with the way that change happens. In the case of human development, such theories address *how* people change over time, from birth to maturity or even death. The "how" includes what drives development; what systems are at play; what is determined by genetics or environment—human and otherwise; what blueprint, pattern, or pathway is involved; and myriad other factors. Moreover, human development involves an array of evolving systems within the individual, such as the body, mental life, and cognition, in conjunction with those that interface with the individual, such as family, subculture, culture, and historical epoch. Among developmental theories, there are differences in conceptualizations of the fundamental forces creating movement, modes of change, and the factors that shape and, in some cases, determine the form of change.

The established developmental progression from infancy to adulthood has been part of educational planning and policy, social institutions and social expectations, protective services, and so on. However, the stage just prior to adulthood has always been ambiguous in the developmental literature. The observable markers of developmental progression that are so prominent in infancy and childhood make early development relatively easy to categorize and, according to some theories, more or less universal, but these markers diminish after puberty and arguably become insignificant. For example, infants are easily identified by their outstanding maturational features, including their lack of motor coordination and language, and by attachment behaviors that uniquely characterize this age group in all societies, even as they may be shaped by culture and family from birth. In contrast to these clear maturational markers, the steps leading to adulthood have been defined almost exclusively by societal norms and cultural expectations; even what constitutes an adult in any given society is a unique cultural construct. Significant maturational features may operate in late adolescence to establish the adult form, but the pace varies widely from individual to individual and has no marker to show the completion of developmental progression to adulthood. Even the important discovery of ongoing brain changes, often cited as the new biological marker of late adolescence and emerging adulthood, do not correlate with any visible sign of change.

Some developmental theories are organized around age stages (Syed 2015) in a given culture—that is, societal groupings of same-age cohorts by virtue of expectations, educational and vocational requirements, social roles, economic factors, and so on. These are inevitably fluid and, by definition, can be readily adapted in response to social changes. The definitions of stages in such theories are unabashedly social constructs, with no claim to universality. In cultures in which mandatory education extends to age 18, the age stages of the first two decades impose a degree of uniformity on experiences and rites of passage. The cohesiveness of age stages fragments as mandatory educational requirements are completed, despite the reality that cultural expectations linked to age persist to varying degrees. Eventually, some version of adult markers historically confer the social status of adulthood on those who achieve them. In our Western European culture, adult markers have been relatively stable for centuries: financial autonomy, independent domicile, marriage, parenthood, and an established career.

Theories of Human Psychosocial Development

A key feature of Arnett's proposal is that emerging adulthood is a new developmental phase; this assertion joins ongoing controversies about broader conceptualizations of the developmental process and arguably invokes a historical paradigm (i.e., developmental phases) that, despite its wide application, has lost favor in the contemporary scientific literature. In this subsection, we offer a brief survey of ascendant developmental paradigms in our field and consider how theories delimit themselves; frame their scope; and hypothesize mechanisms, series, sequences, and patterns.

Because humans are infinitely complex, consisting of a vast number of components and systems, and because they must be understood in their cultural context, developmental thinking figures into an array of social and biological sciences, including medicine, psychology, linguistics, sociology, and embryology. Given the complexity of the subject and the many scientific disciplines dedicated, directly or indirectly, to its study, it is not surprising that developmental theories are plentiful and varied. Moreover, these theories typically reflect the contemporaneous developmental zeitgeist that is favored by the scientific community, such as linear models.

Like other theories of development, those concerning human psychology typically tackle the problem of causality, not only in terms of developmental forces that propel the individual forward but also regarding developmental outcomes. In this context, theories explicitly or implicitly address the nature-nurture continuum and give greater or lesser weight to genetics versus environmental factors. Both nature and nurture have infinite variations, including the gamut of genetic variation and the range of child-rearing practices, parental psychopathology, subcultures, national cultures, societal upheavals, and traumatic events. Genetic factors also have multiple components because gene expression can be powerfully influenced by intrauterine events and early environment. These complexities can be invoked to explain individual and generational outcomes.

Within the group of theories that focus on human development, there are those that concentrate on one element, such as cognition, learning, motor development, language, or psychosexual development, in contrast to other types, sometimes called *grand theories* (Govrin 2006), which purport to explain all development, often by delineating primary mechanisms or forces. Grand theories of psychological development describe a universal process and engine for development of the mind, more or less sweeping away traditional domain boundaries and binaries such as "nature versus nurture, continuity and discontinuity, modularity versus distributed processes" (Gopnik 1996; Thelen 2005, p. 256). For example, Loewenstein et al.'s (1966) *Psychoanalysis—A General Psychology: Essays in Honor of Heinz Hartmann* proposes to explain the entire sweep of psychological developmental progression, including psychopathology, in terms of psychodynamic mechanisms. Systems theory proposes mechanisms of change that are universal in all developmental domains. These grand theories claim to elucidate developmental pathways by delineating one or more unifying mechanisms that operate across the spectrum of domains.

Critics of such ambitious grand developmental propositions protest that different aspects of development require an array of models. Self-regulation may need a different model than cognitive function; the evolution of object relations may demand a different conceptualization than the development of language. Moreover, according to some thinkers, these divergent theories can coexist, each explaining a different phenomenon. This contrasts with the view that fundamental developmental mechanisms figure into the evolution of all domains (Thelen 2005; Thelen and Bates 2003); in the past decades, this premise has figured prominently in its current incarnation as nonlinear systems theory.

Phase Theories

Phase-sequence development has a long history in developmental science and in psychoanalytic thinking, as in the proposals of Sigmund Freud (1905; psychosexual phases), Gesell (Gesell and Amatruda 1945; maturational phases), Piaget and Inhelder (1969; development of cognition), Hartmann (1939, 1964; ego development), Anna Freud (1936; emergence of defenses), and arguably Erikson (1950, 1959; psychosocial development— also claimed by systems theorists and life span theorists). Different phase theories acknowledge the role of many factors but weigh the role of genetic endowment and the unfolding genetic blueprint (Weil 1970), environment, and experience differently. Most phase theories incorporate some concept of biologically driven maturational advances (as in the evolution of libidinal phases in classical Freudian theory or cognitive capacities in Piagetian theory) and the role of heredity, at least in determining the range of potentials. Increasingly, they recognize that the environment must provide adequate nutriment to cultivate maturation potentials (as described by Vargas et al. 2020; Weiss and Saklofske 2020). A further refinement may be the inclusion of *sensitive periods* (the modified human form of critical periods), in which the organism's maturational state requires coordinated environmental nutriment for the evolution of function. Some studies highlight evidence of recoverability; for example, cognitive performance may improve radically with environmental enrichment (Weiss and Saklofske 2020). Similarly, phase theories may differ in their view of *plasticity*, which describes the possibility of modification of sequence and environmental input and transformation of outcomes.

All such theories are built on models that incorporate the following ideas: Development moves toward maturation and increasing differentiation of function, a conceptualization that supports the notion that developmental processes diminish with the declining force of biological maturation. This maturational emergence of functions drives development forward by introducing novel capacities; these in turn facilitate the comprehensive reworking of prior mental organization (Abrams 1983). These reorganizations represent a predetermined sequence of phases with the following features:

1. *The phases are hierarchical.* This implies that there is an invariant sequence, with each new stage representing a step in the progression; although some of the features of the prior stages remain or can be elicited under certain conditions, the overall organization of the new phase is markedly different.

2a.*The phases are internally coherent and consistent.* The developmental domains under consideration are ideally synchronous—all progress simultaneously. This yields a developmental stage in which various aspects of mental function manifest the same level of maturity. In the most extreme version, there is no internal progression toward full function or gradual accrual of elements required for the next phase; strictly interpreted, there is "a zero-order transition period between the initial appearance of each item and its state of functional maturity" (Flavell 1971, p. 425).

2b. *The items within a phase interface to "form conceptual totalities"* (Flavell 1971, p. 445); that is, they organize into coherent patterns and structures and are "self-regulated" (p. 444).

3. *The phases are qualitatively distinct.* Development is not just more of a given capacity, although no doubt capacities persist, are augmented, and mature. There are qualitative changes in mental organization achieved by quantum shifts in said organization due to the maturational entry of novel elements and the effect of new environmental input.

4. *The phases are discontinuous.* That is, despite recognizable elements from prior phases, the new phase reorganizes and repurposes these and/or reconfigures their role in the current level of mental function; there is "continuity of function and discontinuity of organized phases with their inherent mediating structures" (Abrams 1983, p. 115). Thus, to constitute a new phase in a given cohort of a population, one can readily distinguish the mental organization of individuals within it from the mental organization of individuals in prior and future phases, and such unique qualities serve as a "conceptual landmark" (Flavell 1963, pp. 645–646) in the developmental process. Although some stage theorists insist on "abrupt" or quantum shifts in stages of personality development, most have modified the "zero-order transition" concept: stages are marked by the gradual evolution of new capacities that achieve "functional maturity" only after the stage has concluded and the ascendance of the new set of capacities has occurred (Flavell 1971, p. 450).

As noted, phase-sequence developmental concepts have figured prominently in many twentieth-century theories, including Sigmund Freud's theory of psychosexual development; Piaget's theory of cognitive development; and grand developmental theories such as ego psychology, including Anna Freud's work, in particular her notion of development of defenses and developmental lines. There is by no means a singular phase theory.

Ego psychology, which incorporates the phase theory of psychosexual development, dominated North American psychoanalysis in the United States for decades despite critiques that it is a dry, linear, and one-person (i.e., not interpersonal) psychology (Busch 2013, p. 294). Its developmental model has been debunked as a prescriptive linear progression (Balsam and Harris 2012; Coates 1997) that pathologizes deviations from lockstep evolution. However, some of the developmental ideas proposed in ego psychology, such as conflict-free autonomous ego functions, are implicit in many theories: the presence and unfolding of cognitive capacities or the constitutional foundations of resilience and adaptability (Fajardo 1991) are assumed to be inborn potentials that facilitate the child's movement toward greater differentiation and functionality (Hartmann 1939; Weil 1978). Ego psychology was gradually eclipsed by other models in North American psychoanalytic theory, in which the emphasis shifted away from ego development to the interpersonal world as a powerful shaper of human development and the regulator of self-esteem. These later theories privilege the crucial role of the environment, especially the human environment. Unfortunately, the decline in interest in stages has led to a similar decline in theory addressing development beyond early childhood. Without the unifying principle of maturation-driven emergent capacities, subsequent changes are viewed as individual and idiosyncratic.

Ego psychology was a singularly coherent theory in terms of its approach to the developmental trajectory through adolescence, positing a relatively predictable series of emerging ego capacities that interact with experience, bodily development, and the environment. It was concerned with all phases of active development throughout the first two decades, during which physical maturation is prominent. The premise was that ego capacities follow a predetermined maturational sequence and arise as conflict-free functions, interacting with the ego, body, and environment. Indeed, from their moment of emergence, such interactions lead inevitably to the recruitment of a given ego function into conflict and conflict resolution (Weil 1978). This is exemplified by Anna Freud's pioneering work on developmental lines and on defenses, both of which incorporate such an ego psychological foundation. Her formulation of developmental lines especially, unfortunately misrepresented as a linear model (Coates 1997), is more accurately understood as an early foray into a multisystem approach in which clusters of developmental units coalesce and permit shifts to a higher level (Neubauer 1984).

Life Span Theories

As with all theoretical positions, there are several forms of life span theory in the psychological sciences. In the developmental science literature, life span theories (or life course theories) rest on a specific definition of development that embraces an evolutionary orientation: it is a "selective, age-related selection-based change in adaptive capacity" (Baltes et al. 2007, p. 583). The theory places age-related plasticity and adaptation to environmental requirements at the forefront. A life span perspective endorses "a family of theoretical propositions," including the following (Baltes et al. 2007, p. 596):

- Development extends over the life span or life course, and no period of development is more important than the others.

- Development is multidirectional; changes can vary depending on the category of behavior.
- Gains and losses occur simultaneously; there is no simple movement toward a higher level of capacity.
- Plasticity is an important feature of ontogenesis, as are constraints on plasticity within the individual. There are age-related changes in potential (i.e., rising age increasingly limits potential) and therefore age-related shifts in the role of culture in supporting individual adaptation.
- Ontogenesis is inevitably embedded in its historical-cultural moment.
- The paradigm of contextualism asserts that the interface of complex influences, namely, age-graded, history-graded, and nonnormative factors, determines individual development.
- Development is multidisciplinary; an exclusively psychological viewpoint is inevitably a partial perspective (Baltes 1987, p. 613). Life span theories diverge from traditional phase theories in several important ways, including in the basic assumptions that development continues throughout the course of life and that plasticity is an enduring feature of ontogenesis (Baltes et al. 2007), positions at odds with the notion that mental structure is completed and stabilized at the close of adolescence.

The psychoanalytic developmental literature also has a school of life span developmental theory, popularized during the 1980s, that takes an expansive view of development as a lifelong process (Colarusso and Nemiroff 1979; Emde 1985) rather than harnessing it to physical maturation and the emergence of novel ego capacities. The focus is on the vicissitudes of self-regulatory capacity, beginning with the mother-infant interaction and progressing until autonomy and adaptive function are self-maintained. It is never "finished," because destabilization continues to arise from the environment (including the interpersonal world) and from within the organism. Early gains and losses occur around the child's growing capacity to assume the maternal regulatory role because such steps require gradual renunciation of the mother's auxiliary functioning as scaffolding of the child's self-regulation.

Psychoanalytic life span theories eschew the idea of uniform and homogeneous developmental periods as implied by phase theory. In contrast to phase theory's notion of quantum shifts based on emergent capacities that achieve predictable, hierarchically ordered levels of equilibrium, life span theory offers a concept of development that is continuous, unpredictable, and uneven: homogeneity across domains is not assumed at any given moment, and capacities ebb and flow in importance and salience over the developmental trajectory. Life span theorists are usually interested in adult development (Emde 1985) because postadolescence was not included in the developmental process in classical ego psychology in accordance with their idea about the centrality of biological maturation. To life span thinkers, the later years are active developmental periods in which ongoing reorganization and restructuring occur, instigated by intrapsychic demands, unique and idiosyncratic environmental challenges, and especially relational experience. Although both self-organization and defensive organization undergo continuous renovation (Emde 1985), these theories emphasize that change in the adult is in large part a function of the *transactional self.* This is the self in an interpersonal context that may exert forces leading to defensive reorganization and other forms of fundamental transformation. Some prominent developmentalists, such as Erikson (1959), use a hybrid model wherein stages are loosened from biology and linked to psychological and psychosocial accomplishments. Erikson's eight stages of man extend over the entire life span; although each challenge has its moment of crisis, all prior levels of resolution can be recruited and reworked by the current developmental demands.

Erikson's theory highlights the multiplicity of the concept of *continuity* in a life span approach, which can refer both to the potential activation of past conflicts and solutions throughout the life span and to an emphasis on the subjective experience of continuity and self-sameness within the ever-transforming sense of identity. Continuity does not mean that old patterns of thinking, self-regulation, self-representation, defenses, or adaptations are always prominent. Instead, they are understood to be dormant but available for reactivation over the life span. This approach is exemplified by the reworking of the concept of *separation-individuation*, originally introduced by Mahler et al. (1975) concerning the early childhood process of separation from the mother and subsequently applied by other theorists to adolescence (Blos 1967), adulthood (Colarusso 2000), and disruptive circumstances such as immigration (Akhtar 1995). Continuity is also illustrated by the original idea proposed by Dowling (2004) that mental life is "constantly interactively emerging," a process in which "what is continually rewrites what has been" and "where accessibility is limited by defensive barriers within a 'horizontal' present, not by being buried in 'vertical' layers of varying accessibility" (p. 192).

Life span developmental theories share common ground with systems theory (discussed in the following subsection) because they explicitly recognize multiple systems at work and consider the importance of adaptation to the environment as a developmental force on all levels, including its role in determining some aspects of genetic expression.

Nonlinear Dynamic Systems Theory

Dynamic systems theory is founded on a few central ideas: complexity, continuity in time despite quantum shifts, dynamic stability (Thelen 2005), self-organization, and emergence (Newman and Newman 2009).

- *Complexity* refers to the view that human behavior arises from the interaction of many components, often systems in themselves, none of which can be deemed superordinate.
- The interaction of these components results in the *emergence* of coherent patterns that are determined by prior states and similarly determine future states; they are *continuous*. Patterns that arise differ in regard to their stability and flexibility; stable and universal patterns that characterize certain milestones in human development are not hardwired but reflect attractor states that emerge from the interaction of components, including maturation, environmental expectations and examples, and cognitive advances.
- These attractor states remain *dynamically stable* until shifts in any component—due to changing expectations, internal motivation and striving, the maturationally determined emergence of new functional capacities, or experience, to name a few—ignite a cascade of new interactions.
- These interactions *self-organize* into a new stable state. This represents a move to a new attractor state that constitutes a quantum shift, both recognizably different from but also continuous with the prior one. Examples of such a shift could include the emergence of upright locomotion or the emergence of a new repertoire of emotions in the 2- to 3-year-old child.

Beginning in the late 1980s, systems theory drew the attention of psychodynamic thinkers, including Spruiell (1993), Galatzer-Levy (2004; Galatzer-Levy and Hauser 1997), Harris (2005), Sugarman (2018), Knight (2011, 2017), Mayes (1999), and many others. Some of these principles are present in most contemporary psychoanalytic developmental theories, even if they are conceptualized differently (Gilmore 2008; Mayes 1999). For example, the phases of phase theory have been explicitly recognized as quantum shifts in mental organization due to the interaction of emergent ego functions, neurobiological maturation (Forsyth 1997), environmental affordances and expectations, and other factors (Abrams 1983). Indeed, attractor states have been analogized to stages (Gilmore 2019), although systems theorists might argue that an attractor state undergoes endless adjustments that lead to turmoil and eventually a new organization. As noted, shifts in components lead to a cascade of new elements and interactions that *self-organize* and achieve a new stability. There are also *cascading constraints* that limit the potential of the components of the system because the deleterious effect remains in effect in the mind (Kloep et al. 2016). The new attractor state is different but nonetheless recognizably continuous. The notion of constraints can be applied to traumatic experiences, disabilities, cultural prohibitions, and so on. Examples of a shift could include the emergence of upright locomotion or the emergence of a new repertoire of emotions in the 2- to 3-year-old child; both of these are individualized by previous conditions (e.g., musculoskeletal impairments or maternal neglect) and have the capacity to influence future development but also can be influenced by it.

Dynamic systems theory has elicited its share of criticism. Berman (1996), in a wide-ranging critical examination of its rise to a position of ascendancy, explored its "shadow side" at length. His concerns included its ready recruitment for the maintenance of the status quo (p. 45) via the deceptively neutral concept of self-organization, its minimal attention to conflict (a central feature of psychodynamically oriented theory), and its rise to a position of such prominence that the valuable features of prior theorizing are eclipsed. He objected to the use of systems theory to explain everything, to denounce all linearity and causality, and to neutralize the importance of past and concurrent conditions (but see Kloep et al. 2016). Despite these critiques, systems theory is, for now, the ascendant paradigm and has brought important ideas into the mainstream of developmental psychology.

The study of adolescence (including the late adolescent period that Arnett reframed as *emerging adulthood*) is part of a tradition of approaching a specific developmental period as a unique developmental entity. Adolescence has attracted particular interest, given that it has been on the scene only since G. Stanley Hall's (1904) publication of *Adolescence: Its Psychology and Its Relations to Physiology, Anthropology, Sociology, Sex, Crime, Religion and Education*, which first described the "storm and stress" of adolescence. Over the following 70 years, comprehensive theories of adolescent development (Steinberg and Lerner 2004) were created by the pioneers of the field, including Piaget, Anna Freud, Offer, Laufer, Blos, and Erikson. In the 1970s, developmental scientists began to address the lack of empirical data, producing innumerable studies and spawning a host of journals dedicated to adolescence and youth. The growing interest in life span and systems theory no doubt influenced this phase because much of the research sought to position subjects in their cultural and societal milieu. According to Steinberg and Lerner (2004), such positioning establishes a "relational" field because it understands individuals in context, takes into account multiple systems of organization, and emphasizes the potential plasticity of this cohort.

Our General Approach to Development

Our approach to development is derived from elements of many contemporary theories in the existing developmental literature. For one, we believe that the terminology of phases is so ingrained in the literature and in popular imagination that it is worth retaining, despite its misuses. In addition, as we described in a previous book (Gilmore and Meersand 2015), these phase descriptors can be analogized to attractor states in nonlinear systems theory where there is a momentary pause in transformation.

In our book *Normal Child and Adolescent Development* (Gilmore and Meersand 2014), we distilled our developmental thinking to create a list of fundamentals. These fundamentals, which define our orientation to the entire course of human life and provide a guide to clinical thinking about people in their developmental context, include the following:

- A focus on the *body* and the powerful effect of the maturing body on the mental life of the individual. This was one of Sigmund Freud's seminal and oft-quoted insights: "the ego...is first and foremost a body-ego" (Freud 1923/1961, pp. 26–27). His earliest developmental theory was indeed based on the maturation of bodily drives, called *psychosexual* stage progression. Since that time, the body has been in and out of fashion among psychodynamic theorists; it has lost ground as a fundamental source of mental life in recent contemporary thinking that has minimized the importance of sexuality and, with it, the role of the body, such as attachment theory and relational theory (for documentation of this trend, see Fonagy 2008). However, interest in the body is currently undergoing a renaissance; its central importance in building up the interpersonal world from earliest infancy is now recognized on a neuroscientific basis: mirror neurons and bodily maps that facilitate the baby's imitation of the caregiver in the first days of life are hypothesized to establish the fundamental recognition that "here is something like me" (Beebe et al. 2003; Gallese 2009; Gallese and Sinigaglia 2010; Meltzoff 2007). Moreover, the body has been restored to its rightful position in cognitive psychology, replacing the information-processing computer metaphor with the idea of embodied cognition (Fonagy and Target 2007). The body as bedrock is threaded through contemporary theoretical literature (see also Fonagy 2006; Lemma 2010). It is also central to neuroscientific formulations of consciousness (Damasio 1999).

- A heuristic delineation of *developmental phases and progression*. Although we concur with critics who decry linearity, lockstep progression, prescribed pathways, and the misuses of classical theory in perpetuating the idea that there is a prescribed sequence to health, we find heuristic and pragmatic value in developmental epochs, if only to identify age stages. These are broadly recognizable developmental periods, demonstrable within and across cultures, that rise to the level of recognizable patterns and are associated with recognizable environmental demands and expectations. As noted, nonlinear systems theory would term these *attractor states* that result from the interface of similar maturational progressions of developing systems across individuals. Any given individual's success or failure within these smaller developmental units reverberates throughout that person's developmental trajectory and so becomes another factor that influences its course.

- A focus on the role of *maturing ego capacities* in the mind alongside a recognition of their ready recruitment into conflict, their fluidity, and their idiosyncrasies. Psychodynamic developmental theory elucidates the transformations in the organization of the mind, including changes in cognitive capacities and defense mechanisms, in different developmental epochs. The understanding of the kind of mind that characterizes a given developmental period and the individual's idiosyncratic version of it facilitates an appreciation of their specific mental experience in previous iterations. This inevitably leads to an interest in the dynamics of memory because early experience is developmentally reconstructed throughout childhood and adolescence (Tuch 1999).
- Recognition of the crucial role of the *process of internalization*, which builds mental structure via representations of self and others. This process is central to the gradual establishment of self-regulation and especially of the primary self-regulatory agency, the superego. This agency and its associated affects of shame and guilt are reconfigured and matured over the entire span of development, becoming increasingly self-determined.
- The central importance of the near *environment* and the still larger remote environment, including the cognitive, emotional, and social expectations of each developmental epoch as realized in a given culture. Our viewpoint considers how these affect the individual child as a product of a particular culture in a particular time.
- The contribution of the immediate environment and the powerful role that adaptation between mother and infant and the *family system* play in the individual's unfolding. This viewpoint recognizes the profoundly important experience of early caregiving and how interpersonal engagement and emotional connectedness in infancy contribute to the origins of thought, an awareness of the self, and an understanding of the minds of others (Hobson 2002).
- A focus on certain key areas that are of enduring interest in psychodynamic theorizing and clinical work: the dynamic unconscious; sex and aggression; object relations, including the attachment system; ego capacities, including defenses; and the subjective self-experience or sense of self. This focus distinguishes the psychodynamic developmental viewpoint from other forms of developmental inquiry. Thus, although we are committed to recognizing the influence of environment, this approach considers its purview to be *the world as represented in the inner life* of the individual.

- An open and inquiring posture toward information obtained from *other neighboring developmental sciences*. This can only enrich the fund of knowledge about development, offering new insights and contributing new directions to inquiries (Gilmore 2008).
- An overarching emphasis on the *meaning* that the developmental trajectory and its events accrue in the mind. The individual developmental experience is continuously reinterpreted over the course of life (Gilmore and Meersand 2014, pp. 7–10).

In summary, we take the view that

> the course of individual human development can be best understood as the evolving interface of a complex dynamic process in which biological, psychological, familial, and cultural systems all play a role. The process of mental development is profoundly dependent on the reliable presence of a nurturing human environment, interacts with it, and then loops back to further influence its own evolution; the human environment extends beyond the immediate family to the ambient culture, which in turn influences and is influenced by the interplay between subculture and society at large. (Gilmore and Meersand 2014, p. 7)

Although we are committed to these fundamental and enduring principles involving the basic components and processes that make development happen, we also believe that many developmental theories have value: different models, mechanisms, and conceptualizations rise to importance at different developmental moments or transformations and, in our opinion, do not require the abandonment of other views that may be relevant to other aspects or moments. Our perspective could be seen as a systems view of theory, in which different theoretical conceptualizations interface with our object of study and are invoked to provide the most complex and layered understanding of that aspect of an individual's development. Thus, as included in the previous list, we use phases of development (understood in systems terms as attractor states), the emergence of ego capacities, adaptation, environmental demands, the rise of intrapsychic challenges, evolving object relations, and other conceptualizations as needed in the picture of a given child or even cohort. Instead of forcing the data into a coherent grand theory, we try to let the data advise us as to which theory will help make sense of what facet of development is occurring. This is especially relevant with regard to this novel developmental shift that stimulated Arnett's ideas. We concur in principle with Linda Mayes (2001):

> What a theory of development needs to take into account is, first, the origins of novelty in any developmental progression.... Novelty occurs in any individual's adaptation to a given set of life circumstances, and novelty oc-

curs from the level of cellular metabolism and gene expression to individually unique mental representations of a bodily experience. (p. 151)

Here we take this statement one giant step further to extend it to novelty on a broader canvas—that is, novelty that emerges as a developmental adaptation to a changed world. Given that, the premise of Arnett's theory of emerging adulthood seems a reasonable application of a particular conceptualization to a developmental period in a certain society. Our developmental principles can be adapted to that same decade of interest in the life cycle—that is, the years between high school graduation and adulthood.

Our Developmental Approach Applied to the Period Preceding Adulthood

The fundamentals that follow generally apply to the entire decade but allow us to comprehend each person's developmental trajectory as these tasks ebb and flow in their salience and resolution. In sharpening our focus to address the particular challenges of late adolescence and emerging adulthood, we select fundamental principles that highlight those emerging capacities that have specific relevance to this time of life and add a few that we consider the special challenges of this era.

- *The importance of the body and its maturation.* As in earlier development, we recognize the significance of the body and brain from earliest life as a vital engine of developmental progression and an essential component of identity. Indeed, the body has a lifelong role in the development of the ego, in adaptation, self-representation, and identity formation and transformation. But we do not embrace the idea that development must be linked to physical maturation. In particular, we ascribe to the principle embraced by the life span perspective that active development is the outcome of a lifelong process of adaptation, in contrast to the basic premise of classical phase theory: a biological driver associated with bodily changes is required to merit the term *development*. Nonetheless, in the two periods under discussion—late adolescence and emerging adulthood—the visible biological driver does continue, as evidenced in the physical maturation between ages 17 and 21, but then gradually wanes in favor of ongoing but invisible brain development and its associated changes in mental development.
- *Adaptation as a fundamental capacity and a developmental driver.* Adaptation is both a product of development and a process that propels development forward. We agree with Hartmann's idea that adaptation represents a continuous effort that "establishes a reciprocal relation between the or-

ganism and its environment" (Hartmann 1939, p. 24). Ideally, this capacity is also adaptable to meet the needs of the individual as environmental demands change—whether due to a particular external environmental stimulus or a change in the internal environment where new capacities and new desires and impulses emerge and press for engagement with reality. In the phases we address, environmental demands assume a new prominence because the typical 17- to 18-year-old is leaving home in a way that feels irreversible, even if they return after college. It is the beginning of a process of adaptation to the larger world in which identity, affiliations, goals, guiding moral principles, and so forth are increasingly self-determined. New challenges arise in the wake of this momentous event, such as the need to transform family relationships, specific requirements of college or jobs, the nature of peer structure and pressures, and interpersonal transactions in relationships that require new levels of sexual and emotional intimacy. The internal demands include grappling with important psychodevelopmental tasks that accompany this decade, such as the establishment of individuation and differentiation in relation to the family of origin; the development of an increasingly autonomous and smoothly functioning superego with reverberations in belief systems, interests, and goals; independent self-regulation; ongoing identity formation; maturation of the capacity to love and integration of love and sex; the capacity to think about and plan for the future; and the capacity to make decisions and take responsibility for them. On the wider canvas, adaptation is vital for accommodation to subculture and culture; however, it is also crucial that this generation harness its creative potential to transform that same culture.

- *Identity formation.* Identity development is a lifelong process, beginning in infancy and reworked through the life span. It becomes a central concern in our time frame because late adolescence and emerging adulthood are dominated by the need to determine one's own course, to embrace one's own values, and to sustain these in the context of interpersonal (especially familial) and environmental demands. The reconciliation of inner representations and external attributions requires an array of ego capacities, including the capacity to integrate discordant elements and synthesize a self-representation that provides "selfsameness and continuity in time" (Erikson 1959, p. 22). Identity formation addresses the questions "Who am I?" (the self as subjectively experienced) and "What am I?" (the self as object, arising from genetic, familial, and cultural sources in interaction with ongoing environmental input). The result is woven together to create a "quintessentially psychosocial entity that is the crowning achievement of the ego's synthetic capacity" (Gilmore 2019, p. 639). As we discuss at length in Chapter 5, "Identity in Emerging Adulthood," identity development in today's world is not settled by the identity crisis of late adolescence but actively continues through emerging adulthood and possibly through adulthood as well.

- *Gradual emancipation of the superego.* The superego performs direction-giving, limiting, and punitive functions (Milrod 2002) that originate with parental injunctions and evolve over the course of life. It has its own developmental progression that continues in late adolescence and emerging adulthood, in which its individuation from received goals and standards of authorities or transient influencers—from parents and religious leaders to youth culture—is questioned in the context of the important step of moving out of the parental orbit followed by the even more important step of moving into the real world. The growing autonomy in decision-making and the capacity to accept responsibility, two features identified by emerging adults as signifiers of adulthood, reflect the maturation of the superego and its independence.

- *The capacity to experience romantic love and to integrate romantic love and sexual desire.* Puberty ushers in a period of unprecedented velocity in bodily transformation with a broad range of associated challenges: the emergence of the gendered and sexual body, the management of the newly matured and reproductively capable body with its unfamiliar vulnerabilities and requirements for care, the upsurge in sexual feelings and desires, the emergence of the postpubescent version of the masturbation fantasy with roots in the oedipal phase, and the dawning capacity for romantic love. Ideally, this last one is fully developed in late adolescence and emerging adulthood and is realized in the first experience of falling in love. Although romantic love has been described as involving both the sexual and the attachment systems (Yovell 2008), it is also, remarkably, a profoundly altered state of consciousness (including disturbed sleep, loss of appetite, inattentiveness to daily life, and an altered sense of time) that marks an inflection point in the experience of "boundaries of the self" and indeed "one's sense of oneself" (Glick 2008, p. 147) that has reverberations in evolving self-representation as an adult. Given its remarkable transformative potential, it must be granted an important role in identity development.

- *Self-representation as an adult in the broader context of culture and society.* Perhaps the crowning indication of successful passage through this preadult period is the capacity to position oneself vis-à-vis the family, the culture, and global issues and to establish one's own direction. Embarking on a path to a committed, self-selected role and/or field of interest is the ideal outcome that contains a vision of a future and establishes individual standards for affirmation, both internal and environmental.

These tasks are continuous throughout late adolescence and emerging adulthood, but they ebb and flow, resolve idiosyncratically, and take on different forms and levels of importance on an individual basis at different times. Even before emerging adulthood burst on the scene, late adolescent developmental challenges were recognized as evolving throughout the 20s, taking on different significance as the young person moves toward 30. However, the same issues of identity, superego autonomy, the evolving capacity to engage in serious love relationships, and deepening interests in and commitment to a sector of society change recognizably over these years, sometimes gradually and sometimes by quantum leaps in their urgency, gravity, or salience in the mind. Each individual's progression is greatly affected by their circumstances: access to education or vocational training, socioeconomic status, race/ethnicity, and so on. With movement out of the mandatory circumstances of high school, a fragmentation of pathways occurs as young people enter the workforce, attend vocational school, or pursue a college degree. Inevitably, the process of grappling with the psychological issues of late adolescence and emerging adulthood and, if desired, the achievement of the traditional signifiers of adulthood proceed at a highly individualized pace that defies neat categorization or standardization. That said, we intend to show the heuristic and clinical value of seeing this decade as inclusive of 1) early emerging adulthood or late adolescence and 2) late emerging adulthood.

Value of Maintaining the Concept of Late Adolescence, Albeit Modified

Critics of the theory of emerging adulthood come from a variety of disciplines and include sociologists, psychoanalysts, social commentators, and developmentalists. Our primary critique may seem semantic or harken to quibbles over dividing adolescence into phases, but we believe it highlights a fundamental error. Arnett's decision to sweep away decades of study and theorizing about late adolescence to rebrand it as emerging adulthood blends it in with a 12-year stretch of development, thereby losing the distinct features that are well documented in the extant literature. Late adolescence is dedifferentiated by the expansion of emerging adulthood to age 29.

The awareness of a looming future is only dawning in late adolescence or early emerging adulthood, which makes it preliminary to the late emerging adult experience. Members of this group are aware of and have grasped the significance of demographic data that invite them to disregard conventional expectations (e.g., to marry or commit to a career) and take the time they need to make enduring decisions. Decision-making has risen to a level of achievement that signifies adulthood more than the classic markers (even if they are intrinsically related). Meanwhile, this cohort is free to explore who they are, try on roles, experiment with sex and relationships, and enjoy their passionate interests, even if the latter do not provide a pathway to an adult future.

The real change in the developmental process of late adolescence is the growing awareness of what comes next; the pressure of the future begins only somewhere in the mid- to late 20s (around ages 23–29), when the active continuation of role exploration that includes identity, gender, and values and the actual uptick in risk behavior, instability, and erratic direction are remarkable. It is protracted in a way that was unprecedented in previous generations. And the delays in the so-called markers of adulthood are only growing; the demographic data that inspired Arnett to create the emerging adulthood concept are trending later and later. For example, the age of marriage has climbed to 28–30 (30.4 for men and 28.6 for women; U.S. Census Bureau 2021). This highlights the fact that ages 23–30 are now the real time for the emerging adult agenda because it is wide open for ongoing identity formation, sustained risk behaviors, instability, and so on. If emerging adulthood ends (arguably) with the embrace of adult roles, then it is at 30 when most of that happens. We address this supposition repeatedly throughout the book, given that emerging adults themselves do not consider the achievement of adult markers a sign of adulthood.

Although there is no question that the traditional period of late adolescence is altered by the presence of the new phase of emerging adulthood that follows, it still retains its important role in the *adolescent* process. We have no objection to conceptualizing it as early emerging adulthood, understanding that many of the tasks of late adolescence are not fully resolved and that role exploration, superego stabilization, and personality consolidation continue into late emerging adulthood. Indeed, we consider the designations of late adolescence and early emerging adulthood at least superficially indistinguishable, if it is understood that this period involves considerable mental transformation and adolescent work on issues such as autonomy, identity, superego maturation, and separation-individuation. It could be said that this period from ages 18 to 23 serves a vital role in both developmental periods. We look more closely at these two segments of emerging adulthood in the chapters that follow.

KEY POINTS

- There are many theories of development, including phase theories, life span theories, and nonlinear dynamic systems theories. Although their approaches to "how change happens" differ, they are used in composite or integrated combinations in the thinking of many developmental theorists.

- Our approach is primarily informed by psychoanalytic, life span, and systems theories.

- The period designated "emerging adulthood" is best understood as inclusive of late adolescence (or early emerging adulthood) and late emerging adulthood.

References

Abrams S: Development. Psychoanal Study Child 38:113–139, 1983 6647649

Akhtar S: A third individuation: immigration, identity, and the psychoanalytic process. J Am Psychoanal Assoc 43(4):1051–1084, 1995 8926325

Arnett JJ: Emerging adulthood: a theory of development from the late teens through the twenties. Am Psychol 55(5):469–480, 2000 1084426

Balsam R, Harris A: Maternal embodiment: a conversation between Rosemary Balsam and Adrienne Harris. Studies in Gender and Sexuality 13(1):33–52, 2012

Baltes PB: Theoretical propositions of life-span developmental psychology: on the dynamics between growth and decline. Dev Psychol 23(5):611–626, 1987

Baltes PB, Lindenberger U, Staudinger UM: Life span theory in developmental psychology, in Handbook of Child Psychology, Vol 1: Theoretical Models of Human Development. Edited by Lerner RM, Damon W. Hoboken, NJ, Wiley, 2007, pp 569–664

Beebe B, Sorter D, Rustin J, et al: A comparison of Meltzoff, Trevarthen, and Stern. Psychoanal Dialogues 13(6):777–804, 2003

Berman M: The shadow side of systems theory. J Humanist Psychol 36(1):28–54, 1996

Blos P: The second individuation process of adolescence. Psychoanal Study Child 22(1):162–186, 1967 5590064

Busch F: Creating a Psychoanalytic Mind: A Psychoanalytic Method and Theory. London, Routledge, 2013

Coates SW: Is it time to jettison the concept of developmental lines? Commentary on de Marneffe's paper "Bodies and Words." Gender and Psychoanalysis 2(1):35–53, 1997

Colarusso CA: Separation-individuation phenomena in adulthood: general concepts and the fifth individuation. J Am Psychoanal Assoc 48(4):1467–1489, 2000 11212197

Colarusso CA, Nemiroff RA: Some observations and hypotheses about the psychoanalytic theory of adult development. Int J Psychoanal 60(1):59–71, 1979 457343

Damasio AR: The Feeling of What Happens: Body and Emotion in the Making of Consciousness. San Diego, CA, Harcourt, 1999

Dowling AS: A reconsideration of the concept of regression. Psychoanal Study Child 59:191–210, 2004 16240612

Emde RN: From adolescence to midlife: remodeling the structure of adult development. J Am Psychoanal Assoc 33:59–112, 1985

Erikson EH: Childhood and Society. New York, WW Norton, 1950

Erikson EH: Identity and the Life Cycle: Selected Papers. New York, International Universities Press, 1959

Fajardo B: Analyzability and resilience in development. The Annual of Psychoanalysis 19:107–126, 1991

Flavell JH: The Developmental Psychology of Jean Piaget (The University Series in Psychology; McClelland D, series ed). Princeton, NJ, Van Nostrand Company, 1963

Flavell JH: Stage-related properties of cognitive development. Cogn Psychol 2(4):421–453, 1971

Fonagy P: The mentalization-focused approach to social development, in Handbook of Mentalization-Based Treatment. Edited by Allen JG, Fonagy P. Chichester, UK, Wiley, 2006, pp 53–99

Fonagy P: A genuinely developmental theory of sexual enjoyment and its implications for psychoanalytic technique. J Am Psychoanal Assoc 56(1):11–36, 2008 18430700

Fonagy P, Target M: The rooting of the mind in the body: new links between attachment theory and psychoanalytic thought. J Am Psychoanal Assoc 55(2):411–456, 2007 17601099

Forsyth DW: Proposals regarding the neurobiology of oedipality. Psychoanalysis and Contemporary Thought 20(2):163–206, 1997

Freud A: The ego and the mechanisms of defense, in The Writings of Anna Freud, Vol 2. New York, International Universities Press, 1936, pp 3–191

Freud S: Three essays on the theory of sexuality, in The Standard Edition of the Complete Psychological Works of Sigmund Freud, Vol VII (1901–1905): A Case of Hysteria, Three Essays on Sexuality and Other Works. Translated and edited by Strachey J, Freud A. London, Hogarth Press, 1905, pp 123–246

Freud S: The ego and the id (1923), in The Standard Edition of the Complete Psychological Works of Sigmund Freud, Vol 19. Translated and edited by Strachey J. London, Hogarth Press, 1961, pp 12–66

Galatzer-Levy RM: Chaotic possibilities: toward a new model of development. Int J Psychoanal 85(Pt 2):419–441, 2004 15142293

Galatzer-Levy R, Hauser ST: Psychoanalytic research: an investment in the future. J Am Psychoanal Assoc 45(1):9–12, 1997 9112609

Gallese V: Mirror neurons, embodied simulation, and the neural basis of social identification. Psychoanalytic Dialogues 19(5):519–536, 2009

Gallese V, Sinigaglia C: The bodily self as power for action. Neuropsychologia 48(3):746–755, 2010 19835895

Gesell A, Amatruda CS: The Embryology of Behavior: The Beginnings of the Human Mind. London, Harper & Brothers, 1945

Gilmore K: Psychoanalytic developmental theory: a contemporary reconsideration. J Am Psychoanal Assoc 56(3):885–907, 2008 18802135

Gilmore K: Is emerging adulthood a new developmental phase? J Am Psychoanal Assoc 67(4):625–653, 2019 31604388

Gilmore KJ, Meersand P: Normal Child and Adolescent Development: A Psychodynamic Primer. Washington, DC, American Psychiatric Publishing, 2014

Gilmore KJ, Meersand P: The Little Book of Child and Adolescent Development. New York, Oxford University Press, 2015

Glick RA: Commentary on: "Is there a drive to love?" Neuro-Psychoanalysis 10(2):145–149, 2008

Gopnik A: The post-Piaget era. Psychol Sci 7:221–225, 1996

Govrin A: The dilemma of contemporary psychoanalysis: toward a "knowing" postpostmodernism. J Am Psychoanal Assoc 54:507–535, 2006

Hall GS: Adolescence: Its Psychology and Its Relations to Physiology, Anthropology, Sociology, Sex, Crime, Religion and Education, Vols 1 and 2. New York, D Appleton & Company, 1904

Harris A: Conflict in relational treatments. Psychoanal Q 74(1):267–293, 2005 15766045

Hartmann H: Ego Psychology and the Problem of Adaptation. New York, International Universities Press, 1939

Hartmann H: Essays on Ego Psychology: Selected Problems in Psychoanalytic Theory. New York, International Universities Press, 1964

Hobson P: The Cradle of Thought: Exploring the Origins of Thinking. London, Pan Macmillan, 2002

Kloep M, Hendry LB, Taylor R, et al: Development From Adolescence to Early Adulthood: A Dynamic Systemic Approach to Transitions and Transformations. London, Psychology Press, 2016

Knight R: Fragmentation, fluidity, and transformation: nonlinear development in middle childhood. Psychoanal Study Child 65:19–47, 2011 26027138

Knight R: Emerging adulthood and nonlinear dynamic systems theory. Psychoanal Study Child 7:74–81, 2017

Lemma A: Under the Skin: A Psychoanalytic Study of Body Modification. New York, Routledge, 2010

Loewenstein RM, Newman LM, Schur M, et al (eds): Psychoanalysis—A General Psychology: Essays in Honor of Heinz Hartmann. New York, International Universities Press, 1966

Mahler MS, Pine F, Bergman A: The Psychological Birth of the Human Infant: Symbiosis and Individuation. New York, Basic Books, 1975

Mayes LC: Clocks, engines, and quarks—love, dreams, and genes: what makes development happen? Psychoanal Study Child 54:169–192, 1999 10748632

Mayes LC: The twin poles of order and chaos: development as a dynamic, self-ordering system. Psychoanal Study Child 56:137–170, 2001 12102010

Meltzoff AN: "Like me": a foundation for social cognition. Dev Sci 10(1):126–134, 2007 17181710

Milrod D: The superego: its formation, structure, and functioning. Psychoanal Study Child 57:131–148, 2002 12733129

Neubauer PB: Anna Freud's concept of developmental lines. Psychoanal Study Child 39:15–27, 1984 6514888

Newman BM, Newman PR: Development Through Life: A Psychosocial Approach. Belmont, CA, Wadsworth/Cengage Learning, 2009

Piaget J, Inhelder B: The Psychology of the Child. Translated by Weaver H. New York, Basic Books, 1969

Spruiell V: Deterministic chaos and the sciences of complexity: psychoanalysis in the midst of a general scientific revolution. J Am Psychoanal Assoc 41(1):3–44, 1993 8426056

Steinberg L, Lerner RM: The scientific study of adolescence: a brief history. J Early Adolesc 24(1):45–54, 2004

Sugarman A: Conflict theory, nonlinear development, and mutative action with cases of cumulative trauma: commentary on Fischer. J Am Psychoanal Assoc 66(1):103–114, 2018 29543094

Syed M: Emerging adulthood: developmental stage, theory or nonsense? in The Oxford Handbook of Emerging Adulthood. New York, Oxford University Press, 2015, pp 11–25

Thelen E: Dynamic systems theory and the complexity of change. Psychoanalytic Dialogues 15(2):255–283, 2005

Thelen E, Bates E: Connectionism and dynamic systems: are they really different? Dev Sci 6(4):378–391, 2003

Tuch RH: The construction, reconstruction, and deconstruction of memory in the light of social cognition. J Am Psychoanal Assoc 47(1):153–186, 1999 10367275

U.S. Census Bureau: Census Bureau releases new estimates on America's families and living arrangements. November 29, 2021. Available at: www.census.gov/newsroom/press-releases/2021/families-and-living-arrangements.html. Accessed April 5, 2022.

Vargas T, Damme KSF, Mittal VA: Neighborhood deprivation, prefrontal morphology and neurocognition in late childhood to early adolescence. Neuroimage 220:117086, 2020 32593800

Weil AP: The basic core. Psychoanal Study Child 25(1):442–460, 1970 5532125

Weil AP: Maturational variations and genetic-dynamic issues. J Am Psychoanal Assoc 26(3):461–491, 1978 701734

Weiss LG, Saklofske DH: Mediators of IQ test score differences across racial and ethnic groups: the case for environmental and social justice. Pers Individ Dif 161:109962, 2020

Yovell Y: Is there a drive to love? Neuro-Psychoanalysis 10(2):117–144, 2008

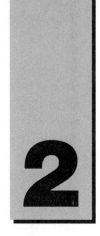

Development in the Period Between Adolescence and Adulthood

The Concept of Emerging Adulthood

Two decades after its formal introduction, the concept of *emerging adulthood* has achieved wide recognition and legitimacy among developmental scientists and the lay public. Arnett's (2000) theory of emerging adulthood arguably revolutionized and certainly invigorated the study of human development, stimulating a massive body of research and stirring controversy and debate. In seeking to answer the question "What makes a person an adult?," Arnett (2004) brought together recent demographic shifts in the achievement of classic adult markers and his findings from surveys of people in their late teens and 20s about their current experience and what adulthood meant to them. This juxtaposition confirmed his hunch that something had changed in the progression to adulthood: a new, prolonged interlude had appeared on the way, characterized by liberation from normative expectations and a freedom to explore roles and identities (Arnett 2000).

Arnett observed that every society determines the nature of the momentous step from adolescence to adulthood by virtue of the culture-specific versions of adulthood and the pathways and rituals that lead the way. He positioned his discovery in the cultural context of the digital age and Western techno-scientific-informational societies: old pathways to adulthood have been disrupted, delays in marriage and childbearing are facilitated by advances in technology, and new levels of education are now required for entry into the job market. Different from adolescence or adulthood, this period, originally designated as ages 18–24 but subsequently extended to ages 18–29, is distinguished by its own sensibility and developmental tasks that justify its recognition as a developmental phase. This is the basis of Arnett's new developmental theory.

In this chapter, we review the features of Arnett's theory and its subsequent application in the enormous body of research that followed his discovery. We elaborate our concerns about the nature of the extant literature and the decision to reframe the phase historically known as late adolescence as part of emerging adulthood; this shift in designation unfortunately homogenizes a 12-year period of active development, one that accounts for a remarkable transformation of the 18-year-old high school graduate into a 30-year-old adult. We discuss the demographic data that alerted Arnett to this new interlude of emerging adulthood. Then we examine what develops during this period such that it merits the status of a new phase. Despite Arnett's warning that this phenomenon is culture specific, the literature generated by his discovery tends to refer to its presence in many societies. Whether it is a (relatively) universal and recurrent process marked by the emergence of new ego capacities and a new level of identity formation, cognition, object relationships, superego development, and purpose akin to other developmental epochs remains an open question. Alternatively, it may be idiosyncratic to Western techno-informational culture.

Arnett's Theory of Emerging Adulthood

Arnett invoked several changes in our society that contributed to the widening of the interval between adolescence and adulthood, as marked by delays in the achievement of the former adult markers. First, changes in attitudes toward sexuality facilitated by reproductive science and technology and the liberalization of access to abortion from 1973 to 2022 significantly reduced the consequences of sexual activity and allowed women to exercise control over pregnancy and childbirth, especially in regard to interruptions in educational and career pursuits. The available technology delinked sex from marriage commitments, which amounted to a shift in the meaning of sexual activity from family building to pleasure pursuit. Second, the demands of the modern workplace and the requirements for technical education were now within reach for men and women, and career building was a new process without historical models. The demographic shift that Arnett highlighted—with delays in marriage, childbearing and child-rearing, and independent living—is a product of these changes: career pursuits, tertiary education or lengthy apprenticeships, delayed marriage and child-rearing, and the reduced pressure to renounce risk behaviors all figure in the delay of the former prerequisites for adulthood. The role of parental support in funding this delay is a noteworthy factor, although it is not universal; clearly, it is most characteristic of the relatively affluent, but members of other socioeconomic strata may receive support in the way of housing, repaid by household contributions.

Arnett (2000, p. 469) described emerging adulthood as the "most volitional years of life," in which young people are released from the requirements of mandated education and not yet tracked into adult roles. This period is characterized by the continuation of role exploration and risk behaviors (impulsive actions undertaken without consideration of consequences), including excessive drinking, unprotected sex, and driving while intoxicated. Young people continue to experiment with substances. They participate in youth cultures, which can be associated with any or all risky behaviors. They return to live in their childhood homes or move in and out of them depending on their circumstances. They remain uncommitted to careers or relationships. Arnett proposed a set of features or developmental agendas that characterize this phase:

1. *Role or identity exploration:* Role or identity exploration has been described as the "heart of emerging adulthood" (Arnett 2000, p. 478). Identity formation, formerly viewed as the major task of adolescence, is now stretched out over another decade. Among the many possible contributors to this new reality, we include the fragmentation of traditional pathways to adult life, an adaptation to the revolutionary changes in the concept of identity in contemporary society associated with disillusionment in clearly defined, binary, and predictive identities. As a consequence, this group spends much of their 20s traversing the "winding road" to adulthood (Arnett 2004).

2. *Instability:* Considerable flux in terms of job and domicile is a concrete manifestation; in addition, researchers have documented psychoemotional instability linked to problematic childhood history (Teicher et al. 2015), increased risk-taking and criminal behaviors (Salvatore 2018), relationship churning (Halpern-Meekin et al. 2013), and other evidence of volatility. Arnett (2016) nonetheless insisted that this group has considerable optimism and a sense of well-being, even if the variable of social class and the associated access to higher education begin to stratify it.

3. *Feeling in-between:* Emerging adults feel themselves to be neither adolescents nor adults. Moreover, they do not ascribe to the traditional markers of adulthood, with the exception of financial self-sufficiency. Their subjective experience of adulthood relates primarily to autonomous decision-making and responsibility-taking.

4. *Self-focus:* Not to be confused with narcissism, at least according to Arnett (2004), the self-focus of emerging adults is intrinsic to their efforts to discover themselves; it contributes to their many efforts to figure out who they are and what they are.
5. *Wide-open possibilities:* This phrase refers to Arnett's appraisal of the future outlook of emerging adults: the world is full of opportunities, novel options, and possibilities unthinkable to the parent generation; this outlook is associated with considerable optimism.

These five features, faithfully reiterated in almost all the publications on this topic, clearly capture something about the mental lives of this cohort. However, we have some concerns about them. First, they are all-purpose descriptions but leave out several important dimensions: for one, they do not illuminate the emergence of new capacities (development's sine qua non) or the shift in the mental lives of individuals in this extended phase. Second, the effect of globalization and the digital world on *psychological* development and the challenges to identity formation and meaning as young people stand on the threshold of an uncertain adulthood are new demands that occupy the minds of contemporary emerging adults. Third, these features do not reckon with the meaning of *late adolescence*, which in our view encompasses the 4–5 years after high school graduation and which is associated with its own developmental agenda. This period deserves recognition and differentiation from the years between 24 and 30, a stretch that is significantly altered from the past.

Most problematic, these features have become the definitive descriptors of emerging adulthood, unquestioned, unmodified, and static over more than 20 years of research. They are now gospel, readily passed along as givens in more than two decades of research and scholarly writing, often appearing without interrogation, updating, or further exploration; this is all the more remarkable because these two decades have seen a radical change in our society with the ascendance of the informational-technological economy and the emergence of the powerhouses of digital communication and social media networks. Platforms such as LinkedIn (2002), Myspace (2003), Facebook (2004), YouTube (2005), Twitter (2006), and Instagram (2010) have had and continue to have powerful influences on the mental lives of people in this age group. Emerging adulthood has been profoundly altered by such developments in communication, which offer immediate access to peers and the planet; this is a world that is less hierarchical and more horizontal, unregulated, and unpoliced by authority, with only a brief history and little heritage. The global culture of emerging adulthood is like no other that came before it; the cultural breach between the digital generation and prior generations is unprecedented because it represents a massive paradigm change wherein communication, personal assets, creativity, and subjectivity are sharply different from what came before (Strenger 2004).

The reification of Arnett's descriptors has limited our understanding of the mental lives of emerging adults. Emerging adult researchers have only begun to examine the massive developmental consequences of a digital society, in which identity formation occurs in a world without roots in the past; without heritage or hallowed roles; without universally recognized defining boundaries, such as gender, nationality, or religion; and without the meanings provided by centuries of tradition (Knafo 2022). The case vignette of Eric later in the chapter describes a young man bereft of the guide rails provided by his family, struggling to establish his own direction and values.

Arnett's original description of 18- to 24-year-olds had such a far-reaching effect that the age range of 18–24 determined the cohort, even after most investigators extended the interval to age 29. The first wave of research that followed seized on the original age range, and almost all the subjects of study were drawn from college populations. This shaped the empirical research and continues to do so, ensuring that the bulk of the information is derived from late adolescence. Even when emerging adulthood was more consistently expanded to ages 18–29, the subjects of study remained predominantly college students. Only in papers specifically dedicated to the late 20s is the cohort selected in the later age range. Unfortunately, the high frequency with which college student samples are studied as emerging adults has made late adolescents the exemplars of the phase. In response to objections to this tendency, Editor-in-Chief Manfred H.M. van Dulmen promised, in the very first issue of the journal *Emerging Adulthood*, to accept findings from college student samples only if there was a "clear rationale" (van Dulmen 2013, p. 3) to justify that choice. (There are certainly some exceptions to this practice—see, e.g., Arnett and Mitra 2020, Grosemans et al. 2020, and Pennington 2016—but much of the work on emerging adulthood is, from our point of view, focused on late adolescence.) Although his admonition eventually had the effect of focusing more attention on the older emerging adult group in recent years, many studies still rely on college students or individuals younger than 24 as subjects. Such tendencies lead scholars to 1) erroneously generalize from what we differentiate as the *early emerging adulthood* or *late adolescence* time frame and/or 2) merge the two periods so that identifying their differences is more difficult.

Another blurring of specificity arises from a different source: the literature intending to test the validity of Arnett's hypothesis in other cultures mostly bypasses the issue of the five features and relies on age parameters. These studies primarily use age ranges to define emerging adulthood (Côté 2014; van Dulmen 2013), in contrast to the application of even Arnett's limited developmental criteria. As noted, the five features (role exploration, feeling in-between, instability, self-focus, and wide-open possibilities) are listed in these publications as givens, whether or not their samples are selected accordingly. In addition, the age criterion is frequently encountered in reports that examine populations from different cultures or subcultures with vastly different opportunities, educational options, social expectations, and economies. For example, in a special issue of *Emerging Adulthood* on "Care-Leaving Processes and Services in Africa" (Volume 8, Issue 1, 2020), the placement of subjects in the category of emerging adulthood is determined by virtue of their being 18 years old rather than by using Arnett's or other developmental criteria. (It should be noted that this special issue uses a legal marker to define the age of the cohort [18, the age at which young people are released from various forms of foster care in South Africa] to define the population of study; the "graduation" does create a real age stage.) The articles in this issue make a strong case for the specificity of populations in terms of being "situated, context-bound and indigenous" (van Breda and Pinkerton 2020, p. 8). Similarly, studies in the special section titled "Decent Work and the Future of Youth" (Volume 10, Issue 1, 2022) collected data from informants 20–25 years old in low-wage sectors; even though some articles delineated Arnett's five features, these were not used as entry criteria. Yet, throughout, the cohort was called "emerging adults." Using age range alone as the criterion for selecting emerging adult cohorts and then drawing conclusions from their study further confuse the meaning of emerging adulthood as a *developmental* concept in which mental development and new capacities play a role. Indeed, the developmental concept seems to be most prominent in samples from Western postindustrial societies.

To add to the confusion, Arnett's stated position is that the idea of a universal developmental progression is misguided and should be regarded with skepticism. Arnett (2007) placed his developmental theory onto a broader canvas and seemed to diminish the role of biology in favor of culture: "Human development takes place within a historical and cultural context that profoundly influences the course it takes. As cultures change across historical time, development, too, changes" (p. 81). Thus, although Arnett (2000) called emerging adulthood a "developmental phase," he simultaneously asserted that emerging adulthood is "culturally constructed" (p. 470) and has been unveiled or created by the "demographic shift" that pushed the achievement of the traditional adult markers (i.e., independent domicile, financial independence, marriage, children, an established career path) into the third decade. He embraced a different conceptualization than the one familiar in the traditional psychoanalytic and developmental psychology literature, reframing phases of development as neither universal nor immutable but rather as strongly embedded in historical time and cultural milieu. The theory of emerging adulthood is intended to apply to this extended passage between the end of compulsory education and the achievement of adulthood in this era, without claims that it will remain unchanged over the centuries.

Arnett did contextualize his discovery in the rapid shift of our culture to a digital, techno-informational society; surprisingly, the effects of technology-mediated experience, globalization, and the major pivot in society are not prominently featured as developmental shapers—they are entirely absent from the five features. One determinant of this relative neglect must be due to the chronology; the generation that became emerging adults at the turn of the twenty-first century, the date of Arnett's (2000) momentous first publication, were digital immigrants and digital pioneers rather than the digital natives of today, and the parents of that era barely spoke the new language. That circumstance was undoubtedly a major factor in the loss of mentorship for that group. Today, as the founding emerging adults have become adults and now have children of their own, the gap between generations has narrowed, but it appears that it cannot close entirely given the pace of technology.

The effect of this new reality on the developing personalities of late adolescents and emerging adults is unmistakable on many different levels; beyond contributing to the sense of wide-open possibilities, it has repercussions for their mental lives. The role of the digital world in shaping personality and its effect on superego organization, including conscious values, worldviews, the dissolution of boundaries, and the normalcy of plasticity and transformation, cannot be underestimated. And identity formation, the major developmental agenda for this age group, is inevitably affected by the new unfettered access to peers of the world and other cultures. The effect of these influences and this exposure to the experience of personhood across cultures can only grow over time. Moreover, given that technology is evolving at breakneck speed and mediated environments are ubiquitous and undergoing rapid transformation, the shape of future generations is difficult to predict.

Developmental Process From Early Through Late Emerging Adulthood

Chapters 3 ("Late Adolescence") and 4 ("What Is Distinct About the Second Part of Emerging Adulthood?") examine the two parts of emerging adulthood in depth. Here we highlight the overall sweep of development and the palpable transformation that is accomplished in this lengthy period. The current cohort is distinguished by the presence of a global pandemic; its effect is only beginning to make itself known, but it is clear that it has altered temporarily or indefinitely the experience of the world and the anticipation of adult life.

What Makes Early Emerging Adulthood (Late Adolescence) Different From Late Emerging Adulthood?

The continuity of developmental themes between early emerging adulthood and late emerging adulthood contributes to the consistent blurring of their differences and even the loss of their dividing lines, as just described in the emerging adulthood literature. This inherent difficulty is compounded by methodological issues in gathering data to study this population.

Despite these complications, our intention throughout this book is to explain the heuristic, therapeutic, and pragmatic value of highlighting what distinguishes the two parts of emerging adulthood—teasing apart apparently indistinguishable developmental challenges and forward movement toward the cognitive and psychosocial maturation of personality that takes place throughout the 20s. Whether Arnett's five features are applicable and informative throughout the 12-year stretch is also explored to assess his claim that these features are the grounds for designating this period a developmental phase.

In the chapters that follow, we explain in greater depth why we prefer the idea of separating emerging adulthood into two segments; we believe that traversing the step from early to late is subjectively recognized and meaningful. It is worth noting that much like the visible alterations that occur from early to late adolescence, the distinction between a late adolescent or early emerging adult and a late emerging adult—for example, between an 18-year-old and a 29-year-old—is fully evident in the eyes of any observer and to society at large. Although it is gradual and incremental, maturation of the face; body; and cognitive, emotional, and interpersonal capacities through the 20s is nonetheless discernible. But even more evident to the lay observer are the different levels of social expectations, pressures, and obligations in the two phases, with each requiring a different, progressive adaptation.

The specificity of adaptation relates to the circumstances and challenges that each era presents to a young person. Even though access to information, cultures, and individuals across the globe is now part of everyday life, many recent high school graduates are embedded in family, high school friends, and the local community despite moments of connecting across the globe through social media and the internet. With the move into college or the workplace, they have only just been freed from the constraints of their established reputations in family, community, and friend groups all shaped in their hometown. Late adolescence is the first step toward individuation; among those attending a 4-year college, this step is usually associated with a geographic move out of the parental home to a residential campus, which thrusts the young person into a new environment in which an identity assigned by high school and family can be consciously shed (or diminished by lack of recognition or a jump in the intensity of competition), opportunities to freely choose people and interests flourish, and a new construction of the self is possible.

Campuses typically offer a vast array of possibilities and directions that fortunately have few serious consequences for wrong turns or failed experiments. This is indeed what Erikson meant when he coined the term *psychosocial moratorium*. Colleges enact their own sequential pattern of age stages, imposing similar pacing and expectations on those late adolescents fortunate enough to enroll in the years after high school graduation. However, the tyranny of the canon and the classics is markedly diminished relative to the past, and the opportunities for self-invention along contemporary lines are amplified.

Moreover, although most high school graduates have some form of college experience, only a small minority of graduates attend a 4-year residential college all the way through to graduation. The 6-year graduation rate was 63% at public institutions, 68% at private nonprofit institutions, and 29% at private for-profit institutions and was 67% for females and 60% for males. It was higher for females than for males at both public (66% vs. 60%) and private nonprofit (71% vs. 64%) institutions; however, at private for-profit institutions, males had a higher graduation rate than females (31% vs. 28%) (National Center for Education Statistics 2022). Many high school graduates go on to 2-year programs or vocational training or go directly to an entry-level job—sometimes called a "McJob" (e.g., a job at McDonald's or with DoorDash, Amazon delivery, or another delivery service)—and live at home. These young people make up the forgotten half: the high school students who drop out, the graduates who enroll in but soon leave college, or the graduates who go directly into the workforce. They often experience multiple job changes (averaging seven before age 30; Hamilton and Hamilton 2006) in search of a meaningful and enduring career path; in the best cases, such changes are preparatory to the discovery and eventual choice of a field of interest sufficiently protean to contain the twists and turns of jobs and new projects. But this is no playground of discovery; it is an arduous and often frustrating search.

Why Late Emerging Adulthood Is Not Just Adulthood

As young emerging adults head into their mid- and late 20s, many are still figuring it out, but they increasingly feel the onus of the future. They do not have a settled vision of adult life and may consciously object to the idea of "settled," but their actions are increasingly influenced by the awareness that they need to commit to a vision of their future. Expectations emanating from multiple arenas of life (finances and employment, graduate education, relationships with parents and siblings, sexual preferences and predilections, intimate and committed relationships, affiliations and social roles, interests, and passions) all create a desire to "only connect" (Forster 1910/ 2018)—that is, to draw together a unified, albeit infinitely changeable, life path or at least the first foray into one. Such pathways are accessible to the degree that financial independence is achieved; the foundational importance of financial independence explains its retention as an enduring marker of adulthood. Especially for those who precociously developed a pathway to adulthood and who have experienced a setback due to a lack of affinity, lack of talent, or loss of interest, the problem of picking up the pieces and seeking other ways to find meaning in life can be daunting and time-consuming. The following vignette, concerning a young man, Eric, illustrates the more privileged pathway of high school to college to a planned career but also shows how it can break down even with a network of supports, considerable opportunity, and preprepared guide rails.

Case Vignette: Eric

Eric began college with a firm vocational plan, well-established moral principles, the requirements for a meaningful life, and a fulfilling vision of the future. An education major, Eric devoted much of his free time at college to volunteering in local schools and after-school programs. His junior and senior years at college were dedicated to researching educational opportunities and limitations in the inner city near his college campus. He had always considered teaching a career goal; both his parents were involved in the school system in his hometown as teachers and now administrators, and he professed a great appreciation and admiration for the stable and attentive family life they had created. He felt that he also benefited from their involvement in their church, which provided him another venue for developing friends and supporting his convictions. He regarded the family lifestyle and his parents' interest in and knowledge of child development to be the pillars of his childhood experience. His major gave him the space to explore other interests in his college curriculum, especially those that he felt would be useful in a teaching career, such as computer science and child development.

Despite or because of this freedom, doubts about a range of childhood assumptions began to trouble him. In regard to his chosen career, his unease escalated as his immersion in his thesis deepened because, to him, it signaled a commitment to a future direction after graduation. In the social arena, Eric felt burdened by his parents' imposition of religious observance and morality; for one, the obligation to attend services on Sunday mornings interfered with late-night partying. Especially after joining a fraternity, he grew increasingly resentful of his family's prohibitions, which he considered inhibiting and moralistic. His romantic interests and sexual confidence blossomed with the status provided by membership in his popular fraternity. His fraternity brothers knowingly ribbed him about his preference for "hot women" who would inevitably elicit parental disapproval because of their sophisticated urban backgrounds and style, their atheism, their sexuality, and their drinking. These doubts and concerns diminished his formerly open exchange with his parents, such that he talked very little about his "dating" life (primarily casual hookups), and when he developed a more serious committed relationship with Tina, he simply did not disclose it to his family.

Despite his growing internal ambivalence about his major and reluctance to complete his thesis, Eric was able to produce a highly regarded paper that won the prize in his major. In preparation for his preordained future, he applied, as his whole family had always assumed he would, to the Teach for America (TFA) program. This plan remained in place until Eric graduated and returned home. Then, his doubts began to escalate in earnest; while conscientiously participating in the TFA summer onboarding program (which he attended virtually from his parents' home because of coronavirus SARS-CoV-2 disease), he felt an urgent desire to quit. On impulse, he decided to drive to Tina's apartment in the city 4–5 hours away where many other friends had moved after college, telling his parents that he would continue online from there. In fact, he discontinued the program at once and then, after a delay fraught with considerable inner turmoil, finally disclosed his relationship with Tina and his resignation from TFA to his parents. He told them that he was going to get a job for a while "to figure himself out."

However, with no other professional preparation or training, Eric found himself directionless and unqualified for any job that appealed to him. After floundering for weeks, he began to peruse the education-related job postings on his college website, feeling somewhat defeated by potentially reverting to a career he no longer wanted. To his surprise, he discovered an "amazing" opportunity to travel with a celebrity musician and family on a tour, serving as a "manny" and tutor for four children, with a 2-year commitment. He spent 2 exciting years with this family, visiting Europe and Asia for the first time with rest stops at their estate, also brimming with activity and interest. He was increasingly steeped in a sophisticated, affluent, and artistic world that was also remarkably "straight" because of the solid character of the star.

Unfortunately, he was still undecided about his next step at the end of this whirlwind adventure; Tina had moved on to a new relationship in his absence, all his friends were settled into living situations, and he had no particular reason to be anywhere. With no other location beckoning, he chose to return to his childhood home. Even though he had been able to put money away from working during the past years and desperately wanted to avoid dependency, his parents insisted on providing room and board, "at least for a while." Left to his own devices, he felt lost: what was he all about after all this? His link to celebrity was not his own identity, and he felt like he had left his childhood self far behind. The few entry-level jobs he found seemed dominated by technology, but despite his courses in computer science Eric felt that his knowledge of technology was insufficient to launch a career.

He decided to discuss his prospects with a close friend from his fraternity, Patrick, whose technological expertise had landed him a great job in a start-up right after graduation. Patrick was happy to help in any way he could and brainstormed with Eric about how Eric could use his experience to appeal to start-ups that were education related. Patrick also encouraged him to beef up his programming skills. As he became more familiar with the role of start-ups in various sectors of the economy, Eric decided to ask for help from his former celebrity employer, whose philanthropic efforts were focused mainly on programs supporting war veterans. Eric spent 6 months in conversation with this network and finally landed a job in a start-up that tracked and made educational services available to war veterans with a variety of brain injuries to prepare them for employment. This work felt rewarding and full of potential to develop in a range of other directions.

This vignette shows the trajectory of a relatively conventional middle-class young man, who arrived at his college campus with a foreclosed identity (Marcia 1966; see also Chapter 5, "Identity in Emerging Adulthood"); that is, his moral and religious beliefs and his occupational plan were already set, apparently the result of unquestioning idealization of his parents' careers, their attitudes, and their lifestyle, all of which were reinforced by his local high school. His conservative religious and moral beliefs made the transition to college life problematic because he was exposed to a more diverse, experimental, risk-seeking, and action-oriented group of students. His fixed occupational plan stood in the way of full exploration of alternative careers in the college setting. Indeed, his participation in Greek life on campus proved to be the most impactful challenge to what he believed was a settled sense of self and life plan. Both his fraternity experience and his first girlfriend led him to question his adherence to his identification with his parents' careers and way of life.

Eric's story is only one of myriad possible trajectories through the emerging adult time frame. Indeed, his college years (late adolescence) showed few features of typical emerging adults. Certainly, some aspects of his foreclosed identity began to show cracks, but the true reckoning was delayed until after graduation. Eric's story highlights the vast difference for this young man between his experience of entry to college at age 18 and his state of mind as he graduated from college at age 22. He was able to make some use of the psychosocial moratorium as his "settled" identity gradually came under scrutiny. But it was only when he took his first steps into his planned career after college that he recognized that he had not given enough thought to what he, Eric, wanted. The renunciation of a well-established pathway to adult life (TFA followed by a teaching career) was the most serious decision he had yet made; he ruefully confessed that the belated revelation to his parents reflected his fear of being pressured to reconsider and his certainty that, even if they accepted his decision, they would no longer be able to guide him.

Many scholars (e.g., Côté 2000) cite the lack of suitable mentors to help emerging adults negotiate the twenty-first-century job market and information economy, although this handicap may resolve when digital natives achieve mentoring status. Nonetheless, Eric was sufficiently open to adult advice, or at least resources provided by adults, to look to his college career office for help. Interestingly, the job he seized on was more glamorous and exciting than it was an opportunity to experiment with different roles. Moreover, it required a renunciation of his autonomy (not so different from the TFA program) and threatened his fragile sense of self by casting him in a role that he wryly described as one-quarter teacher and three-quarters "mother's helper." However, his admiration for his musician boss and the novel opportunity to travel the world were real inducements. And although the job did not further his exploration of his own career direction, it did provide him with experience in the world at large and with a family life vastly different from but also morally similar to his own. The state in which he returned from this 2-year "rock star" experience—with no clear path, no girlfriend, no consolidated relationships with friends new or old, and no settled domicile aside from his childhood home—is a magnified version of the emerging adult life that many 22- to 23-year-olds experience. In Eric's case, his preexisting plan made it a more abrupt regression than it would have been if he had no prior agenda and may have compounded his feelings of failure and confusion.

The following vignette begins in the mid-adolescence of a Black girl from the inner city as she began to think about not going to college. Even for relatively low-income families, the college route has been represented as the pathway to success, with the consequence that vocational training in high school has declined sharply, along with the perceived value of post–high school graduation skills training in a certification program or 2-year vocational college. However, there is a growing realization that college is a costly investment in preparing for a future that is not guaranteed (Rosenbaum 1997); although the parent generation still values a liberal arts education, it is of dubious value to many late adolescents. Moreover, although most high school seniors enroll in college, the dropout rate in the first year is 30%, and the overall dropout rate is 40% (Hanson 2021). Organizations such as the mikeroweWORKS Foundation (2021) have attempted to counteract this trend away from skills training, promoting the value of "dirty jobs" and offering counseling and support to young people who are considering alternatives to college. In choosing not to attend college, Tanya had to buck the pressure in her specialized technology high school to go to college;

she also had to grapple with her guilt at failing to fulfill her mother's wishes. The decision was further challenged by the loss of social status that initially accompanied her decision. This was a very challenging decision point.

Case Vignette: Tanya

Tanya had had to be competitive to get into her specialized technology public high school; when she was admitted, she continued to work hard and did better than average. More important to her, as an eleventh grader, she successfully applied for an internship for her senior year: a for-credit placement as an electrician's assistant or apprentice working on the construction of a new major league baseball stadium, a job that had high status among her classmates and brothers. She was especially appreciative of her supportive boss on the job, Rinaldo, who praised her for her skill and insisted that she was a "natural" and would go far in the field. She initially took this as a flattering joke because Rinaldo knew that she was supposed to be the first in the family to go to college. He himself was a college graduate with an advanced degree in engineering and endorsed the family plan and said that a job would be waiting for her.

Tanya's family was stressed financially, with Tanya and her three younger brothers all living off her mother's income as a radiology technician. The daily anxieties about money made it difficult for Tanya to imagine taking on the debt of a college education. She began to take her boss's compliments more seriously and talked with him about careers in the field and what she could accomplish without college. Despite her good grades, especially in math and computer science, Tanya was not intellectual and much preferred "doing over thinking."

As she began to consider the possibility of not going to college, Tanya dreaded the conversation with the school college counselor because she had the impression that the college route was the preferred plan for everyone (Epperson 2012). The first meeting with her counselor was tense; to Tanya, the counselor seemed to stand for most of the adult world that preached college as the key to success. However, despite her bias, the counselor had been hearing "good things" about programs for plumbers and electricians that offered paid training and job placement. She referred Tanya to an electrical company that was offering minimum wage for those who participated in their 6-month apprenticeship program with certification. Now it was up to Tanya to apply and to come to terms with her mother and her peers, all of whom expected her to go to college.

The pressure of these expectations made Tanya reluctant to share her thoughts with anyone in her circle; she decided to broach the topic with Rinaldo first, even though she was aware of his advanced degree and believed that he would likely encourage her to stay in school. Although he was understandably uneasy and worried that Tanya's mother might blame him, he did recognize the reality of her circumstances. With Rinaldo's support, Tanya approached her mother, hoping to win her over with the financial considerations. As she anticipated, her mother was sympathetic and appreciative but disappointed; her mother was confident that Tanya could repay her college debt over time and had long fantasized that maybe she would end up in medical school. Now, the best her mother could hope for was that Tanya would end up in a job something like her own but lacking the prestigious context; the idea of her daughter working on a construction site seemed like a huge step backward in her family's advancement. In contrast, Tanya imagined nothing but construction sites, envisioning herself in Rinaldo's role as master electrician, ordering around the (mostly male) crew and being the expert, as the stunning new baseball stadium grew up around them.

Tanya met with a version of her mother's disappointed reaction wherever and with whomever she discussed her plan, except, of course, with Rinaldo, who proved to be a steadfast fan of both her and her intentions. She was increasingly enthusiastic about being an expert at something useful and began the program in the summer following high school graduation. She knew she might meet a different kind of problem in this program and on the job because the industry was dominated by white men, with only 5% women and 7% Black people in the field (Zippia 2023). Without her boss to vouch for her, Tanya encountered relentless commentary, ranging from racist to sexist to a mixture of both as the intersection of her race and gender clashed with the ethos and reality of the electricians' world. She would often return home from the training despondent, fearing that she would never be accepted and that her talent would not be tested.

At home, Tanya had to face another peer challenge. With most of her high school classmates now in college, she had few close friends in her neighborhood. In the gatherings she attended when her former classmates were home for fall break, she felt awkward and out of place. Other students she knew who had chosen the workplace over college had gotten temporary positions and seemed to be "killing time" with no sense of the future. Tanya greatly feared their fate, but her uneasiness in both groups led her to feel isolated. She was still determined to complete the program before she "considered reconsidering," but she felt quite lonely.

Tanya maintained Rinaldo in a mentor role and told him regularly of her experiences. He knew the company's stated policy on both racism and sexism was completely at odds with what Tanya was encountering, and he was irate that this could happen to someone he was invested in training. It seemed to him that Tanya was unable to assert herself as he knew she could; he gave her a pep talk and encouraged her to complain to the administration. This was a very difficult challenge for Tanya; she relied on Rinaldo's advice but still was at a loss as to what would be a useful approach but not make her appear a tattletale and a "weak little girl." After she openly confessed her inability to confront the culture at the top, she and Rinaldo talked about a person-by-person approach. Tanya began to seek out the other new apprentices like herself, inevitably mostly men (but not, as Rinaldo joked, "old men"), and worked hard to develop relationships with them. One of these relationships moved on to become a friendship and then a serious romantic involvement. Tanya had no doubt that this relationship improved her standing in the company and also in her family because this man, a Latinx college graduate who intended to return to school for an advanced degree, gave new hope to her mother.

After Tanya had worked under the auspices of the training program for the requisite 2 years, her mentor once again provided an opportunity. He had just

landed a new assignment to provide the electrical infrastructure for a new stadium in another state. He offered Tanya a position on his team and assured her
that her fellow workers would be respectful "or they'd hear it" from him. Much
as she was fearful of leaving her family and her neighborhood, she had faith in
Rinaldo and contracted with him on this job for at least 3 years, with more to
be determined. Rinaldo even offered a part-time job to Tanya's boyfriend, who
was happy to apply to graduate school in the city where this project was located.

This young and talented African American woman chose a path from a
magnet specialized high school to the workplace; many of Tanya's high-
achieving classmates were in college. She had to face the disappointment of
many people invested in her future. Luckily, she had already established a
mentor, Rinaldo, who was very eager to support and guide her. However,
her mother's disappointment, her sense of isolation from her peer group,
and her personal struggles in a profession that retained a degree of racism
and sexism isolated her. She despaired of finding a new social milieu in
which her process was the norm and her growing expertise was appreciated.
Rinaldo's job offer seemed to address much of her current discontent: her
job capital and status as an electrician would be hugely augmented, she
would be temporarily moving to an interesting and vibrant city, and she
would have a beloved father or uncle figure on her team. She was hopeful
that such an adventure would return her home as an established professional.

These two vignettes illustrate the variability in pathways and timing in the
process of emerging adulthood, a point that is emphasized in much of the
emerging adult literature. They both suggest that personal development in the
years after formal education—in Tanya's case following high school and in
Eric's case, college—is crucial in sorting out priorities and assuming agency in
decision-making (Schoon and Heckhausen 2019). Interestingly, Eric's dilemma emerged only after college in the progression from early to late emerging adulthood, although signs appeared as he was increasingly exposed to
college culture, whereas Tanya made a momentous decision in adolescence—
one that was likely to shape her entire emerging adult experience.

Noteworthy in these two individuals is their subjective focus on finding
purpose, concretely represented as a viable career direction but facilitating
unconscious ego integrative functions. This was their adult project, harnessing their childhood fantasies, their identifications, and their actual
aptitudes and assets in the service of a profession, job, or expertise that motivated, mobilized, and, in some cases, inspired them. The stabilization
provided by an experience of competence in useful, interesting, and meaningful endeavors serves an important role in identity integration. Today the
important caveat is that such competence may need to be accompanied by
flexibility and innovative applicability rather than the traditional unitary career paths of the parent generation. In Tanya's case, her skills were certainly
specialized, but as her boss illustrated, a career in construction can lead to
massive projects that require leadership and imagination. Tanya's story also

represents the sequence in which professional identity precedes relational identity, conforming to Erikson's traditional ordering of identity before intimacy (Beyers and Seiffge-Krenke 2010). Although the sequence of identity formation may vary, as the vignettes in the chapters ahead show, it is not unusual for identity coherence, even if not confined to skill or one sector, to facilitate maturation in others and, in contrast, for the splintering of a foreclosed component of identity to alter and disrupt many others, for better or for worse. This was certainly the case for Eric, for whom the dissolution of his project ended up providing extraordinary access to a world of new experiences but no immediate direction. Luckily, his personable nature, skills, and profound investment in service eventually helped him parlay this special experience into a pathway that could lead him to future opportunities to exercise his skills and expertise.

Conclusion

The theory of emerging adulthood was created to explain a palpable shift in the demographics traditionally used as markers of adulthood. Financial autonomy, independent domicile, career, marriage, childbearing, and child-rearing were the sociological markers of a type of adulthood that went unchallenged for half a century. Now all these markers are postponed into the mid- or late 20s and, with the exclusion of financial independence, most have been demoted in importance or dismissed outright. Those defining features of adulthood have lost their regular, predictable appearance and, more important, any meaningful association with maturity. Without guide rails and markers for adulthood, a long period of emerging adulthood has become the norm, characterized according to Arnett (2000) by feeling in-between, instability, self-focus, role exploration, and a sense of wide-open possibilities. By their nature, these features highlight the transitional nature of the period. We have attempted to show that behind these descriptors is a meaningful phase of development that has evolved in relation to a radically changed society and results in a new form of adulthood. Rather than fixed and static markers, this new achievement of adulthood is defined by personal agency, flexibility, adaptability, resilience, and a readiness to grapple with what happens next: a self that continues to experiment (Strenger 2003) and evolve.

KEY POINTS

- The theory of emerging adulthood, originated by Jeffrey Arnett, attempts to explain the delay in achievement of traditional markers of adulthood in twenty-first-century development.

- Arnett proposed that an extended period of development has emerged in our culture between the completion of mandatory education and the arrival at adulthood toward the close of the third decade.

- This phase is characterized by a feeling of being in between adolescence and adulthood. It includes lengthy role exploration accompanied by self-focus, instability, and a sense of wide-open possibilities.

- Discovery of this phase was based on observations in Western postindustrial society, with less convincing evidence of its presence, even in modified forms, in a variety of cultures.

- In a departure from Arnett's theory, we prefer to see this stretch of development in two parts, retaining the concept of late adolescence as an early emerging adulthood period that is dedicated to experimentation and exploration and is distinguished from the second half of this development, in which the demands of adulthood begin to loom large.

- The question remains as to whether the adulthood envisioned by young people in the twenty-first century bears any relation to the adulthood of their parents.

References

Arnett JJ: Emerging adulthood: a theory of development from the late teens through the twenties. Am Psychol 55(5):469–480, 2000 1084426

Arnett JJ: Emerging Adulthood: The Winding Road From the Late Teens Through the Twenties. New York, Oxford University Press, 2004

Arnett JJ: Emerging adulthood, a 21st century theory: a rejoinder to Hendry and Kloep. Child Dev Perspect 1(2):80–82, 2007

Arnett JJ: Does emerging adulthood theory apply across social classes? National data on a persistent question. Emerg Adulthood 4(4):227–235, 2016

Arnett JJ, Mitra D: Are the features of emerging adulthood developmentally distinctive? A comparison of ages 18–60 in the United States. Emerg Adulthood 8(5):412–419, 2020

Beyers W, Seiffge-Krenke I: Does identity precede intimacy? Testing Erikson's theory on romantic development in emerging adults of the 21st century. J Adolesc Res 25(3):387–415, 2010

Côté JE: Arrested Adulthood: The Changing Nature of Maturity and Identity. New York, NYU Press, 2000

Côté JE: The dangerous myth of emerging adulthood: an evidence-based critique of a flawed developmental theory. Appl Dev Sci 18(4):177–188, 2014

Epperson C: The evolving community college model in the Socialist Republic of Vietnam, in Community Colleges Worldwide: Investigating the Global Phenomenon. Edited by Wiseman AW, Chase-Mayoral A, Janis T, et al. (International Perspectives on Education and Society, Vol. 17). Bingley, UK, Emerald Group Publishing Limited, 2012, pp 299–323

Forster EM: Howards End (1910). New York, Minerva, 2018

Grosemans I, Hannes K, Neyens J, et al: Emerging adults embarking on their careers: job and identity explorations in the transition to work. Youth Soc 52(5):795–819, 2020

Halpern-Meekin S, Manning WD, Giordano PC, et al: Relationship churning, physical violence, and verbal abuse in young adult relationships. J Marriage Fam 75(1):2–12, 2013

Hamilton SF, Hamilton MA: School, work, and emerging adulthood, in Emerging Adults in America: Coming of Age in the 21st Century. Edited by Arnett JJ, Tanner JL. Washington, DC, American Psychological Association, 2006, pp 257–277

Hanson M: College dropout rates. Education Data Initiative. November 22, 2021. Available at: https://educationdata.org/college-dropout-rates. Accessed November 22, 2022.

Knafo D: Self-creation and the good life: Carlo Strenger's existential psychoanalysis for our time. Psychoanal Psychol 39:12–19, 2022

Marcia JE: Development and validation of ego-identity status. J Pers Soc Psychol 3(5):551–558, 1966 5939604

mikeroweWORKS Foundation: We've got a PR problem. 2021. Available at: https://www.mikeroweworks.org/about. Accessed March 6, 2021.

National Center for Education Statistics: Fast facts: undergraduate graduation rates. 2022. Available at: https://nces.ed.gov/fastfacts/display.asp?id=40. Accessed May 18, 2023.

Pennington N: Living social: comparing social media use in your 20s and 30s, in Digital Media Usage Across the Life Course. Edited by Nixon PG, Rawal R, Funk A. London, Routledge, 2016, pp 96–106

Rosenbaum JE: College-for-all: do students understand what college demands? Soc Psychol Educ 2:55–80, 1997

Salvatore C: Sex, Crime, Drugs, and Just Plain Stupid Behaviors: The New Face of Young Adulthood in America. Cham, Switzerland, Palgrave Macmillan, 2018

Schoon I, Heckhausen J: Conceptualizing individual agency in the transition from school to work: a social-ecological developmental perspective. Adolesc Res Rev 4:135–148, 2019

Strenger C: The self as perpetual experiment: psychodynamic comments on some aspects of contemporary urban culture. Psychoanal Psychol 20:425–440, 2003

Strenger C: The Designed Self: Psychoanalysis and Contemporary Identities. New York, Routledge, 2004

Teicher MH, Ohashi K, Lowen SB, et al: Mood dysregulation and affective instability in emerging adults with childhood maltreatment: an ecological momentary assessment study. J Psychiatr Res 70:1–8, 2015 26424417 van Breda AD, Pinkerton J: Raising African voices in the global dialogue on care-leaving and emerging adulthood. Emerg Adulthood 8(1):6–15, 2020

van Dulmen MHM: Emerging adulthood: the journal. Emerg Adulthood 1(1):3–4, 2013

Zippia: What is an electrician? Zippia: The Career Expert, April 6, 2023. Available at: https://www.zippia.com/electrician-jobs/#cmp-demographics-section. Accessed May 18, 2023.

PART II
Phases of Emerging Adolescence

In Chapters 3 ("Late Adolescence") and 4 ("What Is Distinct About the Second Part of Emerging Adulthood?"), we consider the concept of emerging adulthood in depth and justify our preference for a two-part developmental process. This is a refinement rather than a refutation of Arnett's discovery; emerging adulthood has resonated with so many researchers and received such widespread recognition that the utility of his insight about the lengthened transition to adulthood is undeniable. Even if the term *emerging adulthood* is applied to this age group simply as an age stage (Gilmore 2019; Syed 2015)—that is, a culturally delineated cohort that shares features that are considered specific and unique—in contrast to a new developmental phase, the lengthened interval before adulthood is now a recognized entity and a subject of intensive study. Arnett's original presentation took only a few years to incubate before it began to be referenced in research studies and scholarly literature; in 2007 alone, more than 1,000 articles were published that referred to the concept of emerging adulthood, and by 2014, this number had quadrupled. Now with more than two decades of study, the ongoing accumulation of data is remarkable.

To our way of thinking, it is no accident that the emerging adult literature is inconsistent with regard to the time frame under scrutiny (ages 18–24 and 18–29); researchers choose one or the other, typically without explanation as to the choice. The original designation of 18–24 begins with the termination of compulsory education in the United States and, depending on the individual pathway, includes entry into and the conclusion of postsecondary education, vocational training, or the first years of employment, presumably ending with the establishment of adult roles. Even as more researchers have extended this time frame to 18–29, emerging adulthood continues to be seen as one continuous developmental era, but we believe that the tasks, achievements, and attitudes of the early half are distinct from those of the mid- to late 20s (Settersten et al. 2015). The first part corresponds to our time frame of late adolescence, whose end is achieved by shifts in consciousness of the future, in the investment in real life (including relationships and occupation), and in further advances in identity formation. Unfortunately, as noted in Chapter 2 ("Development in the Period Between Adolescence and Adulthood"), the problem is that much of the empirical literature that examines the full decade uses only college students as subjects, leaving the crucial second half of this time frame unexamined.

While not intending to reify the categories, we hope to show that ideas from a range of allied disciplines support maintaining this differentiation. Late adolescence has its own intrapsychic developmental process and achievements, as we show in Chapter 3. In contemporary postindustrial society, many of these adolescent tasks remain active through the 20s but take on a different sense of purpose and seriousness. Our segmentation of the process underscores our belief that the concept of emerging adulthood, extending over a decade as it now does, obscures the important developmental step of late adolescence and its palpable difference beginning in the mid-20s, when important steps in identity formation, meaningful choices about adult life, and movement toward true autonomy occur. Dividing emerging adulthood into an early and late iteration provides the opportunity to differentiate these challenges.

The five features of emerging adulthood first identified by Arnett are widely accepted as the developmental agenda of emerging adulthood; the list has passed from scholar to scholar and been elaborated in various ways, but the following five remain the fixed touchstone of emerging adulthood as a developmental phase: 1) role exploration, 2) instability, 3) self-focus, 4) feeling in-between, and 5) wide-open possibilities. In addition, Arnett's early observations about emerging adults' subjective experience and their views on the meaning of adulthood have been replicated in the literature: emerging adults deny the significance of four of the five traditional sociological markers of adulthood (independent domicile, a stable career path, marriage, and parenthood) and privilege only financial independence as a true sign that adulthood has been reached. By their report, the achievements essential to their movement into adulthood include two related psychological capacities: to make one's own decisions and to take responsibility for them (Arnett 2000). From our viewpoint, these indicators of maturity, no doubt reflections of confidence and agency, do not illuminate the full complexity of intrapsychic development that we address. Many aspects of personality evolve in crucial ways over the course of this period, only some of which are reflected in the empirical literature. Although the contemporary psychoanalytic literature is in the early process of development regarding this new phase, there are nonetheless steady contributions exploring the mental life of the emerging adult, focusing on either late adolescence or the young adult experience.

In what follows, we attempt to elucidate what distinguishes the two parts, highlighting intrapsychic development without, of course, losing sight of the real circumstances of emerging adults in society. The effect of culture and society is never more powerful in human development than in these final stages preceding adulthood, because the interface with culture, always present to some extent, has a more direct and powerful influence on the development of ego identity as it begins to take shape in the early years of emerging adulthood. Indeed, according to Erikson (1956), the evolution of identity (roughly corresponding to Arnett's role exploration) is a product of synthesis at the border of self-definition and social reality; it is a quintessentially *psychosocial* entity.

Some of the broad influences that differentiate the two periods are closely linked to environmental circumstances, such as college attendance, which depends on national education policies in addition to individual and community socioeconomic, racial, educational, and geographic trends. Contemporaneous with the rise of the concept of emerging adulthood, several national initiatives shaped the course of life for young people at the end of high school. Two influential national policy acts, the No Child Left Behind Act of 2001 and the Every Student Succeeds Act of 2015, set an orientation toward college attendance for all high school students, with the idea that the mastery of skills achieved there would further their chances of postcollege employability and success (Smerdon 2018). However, the reality of enrollment without successful completion and the low degree of preparedness for contemporary employment provided by formal education are significant (see Vuleta 2022; Wyn 2017). As the numbers make plain, the orderly trajectory of high school to college to employment as envisioned by the college-for-all policy is not the rule; even if most high schoolers do enroll in college (a figure now estimated at 68%–70%), one-third of them drop out in the first year and fewer than half (41%) graduate in 4 years

(Vuleta 2022). It should be underscored that the two broad categories of young high school graduates in the workforce and those who enroll in college are by no means homogeneous within themselves, nor are they crisply differentiated, because many youths crisscross between them. Indeed, the end of high school marks a moment of fragmentation of the life course for each generation as pathways proliferate, often unguided and unmentored: there is "increasing complexity of pathways through youth" (Wyn 2017, p. 93). Moreover, with so many young people not beginning college, staggering their accumulation of credits, or not graduating, the significance of college as a moratorium and of college graduation as a stepping stone to the real world is diminished. Overall, the loss of predictable demands, steps in progression, and support, in addition to the loss of shared cultural expectations and attitudes, leaves this age group deciding what education will serve their vague employment hopes; they are struggling with an "emerging adulthood gap" (Salvatore 2017) in which the road map into traditional adulthood is neither available nor desirable and the future is unimaginable. Age 30 looms as a deadline, albeit less meaningful than in the past, but for what?

From our vantage point, Arnett's choice to incorporate the two periods into one lengthy emerging adulthood simplifies the issue and neglects to spotlight important developmental differences, changes in legal status, brain maturation, and the psychological significance of moving into the mid- to late 20s. We hope to clarify 24- to 30-year-olds' subjective sense of discontinuity from their post–high school selves, despite many similar developmental issues. We also briefly consider how the second phase of this period concludes and assess the concept of "established adulthood" (Mehta et al. 2020), which appears to mean the later embrace of traditional markers of adulthood; in our view, adulthood has come to mean something far beyond the assumption of historically sanctified social roles.

References

Arnett JJ: Emerging adulthood: a theory of development from the late teens through the twenties. Am Psychol 55(5):469–480, 2000 1084426

Erikson EH: The problem of ego identity. J Am Psychoanal Assoc 4(1):56–121, 1956 13286157

Gilmore K: Is emerging adulthood a new developmental phase? J Am Psychoanal Assoc 67(4):625–653, 2019 31604388

Mehta CM, Arnett JJ, Palmer CG, et al: Established adulthood: a new conception of ages 30 to 45. Am Psychol 75(4):431–444, 2020 32378940

Salvatore C: The emerging adulthood gap: integrating emerging adulthood into life course criminology. International Social Science Review 93(1):1–22, 2017

Settersten RA Jr, Ottusch TM, Schneider B: Becoming adult: meanings of markers to adulthood, in Emerging Trends in the Social and Behavioral Sciences: An Interdisciplinary, Searchable, and Linkable Resource. Edited by Scott RA, Buchmann MC, Kosslyn SM. New York, Wiley, 2015, pp 1–16

Smerdon B: Introduction, in Career and College Readiness and Success for All Students (Research on High School and Beyond). Edited by Smerdon B, Kim K, Alfeld C. Charlotte, NC, Information Age Publishing, 2018, pp 1–4

Syed M: Emerging adulthood: developmental stage, theory, or nonsense? in The Oxford Handbook of Emerging Adulthood. Edited by Arnett JJ. New York, Oxford University Press, 2015, pp 11–25

Vuleta B: Everything you need to know about the college dropout rate. What to Become, August 3, 2022. Available at: https://whattobecome.com/blog/college-dropout-rate. Accessed June 3, 2023.

Wyn J: Educating for late modernity, in Routledge Handbook of Youth and Young Adulthood, 2nd Edition. Edited by Furlong A. New York, Routledge, 2017, pp 1–98

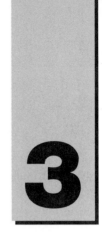

Late Adolescence

The First Phase of
Emerging Adulthood

As described in Chapter 1 ("A Brief Review of Developmental Theory") and in the introduction to Part II ("Phases of Emerging Adolescence"), the blending of 18- to 29-year-olds into a single emerging adulthood cohort obscures highly meaningful distinctions between younger and older individuals within this group. Arnett's (2000) broad approach to a critical decade of development is consistent with the pioneering nature of his work (i.e., identifying and describing a novel developmental phase via widespread trends and general characteristics). As psychodynamic writers, however, we hope to shift the discussion of emerging adulthood toward greater complexity by integrating young people's behaviors and attitudes with less visible aspects of their mental lives; the latter include underlying intrapsychic and relational processes that undergo significant maturation during the late teens and 20s as well as the continuous interaction between the mind and the sociocultural surround. In this chapter, we elaborate the distinctive features of *late adolescence*, the first segment of what we see as a bifurcated decade of emerging adulthood and which we also refer to as *early emerging adulthood*. During this period, 18- to 23-year-olds enter a unique phase of enhanced developmental capacities, expanded social opportunities, and unprecedented challenges as they typically take their first steps away from the structure of secondary school and family life.

Late adolescence, or early emerging adulthood, occupies its own transitional developmental space; it completes the traditional pre-, early, and middle adolescent sequence (described later in this chapter in the section "Late Adolescence or Early Emerging Adulthood as the Final Phase in Adolescent Development") and simultaneously functions as an introductory period to subsequent late emerging adult life. In many ways, the differences between the first and the second segments of emerging adulthood are obvious: images of an 18-year-old recent high school graduate, poised for a first semester of college or an initial full-time job, form an easy contrast to visions of a 27-year-old who has been living independently, conducting relationships, and making lifestyle decisions for several years. The late adolescent feels little urgency about preparing for a distal-seeming adulthood and is just beginning to explore roles, relationships, and interests; the older individual, almost 10 years further along in terms of self-knowledge and self-reliance, experiences a looming sense of the future. At the same time, the presence of common themes and values as delineated by Arnett (2000)—a focus on identity and self-discovery, a sense of possibilities and change, a value placed on self-reliance and independence, and a feeling of occupying a space in between the earlier teenage years and adulthood proper—and the continuity of certain challenges and vulnerabilities (rates of drug and alcohol use, as well as other risky behaviors, that continue to climb through the third decade) position both late adolescents and older 20-somethings within the overarching emerging adult period. We hope that this chapter, together with the next one, which focuses on the 24- to 29-year-old age group, delineates for the reader both the distinctions between and the commonalities between the two segments of this phase.

Introduction to Late Adolescence

Within traditional psychoanalytic theory, late adolescence is viewed as a culminating phase of development in which major components of personality achieve finalization. This process, sometimes referred to as the *adolescent resolution*, marks an integration of defensive style, modes of relating, and personal identity; during this time, childhood identifications are transformed and synthesized with a maturing, individualized self (Blos 1968; Ritvo 1971). The notion of late adolescent personality formation was consistent with the experience of a post–World War II generation, wherein many high school graduates soon entered the workforce, embarked on marriage and parenthood, and only rarely pursued higher education. Within this model of society, late adolescence indeed coincided with making major life decisions; settling down in the overarching arenas of work and love;

and beginning to shoulder adult-size responsibilities for self, spouse, and even children.

In subsequent decades, the powerful effect of technology and globalization transformed the economic and social landscape, ushering in a period in which career paths diversified and increasingly required college-level qualifications (Arnett 2000). A vast increase in university attendance, from around 2 million teenagers in 1959 to around 12 million in 2010, marks the extent to which late adolescence increasingly came to be seen as synonymous with the college experience. This accelerating trend had the effect of prolonging financial dependency on parents; creating a distinct period in between adolescence and adulthood; and contributing to more protracted and wider freedom for exploring aspects of identity, such as personal roles, goals, and interests (Arnett 2000; Malgwi et al. 2013; Schwartz et al. 2013). The college campus functioned for late adolescents as an ideal *psychosocial moratorium*, a term used by Erikson (1968) to describe a unique intermediary setting wherein young people may experiment freely, without the need for binding decisions. A growing generational proclivity toward self-discovery, with deferred commitments to the traditional adulthood markers of marriage and parenthood, was further solidified by the decline of traditional (e.g., manufacturing) jobs; the increased difficulties of achieving financial independence in the late teens and early 20s; and the societal shift toward greater diversity in romantic relationships, family constellations, gender roles, and sexuality (Arnett 2000; Dykstra and Poortman 2010; Savin-Williams 2011; Schwartz et al. 2013).

Changing norms for late adolescent life were presaged by Ritvo (1971), who noted that recent technological advances were encouraging a "more prolonged" preadult period in which the "transition to work and love in the realistic world is a longer process" (p. 242). However, it has fallen to a contemporary generation of writers (e.g., Arnett 2000; Auerbach and Diamond 2017; Gilmore 2019) to reconceptualize this period as a time of far greater internal and external flux, in which foundational aspects of personality (ego strengths, superego functions, identity) remain fluid and continue to evolve despite the lack of clear biological markers that distinguish earlier phases of development. Within this current perspective, the integration of the childhood self with the maturing self requires a lengthy process that achieves ascendance during late adolescence but remains active well into the third decade of life. As described in Chapter 1, these notions reflect a life span approach to development wherein key aspects of personality, in particular in the realm of identity, continue to undergo significant change and growth as they interface with novel environmental and relational challenges and opportunities (Galatzer-Levy and Cohler 1990; Rizzolo 2016).

Autonomous Functioning and Identity Experimentation

The achievement of autonomy and identity exploration, two interrelated processes, form the chief developmental tasks and challenges of the late adolescent period. However, although the late teens and early 20s mark a distinct leap forward in self-reliance, we view as far too general the description of emerging adults as having "left the dependency of childhood and adolescence" (Arnett 2000, p. 469). As psychoanalytic observers, we see the achievement of autonomy as a lengthy, often uneven, and multifaceted process that interfaces with several psychological systems, including cognitive and emotional self-controls, levels of residual middle adolescent conflict with adult authorities, and, crucially, the increasing internalization and independence of a still-evolving superego. Indeed, the contemporary late adolescent's entry into a period of exploration and uncertainty, often without the familiar structures of parental oversight and family routines, exposes novel vulnerabilities and risks with regard to sexual activity, alcohol use, and substance use despite developmental advances in cognitive and emotional self-management (Shulman and Connolly 2013). The 18- to 23-year-old individual is more reflective than the younger adolescent but still feels driven to live in the moment, experience life via action, and test personal powers in the external world; moreover, the higher-level cortical structures needed for mature levels of self-control are not yet fully developed and continue to mature well into the later emerging adulthood phase (Eichler 2011; Spear 2000). Drug and alcohol use increases sharply during the latter years of adolescence and continues to rise during the 20s. The stresses of a more independent life, the struggles to find a place within peer groups, and the urgently felt need for gratification and validation in the external world vie with increased capacities for solid judgment; the late adolescent's relatively greater self-control does not necessarily keep pace with the drive to pursue novelty and stimulation (Conley et al. 2014; Eichler 2011; Harden and Tucker-Drob 2011; Palmeroni et al. 2020; Ritvo 1971; Roberts and Davis 2016).

Nonetheless, compared with the often conflict-laden middle teenage years, late adolescence marks a shift toward relatively greater psychological stability, more consistent emotional self-regulation, and an increasing capacity for independent living; these advances facilitate adjustment to novel environments as the young person often leaves the familiar surround of the family and begins to negotiate the demands of post–high school life, typically college, work, or some combination of the two. Self-governance, although often shaky, begins to expand into domains such as handling personal health and safety, meeting the routine requirements of daily life, making social and moral decisions, affiliating with new friends and mentors, and exploring novel interests. The older adolescent has largely adjusted to the momentous physical changes of puberty but still must learn to assume responsibility for the sexual body and self and for intimate interactions with others. Body responsibility further includes a realization of physical limitations, such as coming to terms with the risks and consequences of alcohol and substance use, a process that often extends into the later emerging adulthood years.

The late adolescent's enhanced facility with self-reflection and tolerance for emotional complexity means that multifaceted social situations can be contemplated in more nuanced ways, with a greater appreciation for subjectivities that differ from one's own. In the realm of intimate dyadic relationships, these subtle but real changes augment both an awareness of the other's needs and an ability to balance caring feelings with self-interest; in contrast to younger teens, early emerging adults more easily integrate sexual desire with tenderness and experience closeness without fearing the loss of their unique individuality and independence. However, although they are more thoughtful and serious about romantic connections than their earlier teenage selves, late adolescents will likely continue to engage in ongoing romantic and sexual exploration throughout the sweep of their 20s, only gradually veering toward more committed relationships.

The following vignette of Ariana, a recently turned 18-year-old who is soon to arrive at college during the coronavirus SARS-CoV-2 disease (COVID-19) pandemic, illustrates her hopes and dreams for personal transformation via anticipated experimentation with new friends, styles, interests, and other facets of identity. At the same time, such desires are tempered by her fears of loneliness, long-standing attachments to a current group of high school friends, and reliance on her parents for help navigating difficult situations.

Case Vignette: Ariana

Ariana anticipated arriving at her college campus 6 months into the COVID-19 pandemic, knowing that some of her former high school friends would be confined to remote classes from their childhood homes. She felt sad about this disruption to the group's usually synchronous experiences. Recently, she had received notification of her university's demand for a complete 2-week quarantine prior to moving into the dorms, and her immediate reaction had been resentment and planned defiance; she knew that complying would mean missing a small previously arranged going-away party in the backyard of a friend's home. Still, she was conflicted enough over this decision to talk it over with her parents, who urged her to follow the school's mandate in order to arrive "with a clean conscience" and a sense of shared responsibility with her new community.

Because many of her junior high and high school relationships had developed out of theater activities, Ariana was concerned after learning that all college extracurriculars were to be offered only via screens. Moreover, she had read the new guidelines about takeout-only dining and dreaded the possibility of eating meals alone in her room. She reassured herself that, via social media, she had already established lively conversations with the other new students who would occupy her suite as well as with several future classmates who had indicated interest in theater, her anticipated major. Via texting and various platforms, these 10 or so young people had maintained an almost constant stream of communication during the summer. Privately, Ariana was hopeful that a certain prospective creative writing major, a young woman whose Instagram postings she admired, would prove to be a close friend; she felt somewhat guilty about her fantasies of spending time with the new acquaintance, feeling disloyal to her current best friend but also longing for the chance to reinvent herself, establish new ways of being with others, and experiment with a different overall style that her current friends would likely pronounce weird or fake. Checking her phone again and finding that the group chat was active as usual, Ariana felt reasonably certain that she would avoid a much-feared sense of social isolation on arriving at her dorm. She had confided some of her private worries to the three of her high school friends who were also leaving for an on-campus experience. As a foursome, they had decided to avoid speaking of these matters with their other high school friends whose colleges were not accepting residential students during the COVID-19 fall semester; such discussions were bound to make those stuck at home feel bad and left out.

In the final days before her parents drove her to school, Ariana was nervous and had trouble sleeping. She took some solace in the notion that she and her mother had purchased all the necessary toiletries in large quantities so she would not run out of the products she preferred to use. Checking in with her mother frequently, she completed packing and added a few extra comfort items, such as an old stuffed animal and a favorite pillowcase. She and her mother went over their various lists—seasonal clothing needs, books that could be preordered for each class, small tasks such as procuring keys and an ID on arrival—multiple times per day. A few months back, when Ariana had found the course selections for first semester to be overwhelming, both of her parents had helped her choose her classes, advising her to fulfill a couple of requirements but also to sign up for one or two fun, interesting options. She did not want to feel pigeonholed as a theater major and had ended up selecting a philosophy class and a music class. Still, she found herself feeling annoyed with her parents and experienced their talk about how much fun she would be having as slightly grating; she conferred with her three campus-bound friends, and they all agreed that their parents were driving them nuts. It was a real stroke of luck that COVID-19 had canceled each of their college's usual family weekend.

Ariana demonstrates an easy grasp of complex thinking and layered social understanding: she tries to keep in mind her own needs and dreams, find ways to protect the feelings of her old friends (both those who are go-ing to and those who cannot attend college in person, whom she perceives as requiring different considerations), and simultaneously integrate herself into a new, unknown social milieu with potential rewards and risks. She is conflicted about competing wishes and urges, ones that pull her forward (self-reinvention, new social and academic opportunities) and other attach-ments that represent her past (comfort items from her childhood bedroom, the guidance of parents, the easy connection with high school friends); her present self feels in transition. She talks to her friends about her insecurities but still relies substantially on her parents for their judgment, advice, and practical assistance. Her transient urge to defy the college's quarantine rep-resents her sorrow over missing an important shared event—especially during a year when so many rites of passage (prom, graduation) were lost to the pandemic—but also a flare of resentment over adult authority and intrusion into her autonomy. Managing this momentary reaction, Ariana is able to make use of her parents' counsel, assess her priorities, and forgo the backyard party. She manages her sadness and anxiety over the imminent separation from home in a few ways, including by transforming these emo-tions into annoyance at her parents, which makes it feel easier and more desirable to achieve distance. Throughout the process of separation, her ac-cess to substantial family and friend support, as well as to the opportunities afforded by her upcoming liberal arts experience, allows her to traverse the final weeks at home with only mild levels of disturbance.

Cognitive and Emotional Development

The late adolescent's increased capacity for reflection and emotional self-regulation, in combination with expanded opportunities for self-reliant behaviors (college, employment), begins to provide the necessary under-pinnings for more autonomous functioning. The need for direct adult over-sight declines as the early emerging adult gains experience and success with managing daily routines, relational conflicts, and academic or work-related responsibilities. Within the psychoanalytic literature, these enhancements in self-regulation are understood as reflecting a gradual transfer of power to the ego; the strengthening and relatively greater cohesion of ego func-tions set late adolescence apart from preceding phases wherein the younger teenager was buffeted by sexual and aggressive impulses and had less steady and more poorly integrated internal resources (Ritvo 1971). Executive functions, or cognitive controls, continue to improve over the course of the late teens and 20s; these varied capacities—directing attention, adjusting flexibly to the shifting demands of novel tasks, organizing personal reactions to complex problems—are instrumental for well-functioning emotional and intellectual responsiveness and develop in tandem with the emerging adult's stronger ability to perceive others' mental states, make links between behavior and inner experience, and monitor and manage feelings and actions (Boelema et al. 2014; Crone 2009; Dumontheil et al. 2010). As emotional and behavioral self-regulation improves, the emerging adult's overall affective and mood stability is enhanced (Blos 1968, 1972; Larson et al. 2002).

These various cognitive and emotional advances interface with the late adolescent's increasing immersion in novel experiences (e.g., befriending peers from more diverse backgrounds than one's other friends, hearing professors assert political views not typically espoused by family and community, engaging in new and perhaps first sexual encounters); together, unfolding internal resources and external opportunities fuel the process of exploration and experimentation that is central to identity development (Schwartz et al. 2013). The early emerging adult's self- and other appraisals are more realistic and include comparisons with a wider range of associates; for example, college students may grapple with their relative successes and failures in both the academic and the social arenas, gradually weaving their knowledge about personal strengths and vulnerabilities into future hopes and plans as well as into beliefs about the self. Simultaneously, parents are increasingly viewed as real people with their own struggles and flaws as they are measured against a widening social lens. Feelings and attitudes toward the self and others are further affected by the capacity to contemplate autobiographical events and outcomes in more complex ways; grasping the connections between early experience and the here-and-now self gives rise to more organized personal narratives and an increasingly coherent narrative identity (Habermas and de Silveira 2008; McAdams and McLean 1985). Ultimately, the self and others are more easily understood as people with their own unique perspectives and life stories.

With greater access to fluid, abstract, and future-oriented thinking, and with concomitant exposure to novel environments, the late adolescent can now imagine multiple forward pathways for the self, including those that do not seamlessly emerge from the values and expectations of parents and the community of origin (Eichler 2011; Schwartz et al. 2013). The following personal excerpt, written by a college student looking back on her younger self, illustrates the process of change in self- and other appraisal, along with a beginning reevaluation of personal values and goals that is characteristic of the late adolescent years:

> As a child, I was taught that the unknown was unacceptable. I viewed it as space that had to be filled. In class, when asked a question, I allowed myself no room for confusion, or even deeper thinking, because I feared being penalized. I would cringe when a classmate would start his or her answer with

"This is just a guess" because I was accustomed to responding with an exact and to-the-point answer. Growing up with this way of learning, I thought that's how it always would be, and should be.

To feed the mind that began craving answers, I applied to work in a research lab the summer before my junior year. Where else could I possibly get more straightforward, precise answers? The research papers I read answered a question with a clear conclusion. I thought life in the lab would offer me the same. Arriving at the lab, I was hyperfocused, waiting to prove myself with a quick, correct answer, just like I assumed the postdocs had spent their careers doing. To my surprise, they were waiting for the opposite: a question that no one in the room had the answer to. One postdoc inquired of the group, "Why is the *Them2* gene not showing up in adipose tissue?" After several moments of silence, everyone's head turned to the primary investigator, who said, "I guess we haven't looked into adipose tissue enough. Nori, research it and get back to us." Nori smiled; he wasn't agitated by the ambiguity. Rather, he was eager to dive into this new inquiry. I felt betrayed. Was the learning method I'd mastered not applicable outside the classroom? Looking back, I should not have relied on my technique. I sought straightforward answers but felt confused and insecure. When I thought about God, I quickly assumed that He was made up because science pointed me toward that conclusion. I felt like an imposter in my own synagogue. Until high school, I didn't know any gay people, so I assumed being gay wasn't an option. Women like men; end of story. I didn't necessarily believe these things, but in the classroom, I was rewarded for giving the right answer, no matter my true instincts. Yet, when I saw the postdocs using an exploratory method that brought them to more comprehensive answers, I knew I had to question my own practices.

While rethinking different aspects of my life using this exploratory mindset, I noticed that most facets of my identity exist on their own spectrums. There were no black and white answers. When I recognized these spectrums, in school and otherwise, I realized that my place on each didn't have to be static. Walking into the first day of junior year, I felt a new sensation: freedom for inquiry. I used this freeing mindset when I took over the biology club as a senior. Instead of solely discussing the undisputed concepts of biology, the club now explores controversial research and *not fully understood topics*. By moving away from the idea that every question has an answer, the club now holds more fluid and engaging conversations.

My life outside of school has also gained more meaning since realizing that not everything needs an exact solution. Because I let go of my urge to define God, I was able to enjoy my time in synagogue. Learning that everyone has a different perception of God made me feel more welcome in the sanctuary. After years of badgering myself over not being able to define my sexuality, I learned to appreciate the fluidity of my identity. By simply accepting myself as queer, I felt fewer restrictions on who I was allowed to like and found a community of people who also saw the beauty in not knowing. My identity can change every day, and the word *queer* will still stand true. I am now OK with the unknown, and I feel more complete because of it.

—Reproduced by permission from Bryna J.

Autonomy and the Superego

Blos's (1967) famous conceptualization of adolescence as the *second individu-ation* comprises the momentous process of reworking close ties to and dependency on one's parents. As part of this undertaking, the individual be-gins to differentiate the self from internalized representations of the parents' prohibitions and ideals; the latter marks the superego of childhood that pro-vides moral guidelines and self-regulating functions, serving as a source of positive self-esteem as well as guilt. Whereas school-age children tend to-ward unquestioning acceptance of and compliance with parental authority, adolescents begin to feel less bound by the older generation's preferences and mores; the teenager's strongly felt need to at least question, if not openly chal-lenge, the parents' values increases the potential for considerable family con-flict. Often, in place of the parents, the mid-adolescent begins to identify with and idealize the behaviors and beliefs of peers, groups, and iconic cultural figures. No longer are mothers and fathers the sole generators of standards.

During late adolescence, the process of individuation shifts: more com-fortable with their sexualized bodies, equipped with maturing cognitive and socioemotional abilities, and relatively less threatened by fears of depen-dency and re-infantilization, young individuals in their late teens and 20s feel a diminished urgency toward knee-jerk rejection and defiance of parents and their values. In addition, greater cognitive flexibility and mentalization capacities lead to more sophisticated moral reasoning; old as well as unfa-miliar values and novel ways of thinking are subject to consideration and reassessment and serve as potential sources for emerging personal princi-ples (Lapsley et al. 1984). As part of the lengthy, gradual process of identity and personality formation, late adolescents begin to re-internalize a modi-fied, more self-determined, and less reactive version of the superego; the more mature form integrates the old (familial and cultural guidelines inter-nalized in the earlier years of childhood) with newer values and ideals that are unique to the young person's generation and particular experience (Settlage 1972). This synthetic process begins during the opening years of emerging adulthood, but the dynamic interplay of novel experience, re-flection, and integration continues well into the mid- and late 20s (see Chapter 5, "Identity in Emerging Adulthood," for a more detailed discus-sion of identity and personality development during the later emerging adult years). Ultimately, unlike the superego of the childhood years, the emerging adult's developing ideals and moral standards represent a more autonomous, personalized, and nuanced set of guiding values and self-appraisal that is independent of the physical presence of authority figures.

Access to nonparental mentors and positive role models is extraordi-narily helpful during this developmental period, allowing the late adolescent to respect and emulate adults who are not associated with the childhood self and by whom they are more likely to be viewed as a soon-to-be young adult rather than as a former infant and child (Chused 1987; Eichler 2011). College instructors and advisers, internship supervisors, job trainers, and bosses may all function in this capacity. Such mentoring adults provide interest and support without familial bonds and can be instrumental in helping the late adolescent begin to envision the self in different ways and separate from the parents' powerful wishes and fantasies. In addition, adult guides offer pragmatic advice, teach skills, and expand the older adolescent's fund of knowledge, fostering a sense of competence and capability.

The *ego ideal*, a wishful and aspirational function of the superego, takes shape as the late adolescent integrates an evolving set of ideals and an envisioned, hoped-for future self with real-life experiences that elucidate individual strengths and weaknesses. Increasingly aware of reality, and of the gap between personal frailties and abstract ideals, the young person is exposed to painful self-doubts and threats to self-esteem. Self-dissatisfactions may be projected onto society as a whole, leading to intense feelings of disillusionment with the existing cultural milieu (Settlage 1972). A key developmental task of late adolescence involves softening unrealistically perfectionist standards for the self and others while retaining ideals and optimism; this gradual and sometimes painful process involves coming to terms with the bodily and psychological self (physical imperfections, areas wherein intellectual aptitude is weaker, emotional needs and vulnerabilities), accepting people's limitations, and tolerating disappointing behavior in the self and others.

The Process of Identity Development During Late Adolescence

In Chapter 5, we discuss in more detail the concept of identity and its unique role in development during emerging adulthood. Erikson (1956, 1968) postulated that identity is a lifelong psychological and social process that acquires preeminence during late adolescence, when the young individual starts to grapple with fundamental questions such as: Who am I to myself and others? What do I stand for and believe in? What is my place in this world? (Besser and Blatt 2007; Blos 1968, 1972; Gilmore and Meersand 2014; Meeus et al. 1999; Ritvo 1971; Schwartz et al. 2013). An increasing sense of urgency for answers corresponds with an intensifying need to define a unique, individualized self that is separate from the childhood persona and parental perceptions. This normative identity crisis fuels a process of self-growth that is marked by active exploration of roles, relationships, values, and myriad other identity domains within a social milieu that provides ongoing feedback; the continuous interaction between self and social surround, wherein the young person presents a particular version of the self and seeks and receives (or fails to receive) validation from others, forms the heart of the identity exploration process. Ultimately, identity formation marks an integration of childhood values, identifications, and self- and other representations with maturing, more autonomous versions of the self (Blos 1968, 1972; Erikson 1956; Ritvo 1971). Although Erikson and other psychoanalytic writers have located the epitome of this process in the late adolescent phase, contemporary research suggests that identity experimentation begins in the late teens but continues throughout the sweep of the emerging adulthood decade.

Identity development takes place at the interface of a maturing and increasingly reflective mind, the surrounding society and culture, and the unique generational zeitgeist within which the young person comes of age. For contemporary emerging adults, their status as digital media natives vastly expands their access to information and ideas, provides potential interactions with distal as well as immediate communities, and offers varied platforms in which they can experiment with verbal and video self-presentations while receiving copious feedback from friends and strangers. These outward explorations are powerfully shaped by the interior mental components of identity, which function less visibly; thoughts and feelings about the self, unconscious and preconscious fantasies about roles and relationships, personal memories, and habitual modes of self-regulation and defense affect the emerging adult's choice of identity pursuits, openness to new experience, tolerance for uncertain outcomes, and receptivity to others' responsiveness.

Moratorium settings, such as college, facilitate the identity process by offering easy access to novel experience and expansive possibilities as well as a time frame in which binding decisions need not be made; however, many environments can support the young person's need for exposure to new roles, relationships, and ways of thinking. Examples of identity experimentation include the first-year college student who seeks to reinvent the self as a less studious, more sociable partygoer; the previously heterosexual adolescent who starts spending time with new, more sexually diverse friends and begins to feel curious about same-sex liaisons; the young person from a secular background who befriends a more observant coworker and starts attending regular services at that individual's church; or the recent high school graduate who initiates a small dog-walking business to earn money, makes friends with other dog-walker peers in the neighborhood, and begins to discover both a penchant for entrepreneurial endeavors and a love of animals. An example of adjusting to life without parental oversight is shown in Video 1. In this video, a 20-year-old college student who began her studies during the COVID-19 pandemic reflects on the complex ways in which she integrates a close connection to her family with her own emerging interests, values, and sense of self.

 Video 1: Adjusting to life without parental oversight

Identity represents the individual's sense of continuity and *self-sameness* in the presence of others, creating stability even during shifting emotional and social circumstances (Erikson 1956). As a complex facet of personality, it draws together disparate aspects of the intrapsychic, interpersonal, and societal selves, integrating fantasies and feelings, modes of relating to others, and ways of being in the wider world of social community. The late adolescent's developing capacity for narrative identity, which encompasses a grasp of causality (i.e., the way in which earlier relationships and events may affect the present), further consolidates a feeling of personal coherence; the self is increasingly experienced as a recognizable, autobiographical self with a past, present, and future (Habermas and Bluck 2000; Habermas and de Silveira 2008; McAdams and McLean 1985). Fundamental aspects of personhood, such as sexual orientation, ethnicity, and race, are synthesized in more complex ways as the young person gains an expanded sense of shared destiny, integrating self not just with immediate family but also with the history and current status of relevant groups and cultures (Umaña-Taylor et al. 2014).

As a substantial empirical literature demonstrates, the multiple domains of identity (e.g., gender, political views, religious beliefs) do not necessarily develop in tandem (Schwartz et al. 2013). However, the process by which young people explore and ultimately commit to operationalizable identity components appears to follow a fairly consistent sequence of active experimentation (also referred to as the *moratorium period*); reflection and reconsideration; and, finally, identity achievement or commitment; this process begins in adolescence, but the bulk of identity achievements are often deferred until the emerging adulthood years (Becht et al. 2017; Meeus et al. 2010; Schwartz et al. 2013). During the moratorium or exploratory phases, individuals actively sort through various alternatives; temporary commitments are made, during which one option is selected, lived out, reflected on, and often reevaluated.

The possibilities for self-discovery, transformation, and reinvention are exciting and energizing for many young people, but the identity process inevitably involves inner tension, ambiguity, a state of inner flux, and a sense of loss. Foundational aspects of the former, younger self—long ago internalized prohibitions and approvals, the parents' dreams and visions for their child's future, and even the emerging adult's own previous self-certainties—begin to shift. Giving up long-held notions, eschewing familiar guiding principles and set paths forward, and beginning to assume greater self-direction often involve a period of uncertainty, anxiety, and internal conflict. Moreover, even within relatively safe environments, such as the college moratorium, some young people feel exposed and insecure when experimenting before others, particularly within highly public internet platforms that carry a risk of negative feedback. Fears and inhibitions about active exploration, or avoidance of the more reflective aspects of meaningful self-discovery, can lead to problematic identity conditions: *foreclosure* occurs when the young person commits to an aspect of identity without fully engaging in prior exploration and reflection, thereby cutting off the potential for full self-discovery; *diffusion* refers to failures in both the exploration and the subsequent cohesiveness of identity (Marcia 1966; Meeus et al. 2010; Schwartz et al. 2013). Such derailments in the search for personal authenticity can manifest via overconformity, poorly integrated representations of self and others, vague and superficial beliefs, or broader struggles committing to goals and values; often, these difficulties reflect not only problems during emerging adulthood but also cascading issues from prior developmental periods, such as long-standing dysregulation of affect and mood or a history of trauma (Ammaniti et al. 2015). Mental health problems or poor management of alcohol and substances further affect the identity process. We discuss the stresses and potential pathologies of identity development more fully in Chapter 7 ("Psychopathology and Emerging Adulthood").

Relationships During Late Adolescence

The relational lives of late adolescents reflect their maturing cognitive and emotional capacities, increased autonomy and individuation, and expanded opportunities for independent social connection. Ongoing identity exploration is inevitably intertwined with deepening interpersonal capacities as fundamental aspects of self-with-other (social roles and values as well as gender and sexuality) are tried on and modified; indeed, the young emerging adult brings an evolving rather than a consolidated relational self to social experiences. Family bonds may remain close, but a decline in dependency on the parents facilitates new and meaningful nonfamilial identifications and connections. Exposure to relationships beyond the family is key to developmental progression as familiar roles and ways of being with others undergo significant reexamination and alteration (Blos 1968; Eichler 2011; Ritvo 1971).

The late adolescent's improved emotional self-regulation and reflective capacities facilitate more mature forms of empathy and mutuality. Internal pressures from sexual and aggressive impulses are better controlled than in the earlier phases of the teenage years, which leads to greater confidence in self-reliance and availability to focus on the other. A desire for more meaningful, intimate romantic connection begins to emerge; whereas adolescents typically start dating between ages 12 and 14, often in group settings, entry into the period of early emerging adulthood is marked by a growing tendency to pair off and to view relationships as less about recreation than about gaining experience with intimacy and sexuality (Arnett 2000; Padgham and Blyth 1991). The ongoing identity process and increasing sense of a unique, independent self are foundational for more mature relationships in which individuality is increasingly integrated with relatedness and self-interest is balanced with caring for and prioritizing another's needs (Auerbach and Diamond 2017). In a wider context, the older adolescent begins to grasp more fully the connection between self and society, both current and historical, and develop a sense of social purpose and responsibility.

Parents continue to play a significant emotional role in their children's lives; the late adolescent's sense of positive connection and perceived parental support is highly correlated with overall social and emotional adjustment, including good self-esteem (Laible et al. 2004). At the same time, in Western industrialized societies, these primary object relationships are irrevocably altered and realigned as the maturing individual assumes greater responsibility for the self and begins to invest deeply in life beyond the family. Shared respect, less hierarchical parameters, and overall greater reciprocity begin to emerge as key features of the late adolescent-parent bond; although the parents often retain significant financial and other responsibilities and continue to function as loving advisers and guides, their role as the sole voice of authority or main consultants is considerably reduced.

Within attachment theory, late adolescence marks a redefining of balance among the key domains of security, autonomy, and exploration; the quality of attachment to parents does not necessarily change, but proximity is less crucial, new ties and loyalties gain importance, and the drive toward identity experimentation carries the young emerging adult far beyond the parents' purview (Ammaniti and Sergi 2003; Steele et al. 2015). Psychoanalytic theories view the late adolescent-parent relationship somewhat differently, conceptualizing this relatively more harmonious, less dependency-laden bond as a natural resolution of earlier mid-adolescent upheaval. In this view, conflict with parents declines as the young person feels less destabilized by sexual urges and re-evoked oedipal longings and less fearful of passivity and re-infantilization; the need to oppose or rebel in order to deny childhood needs and achieve a sense of separation loses its urgency, giving way to a more stable, secure sense of individuality and diminished embroilment in conflict with authority figures. These developments signal a new openness to connections with adults, such as professors, who can mentor the young individual and help compensate for the loss of former ties (Bonovitz 2018; Chused 1987; Eichler 2011).

A decisive turn toward peer relationships originates in the earlier teen years but acquires new meaning during the phase of late adolescence. Friendships play a crucial role in mitigating the loss of physical and psychological proximity to the family of origin and emerge as a major source of overall self-esteem and psychological well-being. Indeed, perceived social connection is highly correlated with the young emerging adult's well-being and positive functioning across a wide range of variables, including good mental health, academic adjustment, and retention in college settings (Conley et al. 2014; Laible et al. 2004; Manago et al. 2012). The use of social media to enhance in-person connections, as well as to establish and maintain purely digital relationships (such as with video-gaming comrades, who are known only through online play and discussion), can function positively by expanding the contemporary late adolescent's perceived social network (Manago et al. 2012).

The early emerging adulthood years often overlap with the first fully sexualized love relationship. The intensity of such experiences typically includes preoccupations, longings, idealization of the beloved, elevated mood followed by deflation, and dependency on the physical presence of the other that is reminiscent of the earliest parent-child bond (Kernberg 1974; Kulish 1998; Ritvo 1971). Often of limited duration, the first love affair nonetheless serves important developmental functions, marking the young person's initial mobilization of sexual desire and fantasy along with tender, caring feelings for the other. Moreover, experiencing the self as sexually desirous and desirable marks a key component of the late adolescent's emerging identity and serves as a crucial underpinning for adult self-esteem; in this way, even if fleeting, memories of and associations with the earliest love affairs can have an enduring influence on feelings about the self and attitudes toward intimacy. Although frequent, transient sexual liaisons are highly typical of the college social scene, even these brief encounters serve as explorations into the sexual and gendered self-with-other; moreover, they provide practice for managing and expressing sexual urges, fantasies, and other feelings in a situation in which personal desires must be balanced with what the other person wants and needs (Besser and Blatt 2007; Shulman and Connolly 2013).

The following vignette traces a 20-year-old male's first 2 years at a residential college, where he experiences his first sexual relationship and notices shifts in his priorities and in his bonds with family.

Case Vignette: Amir

Amir's close-knit family had celebrated his acceptance into a small liberal arts college a couple of hours away from their home; his parents were happy for him to experience independence via dorm living, but they felt comforted by knowing that he could easily board a train to come home for a visit. Privately, Amir was looking forward to weekends on campus, where he would not have to be so furtive about drinking and getting high, behaviors of which his parents disapproved and that had led to considerable conflict with them during high school. In addition, although he had come out as bisexual in ninth grade to most of his friends, and then gradually to the broader group of high school peers, Amir had not shared this fundamental information with his family; he was fairly confident that his parents would react supportively, but he knew that his mother's extended family members, many of whom lived in the Middle East, were quite religious and traditional, and he worried about creating conflicts. He imagined an easier time of it with his father's family, which he perceived as far more assimilated and Americanized. Ultimately, it had seemed easier to simply avoid disclosing to anyone in the family, including his younger siblings, who were likely to be unfazed but who were not known for their discretion. Besides, he had largely eschewed sexual experience, despite a couple of intense crushes, telling himself that he was very focused on his grades and extracurriculars and did not really have time for such involvements. Because of this, nobody in the family had ever learned anything about Amir's sexual orientation; his parents seemed to assume he was attracted to girls only given their occasional, unwanted comments about young women in his friend group. However, Amir was certain that once on campus and out from under family scrutiny, he would feel freer to indulge in sexual experimentation, perhaps more along the lines of what his high school friends, many of whom had lost their virginity in senior year, were eagerly narrating via social media.

As Amir had hoped, his social life began to change almost immediately on arriving at school. As a freshman, he joined a gender diversity club; he felt extremely engaged in and proud of his work in the club and had developed a few close relationships there. In addition, he had experienced a few brief sexual encounters with students he had met at the club's parties. One of those liaisons, with a young man who was an upperclassman and a leader in the organization, began to assume significance. Marcus, who was from an entirely different background—white working class, raised in middle America—had captured Amir's interest from the outset; despite Marcus's small-town roots, Amir perceived him as the more worldly, sophisticated, and relaxed of the two, and he was also warm, friendly, and attractive. Certainly, Marcus appeared to have far more sexual experience, and he took the lead in initiating physical contact. Moreover, although his immediate family actually sounded less educated and progressive than Amir's, Marcus had come out as gay to his parents in junior high school and often teased Amir about his lingering secrecy.

Amir had never been so at ease in his own body or so invested in the world around him; it was as if his feelings for Marcus made everything more meaningful and exciting. Back in high school, which now seemed like the distant past, achieving the highest grades had dominated his personal goals and guaranteed teacher and family approval. Now, however, Amir made a different calculation: he maintained a decent grade point average, but the bulk of his energies went into the club and his social life; often, he and his friends, including Marcus, worked well into the night brainstorming ideas and interfacing with other organizations online but also joking around, playing video games, and drinking beer. His parents had asked about his grades and had seemed slightly disappointed and surprised when he revealed that they were mostly in the B range, but he had dismissed their reactions with annoyance.

Inner tension began to build around an upcoming spring break because not only his parents but also his close high school friends had planned an active schedule of socializing for Amir. But Amir had already agreed to go home with Marcus, whose parents were reportedly eager to meet their son's college boyfriend. He had no idea how to break this news to the people back home; he could handle his friends' disappointment—they would surely be sympathetic because they had often urged him to initiate something with his previous crushes—but he dreaded his mother's predictable quiet, sad reaction and his father's likely lectures. In addition, he was worried about some Instagram postings by his group that showed him with Marcus in affectionate poses; could one of his siblings or cousins have seen the photos? He did not want to feel like a younger kid who fretted over his parents' feelings and his extended family's beliefs; those were their problems, not his. He fantasized about crushing all self-doubts by making a series of announcements to his parents: he would simply assert that he was spending spring break with his boyfriend; furthermore, he would inform them that they should stop questioning him about grades and future plans for graduate school because these were no longer his priorities. For a few days, such fantasies provided excitement and a sense of efficacy; in these daydreams, he was in charge of his destiny. A couple of his college friends encouraged him along these lines, sharing their own stories of having come out to parents with varied outcomes. Ultimately, however, Amir decided against these moves and instead made a compromise: he would go home for half the week and go to Marcus's for the rest of the time. Predictably, nobody was pleased with this outcome, but Amir still felt that it was the best decision. Over the summer, when there was more time, he would have a conversation with his parents about his sexuality so that such situations would not feel so difficult in the future. Meanwhile, he would manage his guilt and hope that Marcus, his parents, and his high school friends would all be understanding.

This vignette depicts a late adolescent raised within intersecting cultures (his American friends; his mother's more traditional, non-Western family) who embarks on the process of self-exploration and actualization, particularly in the realm of romantic and physical relationships, and allows himself to engage in sexual behavior for the first time in his life. In many ways, his love interest, Marcus, represents novelty: the unfamiliar experience of sex and romance, a slightly older individual from an entirely different walk of life, the freedom to pursue gratification without familial constraints. Although Amir rationalizes his earlier abstemious stance as having been designed to keep the peace at home or as a result of his devotion to his studies, no doubt it also reflects his own deeper conflicts, insecurities, and inhibitions. Amir's own belief system and values are in flux: it is unclear whether he himself leans toward his maternal family's perceived traditional stances, which could pose serious internal tension in terms of his sexual desires and relational fantasies. Once away from home and in the presence of supportive peers, Amir finds himself more ready to seek sexual contacts. He begins to reexamine his priorities, now trying to balance academic ambition with his growing investments in other areas; he considers his parents' disappointment in his grades a burden, but how does he himself feel about a decline in his academic performance?

The conflict over a return visit home causes Amir to consider in a new way his ongoing affection for his parents because it clashes with his strong desire to pursue the relationship with Marcus: he no longer wants to "feel like a younger kid," and his fantasies—of a decisive break with perceived family pressures—mark a wish to see himself as a young man who follows his own path. Yet it is clear that he continues to feel guilt over his family's imagined reaction to his sexual orientation and connection to Marcus, to his slipping grades and shifting priorities, and to his decision to spend vacation time away from the family. The spring break compromise is an attempt to deal with inner conflict; Amir settles himself down by resolving that he will reveal more to his parents during the leisurely summer vacation, for the moment incurring everyone's dissatisfaction but not having to deal with some of the larger issues and worries.

Role of the College Experience

The late adolescent period, between ages 18 and 23, overlaps with attendance (not necessarily through to graduation) at some form of college for approximately two-thirds of youth (Bureau of Labor Statistics 2022). Parents may retain a high level of responsibility for their children's well-being (e.g., providing financial support, intervening in health crises), but they operate across a greater distance for the teenagers who head off to dorms; the young person's daily choices about broad swaths of life—making decisions around sex and substances, figuring out how to balance work and recreation—take place without the immediacy of parental oversight. As we have suggested, despite the late adolescent's evolving capacities for independence, these newfound freedoms potentially unmask long-standing vulnerabilities (e.g., deficits in behavioral control and organization) or as-yet-unidentified problems in the face of diminished structure and risky but immediately rewarding behaviors. Our experience as late adolescent clinicians and supervisors of emerging adult treatments is replete with cases of young people who eagerly embark on the college experience, perhaps even with a history of successful performance in high school, but soon encounter major difficulties managing themselves and maintaining the necessary balance between academic work and recreational outlets. In some cases, these young people are negotiating new or exacerbated psychiatric conditions (attention problems, substance issues, mood disorders); in others, a high level of parental, therapy, and tutoring support may have enabled them to function well enough in high school but did not adequately prepare them for a sudden reduction in scaffolding.

At the same time as it exposes the young individual to unfamiliar challenges, the residential college experience provides access to a true psychosocial moratorium: the student can experiment freely across a wide range of identity potentials, trying on diverse interests, roles, and relationships within an audience of peers while largely eschewing finalizing commitments. Although colleges offer a preliminary step toward fuller self-reliance, these relatively protective milieus—with their provision of scheduled classes, meal plans, roommates, activities and clubs, resident advisers, and other mentors—function as way stations between the home life of mid-adolescence, when parents met needs and set terms, and the more reality-based experience of postcollege life that coincides with the second segment of emerging adulthood. Even at that postgraduation juncture, typically around age 22 or 23, many young people return to living at home or are just beginning to make financial contributions to their own upkeep; some will continue on to additional schooling, perhaps further prolonging a period of parental financial involvement.

As defined in "The Process of Identity Development During Late Adolescence," the psychosocial moratorium represents a setting where the young individual selects, actively experiments with, and reflects on a variety of identity domains, ranging from intellectual interests to sexual orientation, while remaining free from pressure to make final decisions about the future; the college experience, with its innumerable offerings of academics, social connections, and mentoring, serves this purpose particularly well. Meaningful engagement in college life inevitably exposes the late adolescent to new identificatory figures, a more diverse range of influences, and opportunities to fulfill previously untapped potentials. Recognition and validation by classmates and friends, admired adults, and the community at large form crucial feedback during the period of exploration as different aspects of the self are auditioned before others and then reassessed. Internet platforms vastly increase the options for creating identities, posting assertions, sharing one's voice and personal stories, and receiving others' reactions.

In our view, these explorations within the moratorium distinguish the late adolescent's identity searches from those of the 23-and-older group; late emerging adults continue active experimentation within different identity domains but also begin to make decisions and commitments that ultimately funnel them along certain relational and occupational paths. The early emerging adult's identity process is often more playful and generally does not seek to actualize dreams and visions for the future. Typically, the encroachment of time and other realities is deferred until later in the 20s, when the individual encounters a greater degree of reality and consequence and begins to narrow the realm of open possibilities and assume greater responsibility for the self (Colarusso 1991; Gorney 2016).

Late Adolescence and the Non-College-Bound Teenager

What about the sizable number of late adolescents who do not attend college? The *forgotten half* refers to young people who traverse emerging adulthood without attaining postsecondary school credentials, a status known to correlate with higher levels of future financial insecurity (Terriquez and Gurantz 2015). This large group, which represents about 40% of emerging adults, covers the approximately 29% of high school graduates who do not enroll in any further study and also the many students who matriculate at colleges but fail to complete their degrees, often incurring significant financial debt without enhancing their qualifications for work (Bracey 1999; Bureau of Labor Statistics 2010; Rosenbaum et al. 2015). Moreover, there are meaningful distinctions between the groups who pursue community college and those who attend a traditional 4-year university because the former are disproportionately drawn from low-income backgrounds. Research on students who pause their college experience, intending to return at some point in the future, suggests that these young people often are experiencing family financial stress; in addition, those who halt their educational progress are unlikely to return and complete their degrees (Terriquez and Gurantz 2015).

Studies on emerging adult cohorts represent diverse socioeconomic backgrounds, encompassing participants who do not attain college degrees (Arnett 2016). Although young people from more disadvantaged circumstances endorse higher levels of depression and less positivity, Arnett (2000, 2016) suggested that their overall attitudes and beliefs positioned them well within the conceptualization of emerging adulthood theory: they reported optimism about the future, described a sense that their current lives are in flux, and placed value on self-development over specific financial goals. Arnett's (2016, p. 234) conclusion of "one stage, many paths" attempts to capture both the diverse trajectories and the unifying themes of the overarching emerging adult group.

However, we feel strongly that the distinctions among these groups of young people—more privileged, college-graduation-bound late adolescents; those who fail to complete postsecondary programs for a variety of reasons; and early emerging adults who are struggling to support themselves and perhaps also their families—are meaningful in ways that have perhaps not yet been fully captured by existing research. Late adolescents who have access to a true psychosocial moratorium—a form of college experience or some other setting conducive to the young person's playful, nonconsequential exploration—will inevitably experience greater identity options over a more prolonged period than their peers who go directly to work or who are both unemployed and without further educational prospects. Lack of access to novel experience, unfamiliar peers, mentors, and new ideas inevitably affects the late adolescent's visions and fantasies of a potential future self. Indeed, all major identity theories (e.g., Erikson 1956, 1968) prioritize the continuous process of trying on roles, receiving feedback from others, and ultimately making selections. Moreover, the presence of new nonfamilial adult figures, who envision and guide the young person differently from the parents, plays a role in emerging adult development (Chused 1987; Eichler 2011). Although the late adolescent who enters the workforce may find such individuals in the form of more senior coworkers and supervisors, the roles embodied by these older adults are far more defined; for example, a boss's investment in a young employee is likely more specific than that of a college adviser promoting exposure to a range of potential interests and self-discovery. These profound environmental differences suggest that reality-based pressures—often in the form of financial limitations and urgencies—potentially force a large group of late adolescents into decisions and pathways that may constrain both self-exploration and future options, an important distinction from the lengthier, fluid odysseys of their more advantaged age-mates.

Late Adolescence and Cultural Experience

The concept of *youth culture* marks the unique set of shared norms, values, interests, and tastes that tend to differentiate adolescents from other cohorts; defining characteristics include modes of communicating, personal appearance and style, and various art forms as well as responses to wider social issues such as protesting wars, mobilizing action for the environment, and promoting a more inclusive society. Studies into youth culture burgeoned following the 1960s in response to young people's growing role as barometers of societal ills and increasing visibility as drivers of change in broad arenas such as sexual mores, civil rights, and attitudes toward war (Esman 1990; Vanden Abeele 2016). Although early and middle adolescents are avid consumers of popular culture (e.g., they are *digital natives*, often in the thrall of internet personalities and influencers) and are frequently moved by social issues, it is primarily their older, more autonomous counterparts—late adolescents and emerging adults—who occupy the vanguard of cultural experience, interfacing directly with cultural entities and serving as forerunners of social change. We explore youth culture in far greater detail in Chapter 6 ("Youth Culture").

Adolescent culture is not a monolith: huge variations in a group's history, socioeconomic status, and access to resources, as well as the dominant events and overall zeitgeist of a particular era, powerfully shape ideals and forms of youth self-expression. However, certain commonalities of adolescent cultural trends are noted: they tend to involve spaces (including the body but also the internet) that are outside the direct purview of adults; they often mark the young person's search for meaning and authenticity outside adult-dominated conventions and expectations, a quest that can be mistaken for rebellion and defiance; and they capture the imagination of late adolescents who are immersed in identity exploration and discovery, contributing to the process of individuation and self-definition (Esman 1990; Gilmore and Meersand 2014; Smith 1976; Vanden Abeele 2016). Moreover, the symbols, attitudes, and behaviors that are demonstrated often elicit discomfort and confusion in older age groups; the use of the virtual world offers a stark example of adolescents' intense immersion in screen media, which often creates a divide with older generations. At the very least, the older age groups are likely to feel out of step with rapidly emerging new social media platforms; beyond that, older adults may experience a more pervasive sense of ineptitude or feel baffled by the younger generation's ease with public self-representations, dating apps, and virtual friends.

In Video 2, a 20-year-old gamer discusses the multiple ways in which his intense technology-based interests have evolved to open up not only potential career paths but also friendships and romantic relationships.

 Video 2: Finding a place in the gaming world

Socioemotional Challenges and Psychopathology in Late Adolescence

In Chapters 7 and 8 ("Therapeutic Modalities in the Treatment of Emerging Adults"), we elaborate the mental health problems and conditions that are common in emerging adulthood and discuss approaches to treating these problems. Most serious psychiatric disorders are diagnosable by the early years of emerging adulthood. These include the personality disorders, which are typically first identified by age 18 (American Psychiatric Association 2022); as we discuss in subsequent chapters, however, many clinicians familiar with the normative states of flux that characterize the entire sweep of emerging adulthood are cautious about applying this particular category of diagnostic labeling to this age group. At the same time, rates of depression, suicidality, anxiety, disordered eating, substance use, and general distress are significantly elevated. College students, in particular, report a high degree of emotional strain; nearly one-quarter report levels of anxiety and depression that interfere with daily functioning (American College Health Association 2019). Clinical levels of stress are especially prominent in the first year of college, corresponding to the initial adjustment to life away from home; establishing a sense of social connection marks a major source of well-being, and perceived failures in this area lead to pronounced disruption of emotional health (Conley et al. 2014). Rates of identity distress, related to increasing internal and societal pressure for self-definition, also rise during the college years; although normative levels of anxiety are expected to accompany identity experimentations, serious stress in multiple domains of identity can disturb or inhibit the process of self-exploration (Palmeroni et al. 2020). Importantly, the manner in which young individuals cope with the transition to college appears to establish more enduring patterns for managing subsequent stressful life experiences (Conley et al. 2014).

Some of the most potentially derailing conditions appear as young people make their first forays into independent living. These include schizophrenia, which is correlated with an array of etiological factors (genetics, previous childhood and adolescent trauma, excessive use of cannabis and other drugs) and tends to emerge during the late teens and 20s (Jaaro-Peled and Sawa 2020; Kessler et al. 2007). Similarly, bipolar disorder, which carries a higher rate of suicidality than other psychiatric illnesses, is typically first identified during late adolescence (Joslyn et al. 2016).

Several prior vulnerabilities are intensified or more clearly disclosed by the late adolescent's sudden leap forward in autonomy and loss of home-based structure. Released from direct parental supervision, the young person who is living away from family must learn how to devise routines; balance work and play; meet project deadlines; and calculate levels of risk when it comes to sex, drinking, and substance use. Those individuals who enter this period of development with a history of less than solid self-regulation, especially if combined with drug and alcohol abuse, are at greater risk for poor adjustment. The same is true for adolescents who have already experienced low mood and anxiety in the early or middle teen years, although these conditions may also make their first appearance in the context of independent functioning (Prenoveau et al. 2011).

The practice of various risky behaviors increases dramatically from mid- to late adolescence and continues to rise during the later emerging adulthood years; indeed, rates of illicit drug use are highest within the 18–25 age group, and alcohol use in this age group is also elevated. Binge drinking occurs at significantly higher rates among college students than among their noncollege peers (Osberg et al. 2011); similarly, use of safe-sex practices on campuses is reported to be low, whereas rates of casual sexual encounters are high (Scott-Sheldon et al. 2008; Shulman and Connolly 2013). These various findings suggest that despite increased capacities for self-regulation, many emerging adults struggle to manage risks in the areas of personal health and safety.

Additional vulnerabilities affect those late adolescents who continue to be mired in the conflict-laden issues of middle adolescence; these young people often remain enmeshed in parent-child tensions, fear losses of power and control vis-à-vis new authority figures, and dread the feelings of re-infantilization that arise in the context of relating to professors or supervisors at work (Chused 1987; Ritvo 1971). Such conflicts powerfully affect the needed capacity to form new, potentially helpful relationships with older mentors and may contribute to failures to perform well in settings where the young person must meet deadlines, subject the self to evaluation, and fulfill others' expectations. Competitive situations, and the potential for successes or failures, may evoke intense and even disabling feelings of anxiety and guilt, leading to maladaptive defense mechanisms (avoidance, self-defeating behaviors). In Chapter 8, which discusses treatment models, we review possible methods of addressing mood, substance-related, and conflict-laden problems in the emerging adult cohort.

Late Adolescence or Early Emerging Adulthood as the Final Phase in Adolescent Development

To best demonstrate the unique psychological tasks, vulnerabilities, and strengths of the early emerging adulthood period, it is helpful to consider its position as the culminating phase of adolescence. In the following paragraphs, we review major theories of adolescent development and examine the young person's progression through a series of physical, social, and emotional capacities and challenges.

The decade or so of adolescence, from about ages 13 to 23, encompasses a period of momentous psychological and physical transformation. During these years, the young person's daunting developmental tasks include adjusting to the sexually maturing body; loosening dependency on the parents and assuming greater responsibility for the self; navigating the social world of peer pressures and potentially risky behaviors; beginning to engage in romantic and sexual relationships; and beginning to explore identity potentials across an array of domains, which leads toward an increasingly individualized and coherent sense of self. Evolutions in cognitive prowess facilitate far greater capacities for self-reflection, broader understandings of social concepts and issues, and an increasing ability for hypothetico-deductive reasoning.

The widespread acceptance of adolescence as a concept is relatively recent; although promoted by Hall (1904) at the turn of the twentieth century, its full legitimacy as an acknowledged developmental phase was not achieved until around the 1950s (Dahl and Hariri 2005). Hall's original notions about the inevitable "storm and stress" of this period are consistent with many but not all views of the teenage years. Within the psychoanalytic literature, internal upheaval and conflict with authority figures are central to theorizing about this phase: the young person is seen as struggling toward autonomy during a process Blos (1967) labeled the *second individuation*, in which the previously intimate tie to the parents undergoes a degree of necessary rupture (Chused 1987; Freud 1958). Such a view is consistent with the oft-depicted dramatic teenager of Western society's films and stories who rebels against conformity, defies adult-set limits, and renounces the outmoded values and mores of established society.

Other writers, however, espouse conceptualizations of the adolescent phase that do not revolve around Sturm und Drang or around discord with parental figures. Attachment theorists, for example, suggest that high levels of conflict and disturbance are neither ubiquitous nor inevitable. These writers emphasize the reorganization and realignment of key organizing mental systems—that is, attachment security and exploration; in their view, underlying connection to the parents remains strong for the previously securely attached child, despite obvious shifts in the adolescent's socioemotional focus, priorities, and sense of personal authority (Ammaniti and Sergi 2003; Doctors 2000). Researchers (e.g., Beyers et al. 2003) who view adolescence through the lens of other specific constructs, such as agency or an internal locus of control, view the teenager's acquisition of autonomy as potentially unrelated to the parent-child bond.

In our view, a contemporary perspective includes recognition of adolescence as a vulnerable period for parent-child conflict and action-based, risky behaviors. Although dramatic external signs of trouble are certainly not inevitable, and the teenager's potential for disturbance is powerfully mediated by family and community support, there is abundant empirical and clinical evidence for increases in disruptions of judgment, poor emotional self-regulation, more frequent discord with parents, and lapses of behavioral self-control beginning in the early adolescent years (Arnett 1999; Dahl 2004; Doctors 2000; Rutter 2007). We believe that psychoanalytic theory offers a rich view of the teenager's internal world, with complex ways to contextualize the well-known propensity for action, apparent disregard for personal safety, and diminished compliance with adult authorities, even in the presence of essentially stable previous and ongoing relationships with parents. Within this theory, such trends reflect several psychological processes: the teenager's increased sexual and aggressive urges and the concomitant drive toward action; fears of re-infantilization and regression that are associated with passivity in the face of the parent-child bond; the need to divest from internal representations of parental strictures and mores (i.e., the superego) in order to establish a unique, autonomous moral compass; and the lengthy, gradual search for a personal identity that involves active, ongoing exploration and testing of one's mettle in all available realms of the adolescent's life (Blos 1968; Erikson 1956; Ritvo 1971; Settlage 1972).

Given the complexity and lengthy duration of adolescence, we find significant value in retaining the traditional division into early, middle, and late phases; although certain major themes, such as identity and autonomy, reverberate throughout the decade and beyond, each period poses its own unique challenges (e.g., the unprecedented bodily changes of puberty during the early phase), marks a high season for salient emotional issues, and contributes to the ongoing development of personality.

We begin with the phase that directly precedes puberty, forming a bridge between the grade school years and adolescence proper. *Preadolescence*, the period immediately before puberty (typically ages 10–12, but sometimes slightly younger, particularly for girls), brings late childhood to a close with a cascade of both subjective and tangible changes; these include novel sexual and aggressive feelings, accelerations in weight and height, and the appearance of secondary sex characteristics, all of which contribute to a sense of internal upheaval that disturbs the former calm of the grade school years (Erikson 1956; Gilmore and Meersand 2014). Heightened conflict with family, mood instability, and outward signs of restlessness often mark the entry into this period of development as the child struggles to cope with a body that seems unfamiliar and uncontrollable (Besser and Blatt 2007; Paikoff and Brooks-Gunn 1991). At the same time, the preadoles-

cent's cognitive advances contribute to higher levels of self-reflection, social perspective-taking, and abstract thinking (Barkai and Hauser 2008;
Piaget and Inhelder 1969; Spear 2000). Increasingly, the child pursues experimentation with transient new identities that signal distinctions from
the younger self and also from the parents.

The passage through preadolescence often corresponds with the child's
shift from grade school to junior high school, bringing an unprecedented
demand for self-organization and a host of novel social pressures. Peer relationships, often with same-sex youngsters, assume greater importance;
membership in friend groups, as well as in intense and often fleeting best
friend dyads, is eagerly sought (Fischer 1991; Friedman and Downey 2008).
In addition, transient forays into opposite-sex encounters, which may have
been eschewed during the latency years, begin to increase (Sroufe et al.
1993). In this early phase of identity exploration, as the child increasingly
looks to peers and surrounding teen culture for cues and new standards, the
preadolescent experiments briefly with different friend groups, styles,
modes of behavior, gender-based roles, and ways of presenting the self.

The dramatic bodily events of puberty mark the entry into *early adolescence*, typically the period between ages 12 and 14. The first highly visible
physical changes of preadolescence, such as gains in height and weight,
continue at an accelerated pace and are joined by the full range of pubertal
changes in bodily contour and functions. The sense that the body is out of
control leads to a variety of defensive maneuvers that seek denial or avoidance of the corporeal self, including the following: a flight toward intel-
lectuality, which recruits newfound cognitive capabilities; a tendency to
renounce bodily pleasures and lean toward ascetic behavior; the seeking of
a personal style that masks the body and its changing contours; and a tendency to delve deeply into digital media, wherein one can create personas
and experiences that seem to negate the concrete, bodily self (Lemma 2010;
Sandler and Freud 1984). Shame over physical development, secretions,
and smells, along with fears of exposure, are particularly daunting during
this famously awkward and also painfully self-conscious time of life. The
young adolescent whose entry into puberty is delayed compared with the
peer group also suffers; social status and feelings about the self in reference
to the social surround are linked to the timing and pace of physical changes.
Indeed, teenagers whose physical maturation appears out of sync with that
of their peers—via either premature or late development—are at risk for
lowered mood and poor self-esteem (Stice 2003).

Relational changes are highly evident during these years: the young adolescent experiences the heightened allure of the peer group along with a
diminished sense of closeness to the parents, a shift that is often felt by

adults to be sudden and dramatic. Formation of exclusionary cliques, bullying, and social competition and hierarchies are highly characteristic of junior high or middle school life, creating intense social pressures that the young teenager must manage independently, absent the previous support of a familiar head teacher or the involvement of parents and caregivers in younger children's playdates (Espelage et al. 2000). Social outings, as well as internet explorations, are increasingly experienced without adult guidance; with parents at a greater distance, exposure to and participation in risky behaviors increase (Rew et al. 2011).

The years of *mid-adolescence*, roughly covering ages 14–17, correspond with the high school experience. The most dramatic physical disruptions of puberty are likely in the recent past, but the teenager continues to adjust to the possession of a mature, sexualized body and to cope with any perceived disappointing outcomes in appearance; indeed, preoccupation with the bodily self and with one's physical presentation continues unabated throughout the adolescent years. Conflicts with and anger toward parents, often in the context of the older generation's attempts at imposing authority and setting limits, increase in frequency and intensity (Collins and Laursen 2006). A necessary but painful loss of idealization of the adult world, captured in literary classics such as J.D. Salinger's *The Catcher in the Rye*, fuels the mid-adolescent's increasing desire for independence but also creates feelings of loneliness. Decisive turning toward the peer group, along with the elevation of iconic cultural figures, substitutes for the previous reliance on parental strictures and mores; within psychoanalytic theorizing, the process of superego development requires that the internalized representations of the parental voice be jettisoned, to be reevaluated and reintegrated during the subsequent phase of late adolescent development (Blos 1967, 1972). Risky behaviors escalate as the customs and judgments of the peer group eclipse the parents' values and approval.

Conclusion

We suggest that late adolescence forms the first phase of a bifurcated, decade-long period of emerging adulthood; this segmentation is proposed in order to mark the significant distinctions between younger (18- to 23-year-old) and older (24- to 29-year-old) members of the emerging adult cohort. Developmentally and clinically meaningful differences include the novelty of and initial adjustment to often-partial states of autonomy, a remaining dependency on parents for practical and emotional support, very early forays into identity exploration, typical immersion in the moratorium of college life, and the sense of adult-oriented realities and commitments as belonging to a distant future. At the same time, both early and later emerging adulthood are characterized by maturing cognitive and emotional self-regulatory systems, vulnerability to risky behaviors, active engagement in the process of identity experimentation, and a tendency toward instability in the arenas of love and work.

KEY POINTS

- The late adolescent's capacity for increased autonomy represents the interface between intrapsychic developments (ego and superego maturation) and social-environmental expectations and opportunities (increased time away from home and parents, college, or work). The quality of independent functioning continues to undergo significant development during the mid- to late 20s.

- The 18- to 23-year-old is better able than the young adolescent to integrate personal desires with others' needs, grasp multiple subjectivities, and view others as separate individuals with their own histories and complex psychologies. Although late adolescence often overlaps with the first sexualized love relationship, such connections tend to remain casual and are subject to the young person's ongoing identity role explorations.

- In late adolescence, connections with parents may remain close and tend to be less conflict laden than those of middle adolescence; parental support continues to play an important role in the late adolescent's well-being.

- Identity exploration, a major developmental task, involves a process of trying on different roles, ideals, or interests in the presence of others; receiving feedback; and then reconsidering options. Digital media greatly expand the potential for self-expression as well as for receiving feedback. Youth culture is closely intertwined with the identity process.

- The identity process is facilitated by psychosocial moratorium settings, such as college campuses, which provide ample opportunities for experimentation.

- Late adolescence is the final period in the developmental progression of the pre-, early, and middle adolescent phases. It is distinguished by relatively greater adjustment to the maturing body; diminished conflict with parents; and improved capacities for self-regulation and interpersonal intimacy.

References

American College Health Association: American College Health Association–National College Health Assessment (ACHA-NCHA-II) spring 2019 reference group data report. Silver Spring, MD, American College Health Association, August 19, 2019. Available at: www.acha.org/documents/ncha/NCHA-II_SPRING_2019_US_REFERENCE_GROUP_DATA_REPORT.pdf. Accessed November 22, 2022.

American Psychiatric Association: Diagnostic and Statistical Manual of Mental Disorders, 5th Edition, Text Revision. Washington, DC, American Psychiatric Association, 2022

Ammaniti M, Sergi G: Clinical dynamics during adolescence: psychoanalytic and attachment perspectives. Psychoanal Inq 23(1):54–80, 2003

Ammaniti M, Fontana A, Nicolais G: Borderline personality disorder in adolescence through the lens of the Interview of Personality Organization Processes in Adolescence (IPOP-A): clinical uses and implications. J Infant Child Adolesc Psychother 14(1):82–97, 2015

Arnett JJ: Adolescent storm and stress, reconsidered. Am Psychol 54(5):317–326, 1999 10354802

Arnett JJ: Emerging adulthood: a theory of development from the late teens through the twenties. Am Psychol 55(5):469–480, 2000 1084426

Arnett JJ: Does emerging adulthood theory apply across social classes? National data on a persistent question. Emerg Adulthood 4(4):227–235, 2016

Auerbach JS, Diamond D: Mental representation in the thought of Sydney Blatt: developmental processes. J Am Psychoanal Assoc 65(3):509–523, 2017 28899191

Barkai AR, Hauser ST: Psychoanalytic and developmental perspectives on narratives of self-reflection in resilient adolescents: explorations and new contributions. Annual of Psychoanalysis 36:115–129, 2008

Becht AI, Nelemans SA, Branje SJT, et al: Identity uncertainty and commitment making across adolescence: five-year within-person associations using daily identity reports. Dev Psychol 53(11):2103–2112, 2017 29094973

Besser A, Blatt SJ: Identity consolidation and internalizing and externalizing problem behaviors in early adolescence. Psychoanal Psychol 24(1):126–149, 2007

Beyers W, Goosens L, Vansant I, et al: A structural model of autonomy in middle and late adolescence: connectedness, separation, detachment and agency. J Youth Adolesc 32(5):351–365, 2003

Blos P: The second individuation process of adolescence. Psychoanal Study Child 22(1):162–186, 1967 5590064

Blos P: Character formation in adolescence. Psychoanal Study Child 23:245–263, 1968 5759022

Blos P: The function of the ego ideal in adolescence. Psychoanal Study Child 27(1):93–97, 1972

Boelema SR, Harakeh Z, Ormel J, et al: Executive functioning shows differential maturation from early to late adolescence: longitudinal findings from a TRAILS study. Neuropsychology 28(2):177–187, 2014 24364395

Bonovitz C: All but dissertation (ABD), all but parricide (ABP): young adulthood as a developmental period and the crisis of separation. Psychoanalytic Psychology 35:142–148, 2018

Bracey GW: The forgotten 42 percent. Phi Delta Kappan 80:711–712, 1999

Bureau of Labor Statistics: College enrollment and work activity of 2009 high school graduates. Washington, DC, Bureau of Labor Statistics, April 27, 2010. Available at: www.bls.gov/news.release/archives/hsgec_04272010.pdf. Accessed November 22, 2022.

Bureau of Labor Statistics: College enrollment and work activity of recent high school and college graduates summary. Washington, DC, Bureau of Labor Statistics, April 26, 2022. Available at: www.bls.gov/news.release/hsgec.nr0.htm. Accessed May 18, 2023.

Chused JF: Idealization of the analyst by the young adult. J Am Psychoanal Assoc 35(4):839–859, 1987 3693788

Colarusso CA: The development of time sense in young adulthood. Psychoanal Study Child 46(1):125–144, 1991 1788372

Collins WA, Laursen B: Parent-adolescent relationships, in Close Relationships: Functions, Forms and Processes. Edited by Noller P, Feeney JA. New York, Psychology Press, 2006, pp 111–126

Conley CS, Kirsch AC, Dickson DA, et al: Negotiating the transition to college: developmental trajectories and gender differences in psychological functioning, cognitive-affective strategies and social well-being. Emerg Adulthood 2(3):195–210, 2014

Crone EA: Executive functions in adolescence: inferences from brain and behavior. Dev Sci 12(6):825–830, 2009 19840037

Dahl RE: Adolescent brain development: a period of vulnerabilities and opportunities. Keynote address. Ann N Y Acad Sci 1021(1):1–22, 2004 15251869

Dahl RE, Hariri AR: Lessons from G. Stanley Hall: connecting new research in biological sciences to the study of adolescent development. J Res Adolesc 15(4):367–382, 2005

Doctors SR: Attachment-individuation, I: clinical notes toward a re-consideration of "adolescent turmoil." Adolescent Psychiatry 25:3–17, 2000

Dumontheil I, Apperly IA, Blakemore SJ: Online usage of theory of mind continues to develop in late adolescence. Dev Sci 13(2):331–338, 2010 20136929

Dykstra PA, Poortman AR: Economic resources and remaining single: trends over time. Eur Sociol Rev 26(3):277–290, 2010

Eichler RJ: The university as a (potentially) facilitating environment. Contemp Psychoanal 47(3):289–316, 2011

Erikson E: The problem of ego identity. J Am Psychoanal Assoc 4(1):56–121, 1956 13286157

Erikson EH: Identity: Youth and Crisis. New York, WW Norton, 1968

Esman AH: Adolescence and Culture. New York, Columbia University Press, 1990

Espelage DL, Bosworth K, Simon TR: Examining the social context of bullying behaviors in early adolescence. J Couns Dev 78(3):326–333, 2000

Fischer RMS: Pubescence: a psychoanalytic study of one girl's experience of puberty. Psychoanal Inq 11(4):457–479, 1991

Freud A: Adolescence. Psychoanal Study Child 13:255–278, 1958 13614588

Friedman RC, Downey JI: Sexual differentiation of behavior: the foundation of a developmental model of psychosexuality. J Am Psychoanal Assoc 56(1):147–175, 2008 18430706

Galatzer-Levy RM, Cohler B: The developmental psychology of the self: a new worldview in psychoanalysis. Annual of Psychoanalysis 18:1–43, 1990

Gilmore K: Is emerging adulthood a new developmental phase? J Am Psychoanal Assoc 67(4):625–653, 2019 31604388

Gilmore KJ, Meersand P: Normal Child and Adolescent Development: A Psychodynamic Primer. Washington, DC, American Psychiatric Publishing, 2014

Gorney JE: In dreams begin responsibilities: adolescence and potential space. Contemp Psychoanal 52(2):179–200, 2016

Habermas T, Bluck S: Getting a life: the emergence of the life story in adolescence. Psychol Bull 126(5):748–769, 2000 10989622

Habermas T, de Silveira C: The development of global coherence in life narratives across adolescence: temporal, causal, and thematic aspects. Dev Psychol 44(3):707–721, 2008 18473638

Hall GS: Adolescence: Its Psychology and Its Relations to Physiology, Anthropology, Sociology, Sex, Crime, Religion and Education, Vol 1. New York, D Appleton and Company, 1904

Harden KP, Tucker-Drob EM: Individual differences in the development of sensation seeking and impulsivity during adolescence: further evidence for a dual systems model. Dev Psychol 47(3):739–746, 2011 21534657

Jaaro-Peled H, Sawa A: Neurodevelopmental factors in schizophrenia. Psychiatr Clin North Am 43(2):263–274, 2020 32439021

Joslyn C, Hawes DJ, Hunt C, et al: Is age of onset associated with severity, prognosis, and clinical features in bipolar disorder? A meta-analytic review. Bipolar Disord 18(5):389–403, 2016 27530107

Kernberg OF: Mature love: prerequisites and characteristics. J Am Psychoanal Assoc 22(4):743–768, 1974 4423688

Kessler RC, Amminger GP, Aguilar-Gaxiola S, et al: Age of onset of mental disorders: a review of recent literature. Curr Opin Psychiatry 20(4):359–364, 2007 17551351

Kulish N: First loves and prime adventures: adolescent expressions in adult analyses. Psychoanal Q 67(4):539–565, 1998 9820891

Laible DJ, Carlo G, Roesch SC: Pathways to self-esteem in late adolescence: the role of parent and peer attachment, empathy, and social behaviours. J Adolesc 27(6):703–716, 2004 15561312

Lapsley DK, Harwell MR, Olson LM, et al: Moral judgment, personality, and attitude to authority in early and late adolescence. J Youth Adolesc 13(6):527–542, 1984 24306953

Larson RW, Moneta G, Richards MH, et al: Continuity, stability, and change in daily emotional experience across adolescence. Child Dev 73(4):1151–1165, 2002 12146740

Lemma A: An order of pure decision: growing up in a virtual world and the adolescent's experience of being-in-a-body. J Am Psychoanal Assoc 58(4):691–714, 2010 21115753

Malgwi CA, Howe MA, Burnaby PA: Influences on students' choices of college majors. Journal of Education for Business 80(5):275–282, 2013

Manago AM, Taylor T, Greenfield PM: Me and my 400 friends: the anatomy of college students' Facebook networks, their communication patterns, and well-being. Dev Psychol 48(2):369–380, 2012 22288367

Marcia JE: Development and validation of ego-identity status. J Pers Soc Psychol 3(5):551–558, 1966 5939604

McAdams DP, McLean KC: Narrative identity. Curr Dir Psychol Sci 22(3):233–238, 1985

Meeus W, Iedema J, Helsen M, et al: Patterns of adolescent identity development: review of the literature and longitudinal analysis. Dev Rev 19(4):419–461, 1999

Meeus W, van de Schoot R, Keijsers L, et al: On the progression and stability of adolescent identity formation: a five-wave longitudinal study in early-to-middle and middle-to-late adolescence. Child Dev 81(5):1565–1581, 2010 20840241

Osberg TM, Insana M, Eggert M, et al: Incremental validity of college alcohol beliefs in the prediction of freshman drinking and its consequences: a prospective study. Addict Behav 36(4):333–340, 2011 21196082

Padgham JJ, Blyth DA: Dating during adolescence, in Encyclopedia of Adolescence. Edited by Lerner RM, Petersen AC, Brooks-Gunn J. New York, Garland, 1991, pp 196–198

Paikoff RL, Brooks-Gunn J: Do parent-child relationships change during puberty? Psychol Bull 110(1):47–66, 1991 1891518

Palmeroni N, Claes L, Verschueren M, et al: Identity distress throughout adolescence and emerging adulthood: age trends and associations with exploration and commitment processes. Emerg Adulthood 8(5):333–343, 2020

Piaget J, Inhelder B: The Psychology of the Child. New York, Basic Books, 1969

Prenoveau JM, Craske MG, Zinbarg RE, et al: Are anxiety and depression just as stable as personality during late adolescence? Results from a three-year longitudinal latent variable study. J Abnorm Psychol 120(4):832–843, 2011 21604827

Rew L, Horner SD, Brown A: Health-risk behaviors in early adolescence. Issues Compr Pediatr Nurs 34(2):79–96, 2011 21568625

Ritvo S: Late adolescence: developmental and clinical considerations. Psychoanal Study Child 26:241–263, 1971 5163228

Rizzolo GS: The critique of regression: the person, the field, the lifespan. J Am Psychoanal Assoc 64(6):1097–1131, 2016 28899146

Roberts BW, Davis JP: Young adulthood is the crucible of personality development. Emerg Adulthood 4(5):318–326, 2016

Rosenbaum J, Ahearn C, Becker K, et al: The new forgotten half and research directions to support them: summary and key findings. New York, William T. Grant Foundation, January 2015. Available at: https://files.eric.ed.gov/fulltext/ED565751.pdf. Accessed November 22, 2022.

Rutter M: Psychopathological development across adolescence. J Youth Adolesc 36(1):101–110, 2007

Sandler J, Freud A: Discussions in the Hampstead Index on "The ego and the mechanisms of defense," XIII: instinctual anxiety during puberty. Bulletin of the Anna Freud Centre 7:79–104, 1984

Savin-Williams RC: Identity development among sexual-minority youth, in Handbook of Identity Theory and Research. Edited by Schwartz SJ, Luyckx K, Vignoles VL. New York, Springer, 2011, pp 671–689

Schwartz SJ, Zamboanga BL, Luyckx K, et al: Identity in emerging adulthood: reviewing the field and looking forward. Emerg Adulthood 1(2):96–113, 2013

Scott-Sheldon LA, Carey KB, Carey MP: Health behavior and college students: does Greek affiliation matter? J Behav Med 31(1):61–70, 2008 17999173

Settlage CF: Cultural values and the superego in late adolescence. Psychoanal Study Child 27:74–92, 1972

Shulman S, Connolly J: The challenge of romantic relationships in emerging adulthood: reconceptualization of the field. Emerg Adulthood 1(1):27–39, 2013

Smith DM: The concept of youth culture: a re-evaluation. Youth Soc 7(4):347–366, 1976

Spear LP: The adolescent brain and age-related behavioral manifestations. Neurosci Biobehav Rev 24(4):417–463, 2000 10817843

Sroufe LA, Bennett C, Englund M, et al: The significance of gender boundaries in preadolescence: contemporary correlates and antecedents of boundary violation and maintenance. Child Dev 64(2):455–466, 1993 8477628

Steele M, Bate J, Nikitiades A, et al: Attachment in adolescence and borderline personality disorder. J Infant Child Adolesc Psychother 14(1):16–32, 2015

Stice E: Puberty and body image, in Gender Differences at Puberty. Edited by Hayward C. Cambridge, UK, Cambridge University Press, 2003, pp 61–76

Terriquez V, Gurantz O: Financial challenges in emerging adulthood and students' decisions to stop out of college. Emerg Adulthood 3(3):204–214, 2015

Umaña-Taylor AJ, Quintana SM, Lee RM, et al: Ethnic and racial identity during adolescence and into young adulthood: an integrated conceptualization. Child Dev 85(1):21–39, 2014 24490890

Vanden Abeele MMP: Mobile youth culture: a conceptual development. Mob Media Commun 4(1):85–101, 2016

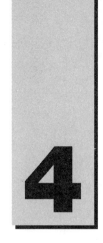

What Is Distinct About the Second Part of Emerging Adulthood?

In this chapter, we elaborate our rationale for proposing a division within emerging adulthood and attempt to better characterize the second half. Although we are aware of the hazards of creating new developmental periods without clear markers, we hope to show the important transformations in mental life that distinguish the relatively neglected second part, making it a critical turning point in development, despite its imprecise borders.

Of course, the usual guidelines apply to any notion of *phases*, a term that is used as shorthand for the strange attractor states of human development that are recognizable as typical developmental configurations, such as toddlerhood or prepuberty (Gilmore and Meersand 2014). Between each state, quantum shifts do occur, but there is always movement preceding the change and vacillations within it, every state has a complex multidetermined etiology, and there rarely is a clear and identifiable moment of transformation even when there may be retrospective recognition of consolidation. In the case of late emerging adulthood, the differentiation rests on the emergence of new attitudes, honed ego capacities, deepening expertise, priorities, and agendas that establish a novel level of gravitas and a notable readiness to reckon with the future. A change in the orientation to the passage of time, to the relational world, and to culture and a new perspective on identity and society are indications of the older emerging adult's maturation and readiness for adulthood; such shifts may amount to a subjectively clear threshold for this stage. The changes in attitudes and agendas interface with changes in social expectations that become increasingly evident toward the end of this momentous decade; the late 20-something is expected to be individuated from family and honing in on a career interest—in other words, "launched," or on the way to it—and assumed to be capable of more mature consideration and decision-making. Light-years from the mental state of the late adolescent straight out of high school, the 28- to 30-year-old shows clear differences in all arenas: evolution of identity, potential for self-reflection, global perspective, confidence in the autonomous self, relational maturity, the diminished allure of popularity in the digital world, and readiness for responsibility in personal or professional life. Societal expectations from the more intimate interpersonal world are also markedly different for that 28-year-old—as conveyed by family, colleagues, and peers, similarly promoting a more mature consideration of adulthood.

The current extension of the time frame of emerging adulthood to age 29, as opposed to the original interval of 18–24 in Arnett's (2000) article, happened gradually and without official acknowledgment. Although this extension has been adopted by most researchers, the change was never fully explained or justified, and the cohorts studied remain predominantly the original 18- to 24-year-olds. In fact, most studies continue to use college students, who as a cohort are reflective of neither the forgotten half (high school graduates who do not attend college) nor the 25- to 30-year-olds. Here we focus on the neglect of the latter group: as noted in Chapter 2, "Development in the Period Between Adolescence and Adulthood," despite the massive accumulation of research and scholarly analysis about emerging adulthood in the past two decades, the second half of this period remains a dark continent—difficult to discern and consequently rarely explored. It is mostly in the awareness of imminent adulthood that some of the mental states and experiences of the late 20s have received attention.

Late emerging adulthood encompasses the years leading up to the realization and recognition of actual adulthood. Even the self-description of "feeling in-between" does not diminish the subliminal awareness that the balance is shifting: a more consequential status is coming, mirrored by the valence of age 30 in the popular imagination. However, even age 30 has lost some of its bite in contemporary culture; it is no longer the same momentous landmark because the tyranny of the biological clock and societal expectations of an established career path have diminished. But without these concrete and socially endorsed threshold accomplishments of the traditional markers, the formerly "uncontested" state of adulthood (Blatterer 2007a) is now in such flux that it remains remarkably amorphous as a project, an identity component, an aspirational ideal, and a social entity (Hunter 2009).

Our understanding of late emerging adulthood is impeded not only by the limitations of scholarship but also by the subjects themselves; they are widely dispersed in every sector of society and only occasionally amassed by design to share the same experiences. Our in-depth knowledge of this group arises mostly from the clinical context and requires further investigation of its neuropsychosocial underpinnings. Thus, although important insights and information can be gathered from the consulting room, from the occasional studies that extend deeper into the 20s, or from studies that highlight aging youths (e.g., the old-timers in music scenes), the problem of creating a coherent picture of mental development remains. What contributes to the persistence of an action orientation into the late 20s? What are the vicissitudes of identity exploration in the real world as opposed to on a college campus? How do values and ideals individuate from those of the contemporary culture and the peer group? Finally, what is the effect of maturing relationships with family, friends, and lovers?

Traditional Markers

In sociology, the traditional description of adulthood included the achievement of markers that were understood to reflect interpersonal and professional maturity as manifested in commitments to social roles and institutions; they were also credited with accelerating maturation. Although we recognize that sudden transformations are relatively rare in development, the attainment of the psychological state of adulthood does occur within the latter part of the 20s and may become conscious with self-reflection. Nonetheless, the data points are difficult to pin down operationally. Even at the turn of the twenty-first century, the young emerging adults (college students) examined by Arnett expressed skepticism about four out of the five traditional markers (Arnett 2000). Financial self-sufficiency was still endorsed, but independent domicile, a career path, marriage, and child-rearing were demoted in importance. These informants instead cited autonomous decision-making and taking responsibility for such decisions as more meaningful than the markers (Arnett 2000). In the two decades since, young respondents have not reverted to the markers but increasingly emphasize personal attributes that appear to be the maturational aspirations of the entire period.

This demographic shift—that is, the delay in independent domicile, marriage, childbearing, and the like—was the initial sign that alerted Arnett to a change in the development of people in this age range, inspiring his new theory. After two decades of subsequent scholarship, the limited collection of studies on *attitudes* (as endorsed by college students) toward achieving adulthood confirms Arnett's original observations that the evolution of commitments to relationships and interests and the capacity to take responsibility (e.g., Dennison 2016; Roupa and Kusendová 2017) are consistently associated by informants with the subjective meaning of adulthood. Adulthood is then the result of a process whereby experience and psychological development gradually yield a more autonomous and self-determined individual with an evolving independent value system (super-ego) and expertise but without the standard stabilizing requirements of independent domicile, marriage, children, and career. Indeed, the minds and actions of the 24- to 30-year-old cohort suggest that emerging adulthood is no longer simply preparatory to traditional adulthood; it is a way station where the narrative integration of the past, a growing capacity to take perspective, and a more deliberate synthesis of an adult project are achieved in preparation for a future that is different from prior iterations.

New demographics and changing attitudes form a kind of feedback loop that seems to gradually expand and extend. In addition to the demographic trends Arnett cited, which were primarily focused on delayed achievements (and continue to drift upward in the two decades since his initial observations), there are others: extended life expectancy, a decline in economic well-being in comparison with the parent generation (Taylor 2015), a decline in marriage rates in the late twentieth and early twenty-first centuries (Curtin and Sutton 2020), and a decline in religious affiliation and participation such that current membership has dwindled to less than half the population (Jones 2021). Although employment among this age group had been trending upward prior to the coronavirus SARS-CoV-2 disease (COVID-19) pandemic, job instability was still much more common and was typically associated with housing insecurity, which led to a boomerang or yo-yo effect (returning home or moving into and out of the parental home; Hill and Bosick 2017) as jobs were gained and lost. Indeed, a linear progression from emerging adulthood to the attainment of adult markers is increasingly uncommon (Hill and Bosick 2017); however, if the destination has unclear value, then the absence of pathways is not the primary issue.

The rapid transformations in digital communication and technology contribute to yet another gap between generations. The famously benighted boomers are now grandparents, and the first wave of emerging adults are presumably tech-savvy parents, but new technology skills begin to bloom in kindergarten. The pace of advances continually creates disjunctions between generational cohorts.

In the section "Markers of Adulthood: How Do They Play Out Today?" later in this chapter, we reexamine these demoted traditional markers of adulthood in today's world and assess whether they add any value to self-representation to individuals as adults. There is, of course, one notable exception to the discredited markers—that is, financial independence. Financial autonomy has always been cited as the rate-limiting step for the achievement of all the other markers—independent domicile, marriage, and children—but currently, it does not appear to be equated with a sure pathway toward an adult life made meaningful by these accomplishments. Indeed, it seems more valued for its potential to support an independent, self-determined life. As long as there is enough money to sustain and stabilize the chosen lifestyle—to maintain autonomous living and to manage geographic, partner, and career changes—the notion of an identity fixed by career, geography, marriage, and children is not a meaningful signifier. One important caveat: As this book was being written, the economy was reeling from the effects of the COVID-19 pandemic—rates of homelessness, unemployment, and crime had increased, and the pervasive disruption of schooling and childcare for all social strata resulted in a critical loss of income for many populations, especially the disadvantaged and poor strata of society. These developments interfered with chances for financial independence, which in turn further delayed independent domicile, weddings, and the prospect of children. COVID-19 pushed the demographic shift that Arnett cited even later.

In Videos 3 and 4, two young men, a 25-year-old architect and a 26-year-old graduate student, present very different versions of late emerging adulthood while grappling with the same issues of career direction. They both convey a strong identification and connection with their parents, even while crafting a more mature dynamic with them.

 Video 3: Creating a professional identity during emerging adulthood

---

 Video 4: Late emerging adult and a creative path forward

Persistence of Late Adolescent Attitudes, Preferences, and Behaviors

Risky Behavior

Studies documenting the persistence of risk behaviors into the late 20s include some data specific to late emerging adults. Although risk-taking behaviors across the globe follow an inverted U pattern, peaking in adolescence and gradually declining in the early 20s, there are a few, including alcohol use (Bray et al. 2019), risky driving, antisocial risk-taking, and risky health-related behaviors (Duell et al. 2018), that remain elevated into the mid- to late 20s.

The neuroscientific *dual systems theory* attributes risk behavior to asynchronous brain development beginning in adolescence. It is now well established that brain development continues through adolescence and into young adulthood (Forde et al. 2017; Spear 2013), beginning with cortical pruning starting at puberty and differentiated by region, especially in the prefrontal area, where it continues until it stabilizes at age 30. Similarly, myelination, which enhances the speed of transmission, evolves throughout development, with a clear spike in adolescence. These findings support dual systems theory as a plausible explanation of the predilection for risk-taking in adolescence: sensitivity to reward and sensation-seeking peak in mid-adolescence, whereas the full development of the prefrontal cortex is achieved only in the mid- to late 20s. Speculating about the protracted development of executive capacities and restraints, Duell et al. (2016) hypothesized that this delay exposes the system to more environmental influence, presumably that of the peer group, subculture, or scene, as well as the culture at large. In a cross-cultural study (Duell et al. 2016), the social expectation of self-control in adolescence appeared to influence the timing and degree to which self-regulatory capacities emerged. These authors proposed that because of the relatively minimal environmental expectations for self-control in North American culture, not to mention the coveted status of flagrant risk-taking within some peer groups and youth cultures, the freedom to pursue sensation and risk continues unchecked, at least in select activities, despite the maturation of the prefrontal circuitry.

Acceptance of risk-taking varies by context, certainly within typical youth cultures but also in many predominantly peer-dominated settings such as college campuses and local hangouts, where substance use, risky driving and sexual behaviors, and antisocial activities continue to be applauded into the late 20s and 30s. For example, health-related risks peak in men at ages 24–25 and continue at about the same level until 30. Risky driving continues to rise until ages 27–28. And ravers continue to search for the next party, where communal trance states, liberal use of methylenedioxymethamphetamine (MDMA; ecstasy), and dance innovation extend well into the 30s, often serving as a kind of weekend identity for the weekday workaday executive (Goulding et al. 2002) (see Video 8 in Chapter 6, "Youth Culture"). Steinberg (2008, p. 27) hypothesized that the problem may be due to the lack of "cross-talk" and "balance" between brain regions governing intellectual capacity and those contributing to psychosocial maturity; these two crucial networks begin to converge only at around age 26. But this idea does not fully explain the persistence of participation in youth cultures and peer groups that reward risk into the 30s.

As mentioned, risk-taking is acutely sensitive to the degree of immersion in a like-minded peer group that rewards audacious behavior. Risk-taking is also hypothesized to be sensitive to changes in social role, such as marriage, but given that the average age at marriage has now stretched to 30 for men and almost 30 for women (U.S. Census Bureau 2021) and that marriage is embraced by less than half the population (Brown and Sheffield 2020), its impact is inevitably reduced. Indeed, many assessments of the desistance effect of marriage on risk behavior used older populations who married before the "divorce revolution" (Zoutewelle-Terovan et al. 2012, p. 5); more recent studies do not show a convincing effect. Instead, some studies point to *parenthood* as the adult experience that mitigates a predilection toward risk (Gorlitz and Tamm 2020). But the effect of parenthood has also been shown to be variable and, in many cases, only a short-lived deterrent (Theobald et al. 2018).

Former Youth Culture

Another factor that sustains some behaviors deemed risky derives from the current or former youth culture of a given individual. As discussed in Chapter 6, many activities associated with risky youth culture continue into the 30s, including among extreme sports enthusiasts, circuit partygoers, goths, ravers, and rappers. Some of these activities are physically dangerous, and some are risky because of substances or illegality. As noted in the previous subsection, some aging youth culture participants straddle two lifestyles: they are weekend warriors dedicated to their youthful behaviors and weekday working stiffs (Goulding et al. 2002); such veteran youth culture participants show sufficient judgment to continue their sustained, albeit selective and intermittent, participation in slam dancing, heavy metal, queer culture, and so on (Bennett and Hodkinson 2012). This enduring identification and dedication not only to the pleasures but also to the sense of self and community gained from youth culture seem to enable some older emerging adults to retain their function—even while they simultaneously face admonitions from others, including the parent generation, significant others, or employers, to settle down. Even among youth cultures themselves, the tyranny of ageism is reflected in critical commentary about aging gay icons (Taylor 2012), rock stars, and ravers—which is all the more striking because these individuals gained their status by defying convention when they first engaged in their cultures. Within a decade, they are not infrequently decried by the rising generations in their cultures as immature and unable to grow up.

Some individuals gradually renounce or diminish the importance of their membership in youth culture, but many in today's world do not. Within the financial constraints imposed by the requirement to earn a living or with the continued support of parents and grants for postsecondary education, there are (and possibly have always been) the aging icons—singers in a range of genres, deejays, extreme sports enthusiasts, and so on—who smooth the way to continued participation. The new model of work, which is removed from the conventional office, allows time to pursue youth cultural interests. The passionate commitment and self-definition attached to these cultures are deeply important; many adherents marry fellow participants and bring their kids along. Some participants develop a vocation or avocation from within their culture, by, for example, managing a band, getting involved in music recording, or taking styles popularized in the culture to the commercial fashion world. The older enthusiasts who initiate their children into their youth culture hope to impart to the next generation the underlying values that attracted them when they first joined the scene and thereby ensure its survival.

Studies of aging youth cultures and the interface with marriage and child-bearing have developed only in the past decade (Little 2018), although research on risks in this age group associated with employment and criminality has a longer tradition. Data remain sparse regarding the effects of family on older emerging adults' continuation of risky behavior. The bulk of the extant literature, which includes risk associated with job demands and crime, shows that willingness to take risks decreases temporarily for men and women alike around the birth of an infant (especially the first) but then within a few years returns to baseline (Gorlitz and Tamm 2020). The power of adult achievements to shape predilections and behavior seems limited at best.

Continuing Psychological Appeal of Risk

The continuing psychological appeal of risk is an arena that merits further research and clinical investigation. The conditions that contribute to the upsurge in risk-taking in adolescence and emerging adulthood presumably are in decline as age 30 arrives, with the synchronization of the neurodevelopmental dual systems. Similarly, the crucial role of *action* in identity formation in late adolescence and early emerging adulthood (Chused 1990) would presumably be less pronounced as young people approach 30. Yet the finding that significant numbers of late emerging adults continue to be drawn to action, with or without substances, may reflect something about the premium placed on identity fluidity and perhaps specifically the complexity of fashioning an adult identity in contemporary culture. Although clues may come from neuroanatomical, sociological, and cultural studies, we believe the psychological counterpart is in urgent need of study. What makes the motor keep running? The extreme sports enthusiasts are perhaps most remarkable and spectacular; some trajectories suggest that the peer group reward diminishes in importance, although other enthusiasts continue to require the peer group for refueling. The extraordinary alpinist Marc-André Leclerc, whose life and death at age 26 were featured in the eponymous documentary *The Alpinist*, eschewed the usual augmentation of public performance and died with a single fellow climber. Perhaps the transmutation of such relentless action into a dedicated life defined by expertise makes sports devotees a unique group, but action and risk-taking pervade other more typical youth cultural activities. For example, some graffiti artists continue into their 20s and 30s and some gay circuit party-goers continue well past age 30.

Importance of Music

Even in cases in which the level of involvement has diminished, connections to youth culture persist. With the pathway forged by the aging icons of various youth cultures who have persevered in their sport or in their music, their similarly aging fans remain avid concertgoers, with deep emotional connections to the musical soundtrack of their scenes. The specific music associated with a culture, whether its main focus or its favored status among adherents, has been recognized as a kind of time machine that restores and reinvigorates the connection to the scene, past and present: "The music is 'the key' to cultural memory" (Fogarty 2012, p. 64). Despite the departure from age-appropriateness and the normative expectation that musical tastes age alongside the body (Bennett and Taylor 2012), entire genres or certain songs, especially one or two that have served as rousing anthems of their youth culture of the past (whether that culture be musical or not; Taylor 2012), are deeply evocative for many former participants.

Markers of Adulthood: How Do They Play Out Today?

Given that emerging adults diminish the significance of traditional markers, a look at the actual trends in their behavior may be informative.

Financial Independence and Employment

Despite the sense among many late adolescents and young emerging adults that their lives are full of possibilities and that personal flexibility trumps stability in terms of their success, their sense of autonomy and diminished tolerance for relying on their family of origin enhance the value of this traditional marker of adulthood. Financial independence has profound significance for many emerging adults who feel infantilized by taking money from their parents and who are keenly aware how the hierarchical parent-child dynamic obstructs progress toward adulthood. Support often comes with pressure to conform to parental expectations, both lofty and mundane, and to parents' views of what is acceptable in regard to object choice, career direction, religious participation, manners, dress code, and the like. As noted in the preface to Part II ("Phases of Emerging Adolescence"), the importance of financial independence is endorsed among younger emerging adults as a condition of adulthood (Arnett 2000), and it appears to be equally important to some parents (Lowe and Arnett 2020) whose recognition provides confirmation. But unless inherited wealth provides the means (a circumstance that itself can undermine feelings of adult efficacy), the desire for financial self-sufficiency must in turn inform the degree of gravitas with which employment is contemplated as the 20s come to completion.

However, in the twenty-first century, instability is not altogether problematic in terms of outcome. Education fluctuation—that is, intermittent participation—seems to be correlated with career success at age 32, which suggests that starts and stops in training and educational options may result in better fit in the final choice; this is the positive side of exploration (Krahn et al. 2015). In contrast, high job instability, termed *floundering*, predicts a less satisfactory future career choice (Krahn et al. 2015).

The pandemic has altered the job prospects of emerging adults from the gamut of socioeconomic strata, which makes it difficult to determine trends. However, well before the pandemic, the emerging adult literature highlighted the loss of predictable career pathways in contemporary society. Many factors contribute to this phenomenon, including the shift to an informational or technological economy, the decline of many traditional societal structures that served to guide the young person into a social role and career over time, the intentional diminution of available vocational training in high school and college, and the tendency to seek higher education in lieu of grappling with the question of a viable career. In this atmosphere, a renewed interest in providing real, concrete skills to young people has emerged. As noted in the vignette about Tanya (Chapter 2), a decision to pursue vocational training instead of a college degree may trouble the parent generation, but for many young people it establishes a solid career pathway and identifies potential excellence within the time frame under discussion.

In the following vignette, Ray, a young man of 23, was groping for the right fit in terms of gratifying work; his family members had all embraced and excelled at traditional professional and academic careers, whereas Ray struggled to come to terms with his childhood conviction that his intellectual and aspirational limitations prevented him from leading a successful life on his own terms. Inspiration arrived just in time.

Case Vignette: Ray

Ray graduated from college at age 23 without a clear plan; he moved back home and took an entry-level job with a magazine. He liked the magazine itself, which was technology oriented, but he was not at all interested in the low-level work he was assigned and had no intention of becoming a journalist; he nonetheless felt that he needed to earn some money to prevent a "total backslide." His parents were minimally intrusive and busy working themselves, but despite their acceptance, it felt regressive to him to be staying in his childhood bedroom. This arrangement put a real damper on his romantic and sexual lives. These had been a source of pride in college, where he had come to realize that he had appeal for a lot of women.

Ray experienced himself as the "black sheep" of his family because his older sister was high achieving, attending a prestigious university for her Ph.D., and his younger sister had just entered an Ivy League college. His parents were both respected professionals (lawyer father and Ph.D. psychologist mother) and professors. Ray had struggled in grade school and had been diagnosed with a learning disability in fourth grade. He began to hit his stride in high school and excelled in his small liberal arts college as a humanities major. Nonetheless, he was convinced he would never be a real (academic) success and would never get the respect afforded his other family members. Behind this was a worry that he had no academic calling. Overall, he was at a loss as to how to manage this knot of self-doubt, career confusion, and sibling rivalry.

Ray's fondest dream was to create a bar-restaurant that would be geared to his age group, with an atmosphere of friendship and warmth. Here he could obliterate rivalry and relax in a world of his own creation among siblings of his own choosing. While working at the magazine, he trolled bars he thought were similarly conceptualized, gathered tips and information, and planned how his place would be different and better. He capitalized on his social skills, which allowed him to win people over with his sincere interest in their stories, his sly sense of humor, and his cultural savvy, and soon collected a pool of potential mentors. Nevertheless, he had few serious investors, no business plan, and indeed no real business experience. After a year of exploring this idea, he was compelled to consider other options. An easy alternative was to apply to the local university and get an advanced degree in English. He thought of this as a preliminary step toward something as yet unclear.

On another front, Ray had recently met a young woman, Bella, who was working on the waitstaff of a popular café while finishing college. She was also uncertain of her direction; she had always wanted to be a dancer but had left her prestigious training school because it had become clear to her that she would never succeed as a ballerina. She struggled to make ends meet but was determined to get her bachelor's degree. She waited tables and occasionally performed in indie dance projects put on by friends and colleagues. Ray teased her about being a diva but confided to his friends and family that he thought she was beautiful and kind. They began to date while he was in graduate school and she was finishing college; they soon cohabited.

Ray completed a master's degree with honors but thought, "Now what?" He was still uninspired by his possibilities. His closest friend from high school had gone to law school, and even though Ray had never before shown interest in the law, he began to think he might give it a try. After all, his father was a successful lawyer, and he had many other relatives who were lawyers, judges, and/or law professors.

The son of a family friend was planning to start prepping for the Law School Admission Test (LSAT) and encouraged Ray to join him. Ray talked this over with his parents, who were concerned but cautiously supportive. They did not want Ray to hit another wall and thought that he might be diving headfirst into a highly competitive world that would not truly interest him without having really tested his aptitude. They nonetheless supported his decision. Ray suppressed his own doubts and decided to join his friend in a course intended to prepare people for the LSAT.

From the outset, Ray was overwhelmed by the memorization, the methodical thinking, and the alien logic of the law. He had learned to work hard in school, but he was simultaneously bored and overwhelmed by the sheer volume of material he was required to learn. He used every resource available online and in person but could not get his bearings. He lasted 4 months and dropped out, feeling disgraced, seriously depressed, and a disappointment to his family. Luckily, he was already receiving treatment and benefited a great deal from a prescription for an antidepressant and from therapy with a person who had already known him for 3 years. He got an administrative job at a hospital with which his mother was affiliated, hoping that when he recovered from this blow, something else would come to him. He was without inspiration or purpose, except in his personal life, in which he felt increasingly committed and certain. He was in love with Bella and knew she was "the one."

Ray's dilemma was made more stark by Bella's evolution; after she graduated from college, she waited tables and worked briefly for Ray's mother in her office. The warm relationship between them sparked Bella's interest in the field of psychology. On Ray's mother's advice, Bella sought a job in the research unit of a nearby hospital and advanced through the ranks to project manager; she took some prerequisite courses and was admitted to a graduate program. This heightened Ray's feeling of urgency, especially because he wanted to propose to Bella. Her support and encouragement were reassuring, but any proposal had to include the statement that he had no prospects but would do his best to deserve her. He was then 28 and she was 25.

The wedding site was to be a farmhouse in the country. Ray decided to join in the preparations for the chosen site and found great pleasure in planting, pruning, and shaping the landscape. By chance, he was present at a luncheon given by his father's colleague that was also attended by the director of a botanical garden and horticulture school; they talked at length, and Ray began to think that the work of planting, caring for trees, and designing landscapes could be very satisfying. On the honeymoon, he raised this possibility with Bella, who reassured him that she would make a good living and that he should follow his instincts.

Ray found horticulture school fun but also very demanding because plant and tree identification seemed like yet another memorization mountain. However, his horticultural work placement put him in a beautiful urban park with hundreds of trees whose names he wanted to know, surprisingly rich and varied wildlife, and real landscaping work to be done. Ray had a more optimistic feeling about the "right fit." He read extensively about the environment and the importance of urban green spaces. He was convinced that despite his lack of a science background, he could learn what he needed from the job and from reading and would maybe even consider a higher degree in the field in the future. When he graduated from the program at age 30, he had a job waiting for him at the site where he had fulfilled his field placement requirements; he felt relieved and happy that he had found the first step in his (possible) career.

Ray's journey highlights the powerful effect of discovering a calling. For Ray, as for other emerging adults, "a career is an integral, active and essential component of a person's life. A career captures individuals' concerns for their occupational futures, confidence to engage in designing their futures, and executing plans to make them real" (Shulman et al. 2015, p. 10).

Stable Work or Career Plan

Ray's erratic trajectory took him through technology, academia, and a brief foray into his father's profession before he arrived at a job in a traditional profession on a historic site. Ray's story is an example of *goal adjustment* (Shulman et al. 2015) and reflects the crucial capacity for *career adaptability* (Savickas 1997). According to Savickas (1997), this capacity should replace the notion of maturity in career development (p. 257). The capacity for adaptability seems especially desirable for today's emerging adults. In addition, Ray's marriage plans, albeit conventional, occurred in a delayed time frame consistent with current trends, although not necessarily in the order Erikson (1979) originally proposed wherein intimacy follows identity.

In contrast to Ray's slow-paced and digressive path, contemporary culture highlights the fabulous "overnight" success of entrepreneurs, technology innovators, internet celebrities, rap stars, influencers, and others: their stories have inspired countless others to self-brand, promote other brands, perform, demonstrate, and teach. The accumulation of "likes" can catapult an internet consumer to internet celebrity; social media platforms have democratized the process by which dedicated posters can enhance their popularity to become influencers, promoting their brand through videos, Instagram stories, YouTube channels, retweets, memes, and the like. Media scholars have focused increasingly on TikTok as the new social media platform as its popularity soars; the app was downloaded 2 billion times in the first quarter of 2020 (Abidin 2021). Interestingly, and in a departure from other popular platforms such as Instagram, "TikTok privileges sounds over images" (Abidin 2021, p. 80). TikTok has evolved into an ever more complex platform, amplified by the forced isolation of the pandemic and reliance on social media. As of March 2021, 22.4% of its users were ages 20–29, surpassed only by the 10- to 19-year-old cohort (25%; Ceci 2023). Internet scholars have taken up the idea of *attention economies* (Goldhaber 1997), in which attention is the currency in an era of information overload: every audience creates potential larger audiences and can be monetized. And indeed, tangible market value has been achieved by many influencers and TikTok posters.

Although the idea of attention economies stirs controversy and debate as a principle of economics, there is no doubt that it has psychological significance for young people. Certainly, the trend of monetizing attention on the internet has been amplified by the lengthy isolation of the pandemic; success on social media platforms is now the setting of the emerging adult project, the opportunity for self-realization tempering adolescent fantasy with real or realistically possible future accomplishment. Indeed, many young people have chosen social media platforms in order to become influencers or celebrities with massive numbers of followers and sponsors rather than seeking conventional employment. With an established following, they hope to parlay their success into more traditional sectors or a stable public persona that can lead to the next gig. Here we see how reliance on the peer group continues virtually, to buoy the process of self-development by likes and eventual endorsements.

More ordinary (i.e., less entrepreneurial) young people are "milling about" (Tanner 2006) in their 20s—even if sitting on their beds—seeking their calling, their opportunities, their envisioned future. Job changes are frequent and require geographic moves, often disrupting relationships and identity components based on regional affiliations (Borschel et al. 2019). Job instability has been especially problematic in the economic downturn created by the pandemic and even in its gradual recovery: "labor market disruption remains a hallmark of the COVID-19 recession" (Parker et al. 2021). The hard-won discovery of a desirable career goal and the stepping stones required to achieve it have been, in some cases, dismantled by job loss, which has led young people to consider different occupations (Parker et al. 2021), especially if the welcoming atmosphere of an interim job in the low-wage sector has proved persuasive. Job insecurity has reverberations in many other choices that are facing the older emerging adult: as noted, domicile and marriage considerations are inevitably influenced by financial stability (Rea et al. 2020).

Independent Domicile

Although establishing a domicile of one's own was not ranked as an essential signifier of adulthood in Arnett's (2000) surveys of emerging adult attitudes, the goal of living apart from parents has been historically deemed fundamental to the growing up process, particularly in studies of the more affluent, college-bound youth whose individuation and independence are facilitated by the intermediate step of campus life and the ready-made array of opportunities it provides. In fact, the processes highlighted by twentieth-century adolescent scholars—individuation and identity formation—were largely derived from observations of middle- and upper-class youths leaving for college. The college experience of grappling on one's own with the change in living circumstances, the many choices available, and the radical diminution of adult supervision was viewed as the backdrop for the early development of autonomy, independent decision-making, the depersonification of the superego, identity explorations, self-regulation, romantic relationships, and progress toward resolution of the "adolescent crisis" (Erikson 1968). Simply in regard to independent living, a 2010 study observed that not only was the subjective experience of adulthood enhanced by having an independent domicile, but also the chances of successfully navigating the series of achievements signifying adulthood were consistently associated with living independently (Kins and Beyers 2010): the effect of independent domicile enhanced the likelihood of "transforming the hierarchical parent-child relationship to a relationship of mutual support" (Kins and Beyers 2010, p. 770) and was correlated with financial independence, the formation of committed relationships, success in role transitions, and the capacity to assume a family role. Clearly, this step has experienced a setback because of the COVID-19 pandemic, even while continuing to follow the direction set in the first decades of the 2000s. In July 2020, 52% of emerging adults (18–29 inclusive) were living at home, the highest percentage since the Great Depression (Fry et al. 2020). There is a noteworthy difference between the two parts of the emerging adult cohort, with 78% of 18- to 24-year-olds living at home and only 28% of 25- to 29-year-olds doing so.

In late emerging adulthood, living with parents after some period of separation is known as the boomerang effect; many college graduates return home directly, joining members of their cohort in their neighborhoods who did not attend college or did so while living at home. The non-college-attending group, ages 25–29 years, has shown the sharpest increase in living in the parental home, up to 25% in a 2014 poll (Desilver 2016). The extension of this situation into the 30s is highlighted by a more recent U.S. Census Bureau report that 17.9% of 25- to 34-year-olds continue to live in the parental home (Creamer et al. 2020). Contributors to this trend, which long preceded COVID-19, include financial constraints in general, college debt, a problematic housing market, job instability, and many demographic delays in the assumption of social roles. By returning to their parents' home in late emerging adulthood, boomerang kids face both shame and censure in taking a step that, however financially helpful, is traditionally stigmatized in North American culture (Abetz and Romo 2021). In these circumstances, mutual efforts to negotiate a shift in the hierarchical parent-child relationship toward greater equality can support emerging adults' steps toward adult identities; such a hierarchical shift promotes the potential for more open discussions of the arrangement, including a timeline and expected contributions to the household (Abetz and Romo 2021). Nonetheless, living at home may highlight how circumstances differ between when parents were starting out and when their emerging adult children are doing so; contemporary emerging adults' immediate prospects and even a hope of achieving anything like their parents' financial success are diminished. According to Taylor (2015) from the Pew Research Center, "on almost every single indicator you might use (e.g., employment, unemployment, income, wealth, debt, poverty), Millennials are the first generation in modern history to start out doing less well than their parents" (p. S10). This trend continues for Generation Z (born 1997–2012).

Of note is that both boomerang and failure-to-launch kids differ by race and ethnicity, with Black, Hispanic, and immigrant (from non-Western countries) youths far less likely than white youths to leave the parental home and more likely to return. A thorough demographic analysis (Lei and South 2016) concluded that these differences are multiply determined, with economics (including macroeconomics), the housing market, role transitions (especially to parenthood), family tradition, and relationships with parents as contributors.

Even as the phenomena of failure to launch and boomerang kids are related to the economics of contemporary emerging adulthood, these general patterns encompass many idiosyncratic factors, such as adverse life events and parental attitudes toward letting go (Livesey and Rostain 2017). Whatever the contributing sources, both parents and adult children may have feelings of failure (Tosi 2020), especially in cultures in which independence and self-sufficiency are valued. Using data from the U.K. Household Longitudinal Study (2009–2017), Tosi (2020) concluded that parental depression increases initially with the return of adult children but gradually returns to baseline.

Given these realities and trends, it is not clear whether the move to an independent domicile will retain any importance as a significant step toward adulthood. However, as the following vignette shows, the failure to move out eventually can be construed by peers as a reflection of immaturity. As this young man's girlfriend noted, "Being in your childhood bedroom is just not hot." This vignette also illustrates a more positive side of this phenomenon: that careers can be launched in ways unknown to the parent generation, even contradictory to their hallowed convictions. It highlights how the opportunity to incubate thoughts and ideas without commitment may provide just the right conditions for developing inspiration. In the vignette, a 27-year-old gamer, Alex, launches a career by gathering notoriety on social media, channeling the inimitable geniuses who came before him and parlaying his talent to make work he loves.

Case Vignette: Alex

At age 27, Alex was a yo-yo kid, moving into and out of his parents' home; he got small freelance jobs as a software designer by advertising on Task-Rabbit and Thumbtack to earn a little money. Alex noted that because he spent his time between jobs playing video games, gaming was all his parents ever saw him do; they were deeply skeptical and worried about his future and hassled him day and night. But his love for video games was unquenchable. He dreamed of being a champion at tournaments but felt he could not face his parents if he gambled his work prospects on gaming. When the nagging turned into arguments, Alex's parents were quick to point out that his undergraduate degree at a prestigious university in computer engineering was too big of an investment on their part to settle for a future of gaming. They noted that it was also a huge investment on his part.

Alex's girlfriend, Louisa, whom he had dated exclusively since their junior year in college, was impressed by his skills in design, engineering, and gaming (which she also enjoyed). She had always been amazed by his spectacular school performance; he excelled in his work without trying. But she knew that that was a deadly "success story" from witnessing its effect on her older brother, Fredo, whose complacency and arrogance made him temporarily unemployable. In Fredo's case, their parents' tolerance dried up almost immediately after he graduated from college. They refused to let him live at home without paying rent, so he was forced to face the workplace and his entitled expectations. Although Louisa thought that her parents had been tough, she saw their response as realistic and growth promoting. And although she could not advise Alex's parents to be more demanding, she openly expressed (to him) her disapproval of his dependency on his parents, his passive adaptation to housing instability, and his unwillingness to think about the future; this was typically under the cover of her complaints that the two of them had no place to themselves, without roommates or parents, where they could be alone and make their own lifestyle decisions, such as getting a dog. She further observed that Alex had the same or better opportunities to work at a start-up developed by their peers as she did, but he disdained having to answer to "some kid from college." She feared pointing out to him that he seemed OK answering to his parents. But he knew without her saying anything that she saw him as childish, like a teenager.

In response to these innuendos and the real possibility that his alternative housing might not be available because his occasional roommate had decided to move in with his girlfriend, Alex was increasingly embarrassed. What would happen if all his friends started seriously cohabiting? As he approached 28, he decided that he had to get serious. The boy genius was (literally) starting to get gray.

Alex then realized that he had been structuring his triumph for a while. In the previous year, he had begun to self-brand as a game wizard on a whim, but recently he had decided to officially launch his brand via his own YouTube channel. On this medium, he demonstrated his ingenious solutions to typical obstacles in moving through the levels of a game favored by people his age, college students, and even some high schoolers. As he accumulated thousands of subscribers, he got annoyed at having to pay the platform half of his earnings. The idea of starting his own company blossomed; he idealized Markus Persson, who invented Minecraft and eventually sold his company, Mojang, to Microsoft for $2.5 billion. Louisa was a little less sanguine about his repeating that success, half wanting it to happen and half not. She certainly appreciated his remarkable talent and was beginning to see some drive flickering when he set his sights on a dream in the sector he loved.

Alex was a big fan of the book *Ready Player One* by Ernest Cline and considered rejuvenating the idea of a virtual world, like OASIS in the book. Doing this would require massive effort and a team. He reached out to certain friends from college whom he thought had talent and ingenuity and enlisted Fredo's business savvy to get investors big and small via GoFundMe and specific appeals to interested parties. Within a year, he and his team had invented a virtual world of astonishing complexity, and everyone believed that it was ready to go live.

What did Alex's parents and Louisa think about this trajectory? Louisa spent time educating his parents; they were of course no strangers to video games but had never really appreciated the depth and breadth of Alex's talents. When Louisa walked them through Alex's world, they said (only a little ironically) that they were "blown away" by its creativity, its endless complexity, and the beauty of its design. They were happy to participate in engaging investors.

As Alex's story illustrates, the extension of the period of role exploration (which can look like lying around and doing nothing) versus conventional employment can bear extraordinary fruit, allowing the time and freedom for talented young people to harness their peak cognitive flexibility and inventiveness (Dougherty and Clarke 2018). It is a version of the kind of "instability" that Arnett designated a defining feature of emerging adulthood. Needless to say, not all emerging adults are exceptional in terms of their innate endowment, which, as Louisa wisely knew, can be an immense gift or a curse.

A more pragmatic question may be how living with parents can be transformed from a continuation of the parent-child hierarchy to a mutually supportive relationship without the aid of a geographic remove, historically seen as the crucial facilitator of Blos's second individuation and Erikson's psychosocial moratorium (Abetz and Romo 2021). In order for emerging adult children to diverge from the value system of the parent generation and figure out what is right for themselves, the parents may need to come to terms with the fact that risk is part of today's world and that flexibility is the only thing a person can really count on.

Many researchers continue to emphasize the importance of role transitions as critical to reaching an adult status (Kins and Beyers 2010). These transitions bear a close relationship to the traditional markers, but they are conceptualized less as attainments in themselves. They are seen as a reflection of an internal readiness to step into adulthood, such as the capacity to make decisions or to make commitments to reliable independent living and the well-being of others. Successfully moving out of the parental home requires that emerging adults be prepared to take care of themselves, assume responsibility for rent and utilities, attend to the usual breakdowns in their environment, and uphold the obligations of the domicile. Today, emerging adults also recognize that risk must be part of their calculations. Clinical work continues to support the psychological importance of this step even if parents must step in as rent guarantors. Although that financial arrangement can feel infantilizing, it can also represent an opportunity to act like responsible adults with parents as witnesses.

Cohabitation, Marriage, and Child-Rearing

Arnett (2014) suggested that attitudes toward marriage and child-rearing have shifted dramatically; just like a stable job and independent living, these two pillars of achieved adulthood are no longer endowed with the same significance, nor do they proceed with a predictable timetable in the early 20s. The splintering of the conventional pathways to adult family life is illustrated by statistical trends in cohabitation, single parenthood by chance or by choice, delayed marriage, diverse family configurations, and a high rate of divorce. Changing views of sex, marriage, and child-rearing (Cilluffo and Cohn 2019) are in sync with the significant demographic shifts observed originally by Arnett. Although attitudes toward sexuality vary in relation to family tradition and religiosity, the trend toward serious, fully sexual relationships without intention to marry has been noted for decades (Rindfuss and VandenHeuvel 1990) and contributes to the statistically significant delay in marriage and older age at marriage for both men and women.

Surprisingly, the U.S. population remains the youngest on average to marry among Western developed nations (approximately 27–28 years old for women and 30 for men) despite increases in cohabitation (Emery 2021; Gurrentz 2018). (According to Mehta et al. 2020, the age at first marriage has climbed even higher: 30 years for women and 32 for men. Despite these varying statistics, the trend is clear.) Indeed, rates of cohabitation exceed those of marriage: among adults ages 18–44 years, 59% have cohabited, whereas 50% have been married (Graf 2019); 66% of cohabitors see cohabitation as a step closer to marriage.

The expansion of cohabitation as a preferred coupling arrangement in the past 50 years stimulated research on the reasons for its ascendance, its demographics, its outcomes, and its correlation with marital dissolution (Kuperberg 2019). The many contributors to its rapid rise include 1) the availability of birth control pills and other forms of contraception, the availability of abortion, and the sexual revolution, which delinked sex and family formation; 2) the trend toward living away from parents (in college dorms or independent domiciles), which diminished parental influence over family forms and over early marriage; 3) the trend toward older age at first marriage; 4) the availability of no-fault divorces, the prevalence of divorce, and the effect of divorce on the children of dissolved unions; and 5) women's greater presence in the labor force and commanding of decent wages, and therefore their greater independence and economic security (Kuperberg 2019, p. 450).

Cohabitation correlates with factors contributing to a *stability gap* compared with married couples; it is associated with less satisfaction and longevity. Despite the availability of birth control, unintended pregnancy is not infrequent among cohabiting couples and is associated with the likelihood of dissolution. For example, two-thirds of cohabiting couples with children separate before the first offspring reaches 12 years as opposed to one-quarter of married couples. In addition, there is a significant racial and class distinction: married couples are more likely to be college educated, to be white, and to have greater earning potential than cohabiting couples (Reeves and Krause 2017). However, any comparison of the stability of cohabiting couples with that of married ones is complicated by the fact that cohabitation occurs at a younger age; age at the formation of a union has an inverse relation to its stability.

Young people's attitudes toward marriage have undergone important changes associated with demographic shifts, individual development, circumstances, and sensibilities. The effect of childhood experience, when parental beliefs and behaviors leave a lasting imprint on minds in formation, is heightened when emerging adults approach role transitions. For example, parents' traditional religiosity, their familial religious observances, and the sanctity of their own marriage may add to the gravity of the path to matrimony, whereas parental divorce and remarriage may cast doubt on the enterprise. Furthermore, young adults' own religious practices, the availability of sexual partners outside marriage, modern birth control technology, easy access to pornography, and the continued draw of youth cultures and many other aspects of contemporary life exert influence on the drive and readiness to marry.

Marital horizon theory (Carroll et al. 2007) suggests that a lengthy marital horizon seems an invitation to persist in risk behaviors, whereas a near marital horizon may hasten maturation, social compliance, and a decline in risk behaviors. The length of the marital horizon has been associated with parent demographics and religiosity; religious observance and belief heighten marital centrality (Willoughby et al. 2015) and shorten the horizon. However, at least in college populations, parents of emerging adults in general (i.e., not assessed for religiosity) favor later marriage (Willoughby et al. 2012), perhaps in the hopes (supported by the literature) that the older bride and groom will achieve greater stability, which may ensure success.

In a study of lower-income emerging adults without college degrees, marriage as aspiration was highly endorsed among men and women alike, but the actual transition was feared because of a loss of freedom and economic strain (Willoughby et al. 2012). Thus, there appears to be a "marriage paradox" (Willoughby and James 2017) wherein marriage continues to be subjectively valued in most populations, regardless of education or income, but emerging adults postpone it so that they can find the ideal soulmate and await the ideal circumstances, including financial independence, before marrying (Leonhardt et al. 2020). Even in countries (such as the Netherlands) where the ostensible incentives to marry—legal and social—have diminished, the "affective evaluation" of marriage persists nonetheless (Billari and Liefbroer 2016). This is consistent with marital centrality theorists' (Willoughby et al. 2015) contention that marriage is still regarded as a goal of high importance for the future. Nonetheless, compared with 1962, when 90% of 30-year-olds were married, in 2019 only 51% of 30-year-olds had achieved that milestone (Kiersz 2020).

Gender, Sex, and Love in Late Emerging Adulthood

Many aspects of twenty-first-century Western culture influence representations of gender and shape the sex and love lives of emerging adults. These factors affect the sensibility of emerging adults regarding their gender identities, their bodies, their valuation of relationships, their capacities or desires to integrate love and sex, and ultimately their attitudes toward marriage. Late-twentieth-century advances in birth control technology and in disease prevention and treatment have effectively delinked an active sexual life from marriage; "possibly for the first time in history, recreational sex became far more important than reproductive sex.... The traditional distinction between marriage markets and sexual markets eroded...and seems to be vanishing in the 21st century" (Hakim 2015a, p. 342). The internet promotes a marketplace sexuality, with apps offering the equivalent of online shopping for dates and continuous access to diverse pornography, escorts, or girlfriend experience services. (The term *girlfriend experience* originated in the 2009 movie of the same name, which depicted a high-priced, cultivated call girl [with a boyfriend] who provided smart, individualized escort services to influential politicians.) It also provides a ready network for exploring like-minded others in terms of sexual identities and predilections. Other diverse influences on sexuality and love include the prevalence of

divorce, especially parental divorce; the college hook-up culture and its facilitators, such as apps and substances; current trends rejecting binary views
of sex, gender, and sexuality in favor of fluidity and self-determination
(Ventriglio and Bhugra 2019); sexual violence; the male deficit (i.e., "the
centrality of sexuality, sexual desire, sexual behaviour and attitudes," which
is greater in men than in women; Hakim 2015b, p. 314); and the #MeToo
movement, its effects, and the resulting backlash.

Divorce

Although the rate of divorce had declined since the early 2000s, in the after-
math of the COVID-19 pandemic, the rate began to rise; the year 2020 saw the
largest single-year increase in many decades (Wilkinson and Finkbeiner Family Law Attorneys 2022). The emerging adults of the current period were born
as the divorce revolution was waning; nonetheless, many of their families ultimately experienced divorce. The effects of divorce on children of different
ages vary; given that momentous events have unfolding sequelae in a developing child, a process-oriented approach (Strohschein 2005) is best suited to assessing the immediate and long-term effects of divorce on young children.

A study that compared children of divorced parents in the 1990s (now
late emerging adults or just over 30) with children of continuously married
parents showed a small but demonstrable effect size in regard to impairments in conduct (especially in boys), academic performance, psychological
adjustment, self-concept, and social relationships (Amato 2001). Many deleterious effects, such as a decline in socioeconomic resources and psychosocial supports, do not necessarily emerge immediately. For children still
living at home even in the best of circumstances, parental separation and
divorce inevitably disrupt the rituals of daily life: pressure, real or imagined,
to choose sides (Shimkowski et al. 2018); forced compliance with the edicts
of a third party; rules about which parent can be seen when; or weekends
hijacked by arrangements made by a judge, by lawyers, or for the parents'
convenience. Children find their time divided up with no regard for their
own scheduled activities, such as birthday parties, games, or performances.
School sports events can be an occasion for tension when warring parents
both attend and, alternatively, can lead to disappointment if one parent
does not show up. There is a corrosive effect on children's evolving portrait
of each parent and on their views of love relationships and attachments
(Lament 2019). Children are perpetually missing one parent; having two
homes only serves to make each one feel unstable and altered, especially
when the parents date or remarry (Gunsberg 2019). The parents' remar-
riages can prove distressing, perhaps especially if they occur after the children themselves begin to date.

As young people progress through late adolescence and emerging adulthood, passing through the rituals of graduations, holiday events, family gatherings, and introductions of friends and current love interests, divorced parents continue to create complications and frequently more serious psychological distress. Importantly, children of divorce have less confidence in marriage commitment—this is especially true of daughters of divorce, whose mistrust exceeds that of sons (Whitton et al. 2008). Interestingly, one factor that has been singled out as contributing to the decline in divorce rates is the contemporary later age at marriage, especially among brides, which, as noted in the subsection "Cohabitation, Marriage, and Child-Rearing," is correlated with marital stability and longevity (Rotz 2016).

In contrast, there is also the phenomenon of late divorcing parents—the parents who wait to separate until their children leave home for college or independent living (Sumner 2013). In fact, according to a U.S. Census Bureau report entitled "Number, Timing and Duration of Marriages and Divorces: 2016" and the 2016 1-year American Community Survey, divorce rates have risen since the 1990s for adults ages 55–64, attributed to the "marital instability of the aging baby boomer generation" (Gurrentz and Mayol-Garcia 2021). These late dissolutions have a progressive effect as well, especially in the current era when many emerging adult children plan or need to return home for periods of vacation or for an interim living arrangement. The loss of a stable home situation, often associated with geographic rearrangements, a decline in socioeconomic status, and parental distress, can be disruptive to emerging adults who are relying on their parents to be there but also to not require special notice. As these young people approach their own commitments, they must struggle with the sequelae of their parents' relatively recent divorce: having doubts about marital stability, vowing to never get married or never get divorced, or, alternatively, seeing divorce as a viable option from the get-go (South 2013). Adult children of divorce show a modest increment in risk for psychological, social, and marital difficulties; this is augmented in adult children of parents who divorce repeatedly (South 2013, p. 138).

Sexuality

Sexuality is an arena that is subjectively considered of great importance to people in their 20s but scarcely addressed in the scientific literature on emerging adulthood, especially the second half, although, as we describe shortly, it has been taken up by popular publications. The previously cited reasons for the lack of solid research findings apply here—the absence of a ready-made cohort, the dispersal of individuals into myriad walks of life and circumstances, the transience of geographic location—and result in the relative inaccessibility of the older group for the purposes of research. Certainly, factors related to college sexual behaviors, such as on-campus Greek cultures and the frequency of sexual assault, have received considerable attention, especially as they bear on the prevalence of hookups and sexual violence. The younger half of emerging adulthood is famously the age stage of heightened interest in, opportunity for, and activity in sexual exploration and experimentation. Such predilections are augmented for many by the removal of familial oversight and the immersion in self-selected peer groups—in college and in the vast range of youth cultural scenes. Moreover, the use of substances, especially but not exclusively alcohol, reduces inhibitions and melts moral constraints; in some youth cultures, alcohol and drugs are critical components of participation in the scene. The sexual trend in colleges is toward hook-up cultures, in which casual sexual encounters without commitment have replaced traditional dating culture. Although at least two surveys (Maida 2018; Monto and Carey 2014) refute the idea of any drastic change in past decades, there are abundant scholarly reports of a different kind of sexual culture on campus. Many of these cite statistics supporting the overriding presence of hookups: between two-thirds and three-quarters of college students report at least one hook-up experience, and many describe repeated hookups (Heldman and Wade 2010). But there is a growing trend, highlighted in a number of lay publications, toward a "sex recession," with an overall decline in sexual activity among youths (Kitchener 2018). This has been confirmed by other commentators (Wooden 2019), including in a feature in *The New Yorker* titled "Down With Love": "People who are in their early twenties are estimated to be two and a half times more likely to be sexually inactive than members of Gen X at the same age" (Heller 2022, p. 54).

These contradictory findings are hard to reconcile, and the pandemic has added an unpredictable variable in terms of the degree to which this age group observed quarantine and limited physical contact with unknown persons. In addition, for the late emerging adult, the additional demands of job, family roles, and avocational pursuits; the loss of a shared physical location; and the absence of the wraparound peer group would seem to make the casual hook-up culture of younger days difficult to sustain (Nievera 2013). However, some contemporary circumstances continue to make it possible. First, the vast improvements in medical technology intended to make sex safe create a (sometimes illusory) worry-free attitude toward sex with unknown partners (debunked by the recent monkeypox epidemic). Second, sustained participation in youth cultures can serve to replace the college campus as a milieu in which like-minded people have frequent contact and hook-up opportunities. Third, the extended amount of time for which 20-somethings are single would seem to invite ongoing sexual experimentation and exploration late into the 20s. However, the pressure to find a mate as 30 approaches gradually concentrates this exploration to a focus on securing a life partner.

Another factor that may figure into the inconsistencies in these reports is the internet. Access to sexual imagery, services, and pornography has altered attitudes toward sex. A developmental perspective suggests that if access is un-impeded and retreat to the internet world of sex becomes a reliable defensive maneuver in the face of real-life sexual frustration, the rigid sexual scripts of pornography tend to replace the adolescent process of self-regulation of narcissism and drive and interfere with superego integration, the evolution of ego capacities, and the development of object relations (Sugarman 2021). Because of the internet's reliable delivery of stimulation and the degree to which it fosters both extreme and recurrent scripts, the pursuit of real re-lationships and real sexual encounters in all their complexity may be sty-mied. In older emerging adults, the internet can serve a different but related function as it perpetuates the hook-up orientation in sexual life; the prolif-eration of dating apps and their gradual specialization into those intended for anonymous hookups versus those that have a relationship goal have cre-ated a veritable department store of sexual opportunity in which specific preferences are pre-established and matched. Some dating apps, such as the gay dating app Grindr, are based on geoproximity, pseudonymity wherein a sketchy profile is provided but other information is deliberately limited, and "quasi-immediate sexual gratification" is readily available (Licoppe et al. 2016, p. 2555). Heterosexual-oriented apps and apps specializing in certain sexual behaviors, queer sexualities, or alternative self-definitions are plentiful; some of these suggest that relationships may develop, but many have the stalemated quality of relentless repetition. Nonetheless, deter-mined and lucky people are known to find their life partners on dating apps.

Clearly, the cultural climate of the twenty-first century has had a variety of effects on the development of sexuality. Indeed, the queer challenge to the heteronormative narratives that dominate the whole enterprise of be-coming an adult have called into question many of the assumptions regard-ing sex and dating. Nonetheless, the fact that marrying and having children remain adult transitions that are achieved by a high percentage of emerging adults, even if these transitions are not embraced conceptually by them, re-inforces the twentieth-century stereotype of the heterosexual couple with two kids, leaving little room for the multiplicity of sexualities, non-kinship groups, and new ways of forming families: the "queer vision of adulthood is one that analytically uproots, interrogates, and thus decenters the (het-ero)normative sexual tropes currently tacitly fused into prevailing scholarly approaches to the transition to adulthood" (Torkelson 2012, p. 135).

Another challenge to these heteronormative tropes is the rise of cancel culture and #MeToo, which have galvanized women and suppressed, if not resolved, the toxic masculinity that nonetheless contributes to sexual assault on campus and in the workplace (Hoffman 2020). Statistics on sexual assault on college campuses, among the familiar and easily accessible cohort, have shown that as many as one in three women and one in six men are victims of assault; the risk to non-college-attending emerging adults is estimated to be 20% greater (Khan et al. 2020, p. 140). The implication is that the societal normalization of sexual violence, epitomized by the acceptance of coercive sexual intercourse as normal, paradoxically may be contributing to recent findings that sexual violence is diminishing in the United States. In other words, violence may be underreported and/or accepted (Armstrong et al. 2018). Even the notion of the male *sexual deficit*, which refers to evidence that men's sexual appetites both exceed and persist longer than women's, may not be entirely explained by evolutionary science and may be a product of socialization. In addition, the intersectionality of risk factors (race, socioeconomic status, gender) for and expectations of sexual violence creates added risks for certain populations.

Relationships With Parents and Parents' Recognition of Adulthood

Parents' reaction to the new careers, living arrangements, and values endorsed by adult children is often puzzlement and worry. Parental pressure to "settle"—that is, to marry, buy a house, and have children—seems to vary according to the parents' recognition that traditional pathways are disappearing or are less attractive and that the twenty-first century has ushered in a very different world. Indeed, the importance of parents' attitudes in facilitating and acknowledging adulthood in their emerging adult offspring has been insufficiently examined (Lindell et al. 2017; Nelson et al. 2007) despite the fact that, with the rejection of socially sanctioned accomplishments, parents and other family members are key sources of confirmation of adulthood. Some familiar methods of parenting that have been shown to affect the development of mature decision-making and autonomy during early emerging adulthood—psychological control, behavioral control, and helicopter parenting—have different sequelae in later emerging adulthood. For example, behavioral control in contrast to psychological control seems to create an enduring scaffolding to limit risk behaviors even when attenuated by lack of daily contact. In contrast, psychological control in early emerging adulthood forecasts a reduced capacity to commit to identity and occupation and overall diminished emotional adjustment (Lindell et al. 2017).

Again, the singular traditional marker of adulthood that confers societal recognition and is highly important to both emerging adults and their parents is financial self-sufficiency. Despite the obligation, even willingness, of parents to shoulder financial responsibility for their emerging adult offspring into the mid-30s (Lowe and Arnett 2020), the tendency toward sustained parental financial support during emerging adulthood is associated with conflict, parental worry that their emerging adult offspring will never achieve adulthood, and parents' ambivalence toward their dependent child. The cutting of financial ties has a range of effects; it can shift the relationship toward greater equality but simultaneously diminish the parents' right to know what their young adult offspring is really doing, potentially creating an impenetrable and unbridgeable barrier. Indeed, despite its merits, financial independence can be a complacent standard that obscures problematic directions such as an irreversible slide into sex work or drug trafficking. Clearly, the diminished potential of lower-socioeconomic youths to achieve financial independence can result in a readiness to pursue illicit activities.

In the following vignette, a 26-year-old woman, Bea, chose sex work, "at least for a while," in order to obstruct parental control and establish autonomy. Her own psychology and the current realities of sex work seemed to irreversibly steer the direction of her identity formation.

Case Vignette: Bea

When she was 25, Bea moved from the suburbs to a large city with a friend from home, Steffi, in order to get a decent-paying job and finish school. Steffi assured Bea that they could board in a house with some other women she knew for very little rent in exchange for some light clerical work in their property owner's business. Bea was satisfied with that information and did not inquire further.

Bea was very eager to get away from her hometown, where her divorced parents, after years of acrimony and negligent parenting, had each remarried and reconciled sufficiently to communicate about their two children. The divorce had occurred when Bea was about to begin high school; her mother abruptly moved an hour out of town to live with another man, whom she eventually married, and was present only intermittently for the next 4 years. Bea's father was a busy, successful businessman who was enraged at his wife's abandonment and openly resented his sudden obligation to single-handedly raise two children. He hired a neighbor, Amanda, also recently divorced and in need of work, to take care of the kids after school along with her own three children. Bea never liked Amanda, was suspicious of her "marriage motives" in relation to her father, and adeptly deflected Amanda's parental ministrations onto her younger brother.

Bea entered high school with an aggrieved conviction of abandonment by both her parents and a defiant attitude toward their "so-called values"; she threw herself into partying, alcohol, drugs, and sexual activity. She was consciously aware that she was testing her parents and Amanda: did anyone notice or care? This behavior did not interfere with her customary good grades, and she was able to gain admission to a college in the area. Suprisingly, she sank into lethargy as her freshman year began. She dropped out before the end of the first semester and convinced her mother to take her in. However, it soon became clear that her stepfather had no intention of putting her up indefinitely. Bea then angrily returned to her father's house, knowing this meant submitting to his relentless badgering to go back to school; to placate him, she took a few classes for credit at a local college and worked as a barista. Under such circumstances, Steffi's proposal was a godsend. Because Bea was able to use a grandparent's address to apply to the local college in their destination community, she enrolled in a low-cost school and took off for the city.

The house in which the two women roomed turned out to be a venue for sex work; most of the young women, who were just starting out, were not well established and/or not earning enough to go out on their own. In casual conversations with these women, Bea learned that they were satisfied with their work and felt safe because the men were vetted by the owners. A few women who were in demand were hoping to go out on their own by creating a base of regular clients who would bring in enough consistent income to pay for an apartment and a classy website, where client commentary would solicit further patronage. The ground floor of the house was a "salon" where men could be entertained before going upstairs to individual rooms or going out for the evening. Steffi and Bea lived in the basement apartment. They were not pressured to participate; rather, their duties consisted of maintaining the salon's appearance and supplies and doing "dispatch"—that is, arranging for liaisons between the regular clients and suitable dates "in the stable."

Bea found living in this situation exciting and entertaining. In contrast, at school she again found herself resentful and defiant. She was especially irritated by her school adviser, who also taught her writing class and, after observing her aptitude, pushed her harder than she liked. Bea began to feel resistant to the whole idea of school and started to sleep through her classes. During the warm days of October, she hung out on the little paved outdoor space in front of the basement apartment and watched the foot traffic go in and out of the upper floors. Despite her loss of enthusiasm elsewhere, she made sure she looked good and was friendly and approachable. Inevitably, she attracted attention and was approached regularly by a few men as they came and went. She recognized their names and knew what they were interested in because she had arranged their prior liaisons.

Bea chatted regularly with a man known as Phil, who was attractive and made no secret of both his affluence and his attraction to her. She was fully acquainted with his interest in dominatrices, which she found intriguing. Their conversations grew intimate until she finally offered to be his "escort" off the books. This began a remunerative arrangement of twice-weekly meetings; Bea ruefully observed that this relationship provided her first regular opportunity to exercise power over a man. When the managers of the house caught wind of this arrangement, they immediately evicted Bea, who luckily was able to rely on Phil to find a place to house her temporarily. In short order, it became clear to her that Phil was married and that this arrangement was unlikely to be permanent. Although she experienced this information, implicitly assumed by everyone else, as a betrayal, Bea was savvy enough not to quarrel with Phil, in the hopes that he would sustain her while she figured out her next steps.

Bea's story shows how a traumatic but common childhood event—a parental divorce in early adolescence—ushered her into high school dominated by her anger at both parents and a deep sense of abandonment and betrayal; it also taught her how to evade interference. Her developmental progression through late adolescence was derailed by her rage, and she spent the first part of her 20s stuck in the feelings engendered by her parents' separation, divorce, and abandonment. She found herself, out of a combination of serendipity, naivete, and excited determination, committed to sex work in her mid- to late 20s, "kept" by a man who was unlikely to keep her indefinitely; she now faced a turning point. Would she attempt to revisit school and/or seek work that was acceptable to her family, or would she follow the path she had begun? She was well aware that the idea of doing sex work "until you got on your feet" was never so simple, but this was nonetheless her temporary solution. Assuming the identity of a dominatrix, more than anything Bea had done before, felt like it completely defined her. However, the identity of sex worker, outside the actual bedroom, was not fully aligned with her sense of self; it felt shameful, nihilistic, full of risk, and like a complete break with her past.

Cognitive Development: Creativity, Connectivism, Innovation, and Depth

Despite the limited evidence of anatomical brain development in the late 20s, there is heightened neuroplasticity during emerging adulthood (Steinberg 2014, p. 9), in which receptivity to experience and augmented adaptability facilitate new ways of thinking and creative possibilities. Aptitudes, both verbal and numerical, peak in this period. Expertise in chosen fields begins to accrue and deepen. Various talents, such as artistic innovation in music, art, and literature or entrepreneurial use of technology for creative purposes ("entrepreneurial alertness"; Obschonka et al. 2017), come to fruition. Especially for those inventors in the digital world, this upsurge, in combination with early exposure to technology, shifts cognitive development toward "distributed cognition" (Dougherty and Clarke 2018, p. 359, quoted in Tapscott 2009, p. 114). Human brainpower interfaces, partners, and functions with machines and human networks to free energy and enhance creativity, entrepreneurship, and innovation.

The theory of connectivism was introduced as a model for learning in the digital age by Siemens in 2004 (Siemens 2004). The core postulate of this learning theory is that today's contemporary technological environment promotes a special cognitive capacity, *connectivism*. Information in the age of the internet is so plentiful and omnipresent that it exceeds any one individual's storage space. Human intelligence is optimized by the ability to know where to find information, how to apply knowledge, and what to connect. Such connection-making is the crucial competence, essential for originating new ideas and generating networks (Corbett and Spinello 2020). The emerging adults of today, backed by early exposure to computers and education in the uses of technology, are fully equipped to exercise connectivity and to create novel and original solutions. These observations support the idea that emerging adulthood is not merely a passage to full adult cognition but a unique phase in mental development (Hall 1904). Once defining interests are determined, it is also a time when proactivity, expertise, and specialized knowledge deepen (Obschonka et al. 2017).

Despite the highly touted success of young entrepreneurs, the age of founders when their innovative companies achieve the highest market value is 40 and older (Azoulay et al. 2018). This finding underscores the reality that business expertise and development benefit from experience. Although entrepreneurial alertness can be observed in late adolescence and may blossom into a variety of small businesses—for example, those homegrown ventures featuring sneakers or streetwear—it is the accumulation of confidence and business savvy during emerging adulthood that produces the enterprises associated with real growth in market presence. Recognition by the larger culture fuels and sustains the drive to make something big happen, from its origins in late adolescence to its full fruition in established adulthood.

The Challenge of the Late 20s

Whether there should be any clear demarcations for the end of the prolonged period of emerging adulthood is doubtful; contemporary adulthood is increasingly individually determined and not tied to traditional markers. Yet its eventual end makes the late 20s the crucial lead-up to and age 30 the target moment when the older emerging adult's experience, self-reflection, and autonomy coalesce to yield an intentional future and a partner (if wanted) for adult life. This is reflected in the observations of life span theorists such as Colarusso (1991), who suggested that the sense of time undergoes a shift as the early exploratory phase comes to a close and, in some cases, is consigned to the past. As 30 approaches and the passage of time accelerates, the serious and consequential effects of behavior and decision-making are heightened; the drive for reward is presumably counterbalanced by the growing capacity for contemplation, commitment, and judgment, resulting in a changed relationship to risk, sensation-seeking, and novelty. In the New Testament, 30 is the age at which dedication to a calling emerges, as in Jesus' founding of his ministry at this age. By age 30, then, the average emerging adult is more focused on the future and more responsible, directed, and serious. At 30, most emerging adults' expectations for themselves are aligned with these qualities. Moreover, the idea of a sustained relationship with a partner is more imaginable, followed by thoughts of marriage or committed cohabitation.

How is age 30 represented subjectively? Certainly, some see it as the beginning of adulthood, when conversations veer toward weddings, children, and future plans and away from favorite bands, party venues, and having fun. The idea of age 30 has retained the capacity to move an individual's attention decisively toward the aging body and maturing beauty. Some celebrities (such as Emma Watson) describe the anxiety around turning 30, sparking a larger conversation about the pressures to be someone or to have done something by that age (Nathanson 2020). This debate reflects the anxiety among celebrities and their contemporaries that age 30 marks a crossroads in their career; if they make the right choices and emerge as more grounded and mature artists, they may be able to move forward with their advancing age. The focus on age 30 in the popular press highlights how it continues to loom as an important finish line for youth and a threshold to some version of adulthood.

However, Paul Taylor (2016), senior fellow at the Pew Research Center, demurred, showing how demographic trends suggest that the signifiers of having arrived—the so-called markers of adulthood—are actually not on the horizon for many people approaching 30; however, he concurred that their sensibility in regard to adult life has undergone considerable alteration. According to his informants, age 30 no longer signifies a turning point at which the adult milestones set in the twentieth century should be met or set for the future. It may still serve as a *platform* for the future, created by experience and self-reflection (Taylor 2016), but it may not be a future in which adulthood resembles anything like the twentieth-century image. If, as Michael (1980) suggested, adulthood is a process of *becoming*, then the achievement of adulthood implies flexibility, adaptability, and a sense of ongoing transformation. Especially in the era when identity is what you are doing now, there is no intrinsic value in being "settled."

Such findings illustrate how expectations regarding the stereotypical, standardized versions of nuclear family, careers, and living situations (Taylor 2015) have been reduced. Components of those outcomes do gradually emerge, but not necessarily by age 30, not in all sectors, and not by emulating the parent generation. Before the COVID-19 pandemic, marriage rates in 2018 were at an all-time low (Brown and Sheffield 2020), and birth rates were declining as well (Barroso 2021; Stone 2020). Whether these statistics are harbingers of a more fundamental change in the meaning and accoutrements of adulthood as the twenty-first century unfolds is, according to Blatterer (2007b), obscured by the fact that adulthood "as a stage of life, remains conceptually fixed, unproblematic, and thus escapes articulation, let alone analysis" (p. 778). That is, the definition of adulthood is still embedded in mid-twentieth-century values (Gilmore 2019), and no one (including Arnett, whose paper with colleagues on "established adulthood" relies on the old milestones; Mehta et al. 2020) has bothered to truly interrogate the latter (Blatterer 2007a). This most certainly contributes to the end point of emerging adulthood, originally set at 24 and within just a few years extended to 30. Clearly, the lack of concrete markers requires reliance on idiosyncratic subjective experience. Arnett's original conclusions about conceptualizations of adulthood were based on interviews with young emerging adults (i.e., college students), who denied the significance of conventional milestones and identified subjective feelings—the sense of autonomy and responsibility for one's own life. Is it possible to pinpoint when this state has arrived?

The status and conviction of adulthood may now be individually determined, but inevitably, identity requires affirmation by society, even if in nontraditional ways. Like other components of identity, the social surround is essential for supporting the feeling of adulthood. Adulthood, by contemporary definition, is not a collection of achievements or an assumption of social roles, nor is it only a state of mind—it is equally importantly conferred by others. As an important component of identity, adulthood illustrates the centrality of cultural context. This idea is the legacy of one of Erikson's key contributions (Erikson 1946, 1950b, 1956) regarding identity development, that is, that it is a *psychosocial* creation in which the affirmation of others and of society at large is essential to consolidating one's self-experience. Indeed, many identity theorists emphasize the degree to which identity is drawn from cultural and historical resources without the subject's conscious awareness of its origins. Note sociologist Blatterer's (2007b) definition of adulthood: "a dynamic, intersubjective process of social recognition in which collectivities and individuals are inescapably implicated" (p. 2). Social, personal, national, historical, cultural, and familial systems are all brought to bear on how adulthood is conceptualized and conferred. There is no objective threshold, no set of descriptors established in one epoch that can last decades, much less centuries. Blatterer (2007a) suggested that adulthood can be claimed only if society proffers its people equal "personhood" and full membership in the social system. Of course, this definition makes clear that marginalized groups are denied such affirmation:

children by definition, but also minorities of all types and other sectors of society, which, in the collective view, are deemed "immature."

These conceptualizations are primarily sociological; for the individual emerging adult, the granting of personhood arises from an array of contexts and has a complex history in each of the sectors that contributes to the recognition of adulthood: school, family, social circle, and employment. In all settings, from domestic to the workplace, the accumulation of expertise and opportunities to demonstrate leadership and decision-making promote recognition from others that adulthood is achieved.

In large part, context determines the nature of adult recognition of personhood. In the twentieth century, social approbation was linked to whether choices conformed to traditional measures of adulthood. Increasingly, in Western cultures, such decisions are liberated, at least to some extent, from those constraints; the value placed on stability is now thoroughly contested and replaced by the values of flexibility, fluidity (Ventriglio and Bhugra 2019), freedom to choose, and freedom to change one's mind.

The loosening links between chronology and stage categorizations in contemporary society are increasingly portrayed in the media, in which youthfulness as a descriptor is qualitative rather than quantitative. In fact, youthfulness has been leveraged to the status of a market commodity available to those who can afford it. But what of the body? The body's transformation into its mature form is a process of great interest to adolescents and emerging adults (Omelchenko et al. 2018), and its early achievement can trigger depression and anxiety, especially in girls, whereas its delay is often considered an impediment to feeling like an adult. The timing of maturation has proved to have a significant effect on psychosocial development (Mendle et al. 2007; Stice et al. 2001). Thus, the body can precociously confirm or deny adulthood. However, the body is not static; as emerging adults move through their 20s, their bodies can begin to unveil early indications of changes that are associated with aging, despite access to a vast array of youth-preserving interventions. For example, hair loss, waist thickening, and graying can launch a dive into the market of youth-preserving products, dieting, exercise regimens, surgeries, and other medical interventions. Evidence of aging is usually minimal in the 20s but nonetheless is detectable to peers, threatening emerging adults with the loss of full personhood in their preferred social settings. The aging body may feel increasingly at odds with the internal conviction of youth and come to be experienced as "the mask of aging" (Bennett and Hodkinson 2012, p. 3).

Achieving Adulthood

> [A]dulthood is just as much as childhood a process of becoming, of progressive transformation from one state to another, with critical periods of change and of consolidation: it is not only a state of being.
>
> —*Robert Michael (1980, p. 27)*

> Young adults are forging a new adulthood that involves strong ties of interdependence between parents and adult children, increased precarity, creating ongoing practices of improvisation, a sense of temporal disjuncture as older patterns of transition are disrupted...foster[ing] new approaches to imaging the future.
>
> —*Johanna Wyn (2020b, p. 487)*

With the growing interest in adult development in the past decades, the idea of adulthood as a state of *becoming* or *improvising* rather than a static achievement has been supported by social commentators and developmental researchers (Mehta et al. 2020; Wyn 2020a). Of course, such a formulation makes the threshold to actual adulthood very difficult to pinpoint and the state of adulthood equally difficult to define. Because the traditions have been cast aside, the main sociological interest in adulthood centers on its "reputed deferral or rejection" (Blatterer 2007b, p. 776) of the markers; alternative definitions are poorly delineated. The image of adulthood established at the mid-twentieth century, captured by the familiar roles and rituals and epitomized by the normative nuclear family, is no longer the psychological goal of today's young people or the actual outcome of the development achieved during their 20s. It is not just a question of the loss of traditional pathways; the meaning of adulthood to individuals and social scientists alike has become obscure. Even if we put aside the heteronormative conventionality of the historical picture, the *settled* quality (i.e., stable relationships, jobs, and child-rearing) is no longer an agreed-on or desirable feature among twenty-first-century adults. In fact, *situational living* is the optimal adaptation; decisions are taken moment to moment depending on circumstances, flexibility is the key to success, and mobility is consecrated. Such fluidity has replaced the idea of a linear trajectory over the course of life (Blatterer 2010). Beyond these descriptors, the features of adulthood are indistinct and have become difficult to generalize and impossible to count on.

Conclusion

Late emerging adulthood is, in our view, the period when changes in culture and human development have yielded a new entity. It is when 20-somethings notice that there are no guide rails leading them to a predictable life and that they need to craft an approach to wide-open possibilities, ideally tailored to their interests and talents. It may be that a survey of late emerging adults on the cusp of 30 would take a slightly softened position on the meaning of traditional markers, even beyond financial self-sufficiency. It seems clear that one thing leads to another in this arena too: money allows emerging adults to obtain housing, housing makes cohabiting possible, and in these circumstances desires for parenthood may appear.

Even when taking on these roles, emerging adults are not abandoning their convictions that these steps are not what makes a grown-up. Mental development permitting perspective-taking and introspection, deepening expertise, and greater self-direction is highly endorsed.

KEY POINTS

- The extension of the time frame of emerging adulthood to include the mid- to late 20s has been widely accepted, but the second half of this period is rarely studied on its own.

- The second part of emerging adulthood is nonetheless critical: it is the period when adulthood is imminent, when future time begins to shrink, and when decisions must be made about one's place in society.

- With one exception, the traditional markers of adulthood are no longer equated with adulthood; only financial independence is acknowledged as a meaningful sign. Despite the rejection of these markers, aspects of those traditional accomplishments facilitate steps that enhance the internal conviction of adulthood. Nonetheless, emerging adults recognize responsibility, flexibility, and decision-making as truer measures of adulthood.

- These findings suggest that the state of adulthood is now in flux in our culture; indeed, adulthood itself is conceptualized as more fluid and changeable, requiring adaptability and resourcefulness.

References

Abetz JS, Romo LK: A normative approach to understanding how "boomerang kids" communicatively negotiate moving back home. Emerg Adulthood 10(5):1095–1107, 2021

Abidin C: Mapping internet celebrity on TikTok: exploring attention economies and visibility labours. Cultural Science Journal 12(1):77–103, 2021

Amato PR: Children of divorce in the 1990s: an update of the Amato and Keith (1991) meta-analysis. J Fam Psychol 15(3):355–370, 2001 11584788

Armstrong EA, Gleckman-Krut M, Johnson L: Silence, power, and inequality: an intersectional approach to sexual violence. Annu Rev Sociol 44:99–122, 2018

Arnett JJ: Emerging adulthood: a theory of development from the late teens through the twenties. Am Psychol 55(5):469–480, 2000 1084426

Arnett JJ: Emerging Adulthood: The Winding Road From the Late Teens Through the Twenties, 2nd Edition. New York, Oxford University Press, 2014

Azoulay P, Jones BF, Kim JD, et al: Research: the average age of a successful startup founder is 45. Harv Bus Rev, July 11, 2018. Available at: https://hbr.org/2018/07/research-the-average-age-of-a-successful-startup-founder-is-45. Accessed November 29, 2022.

Barroso A: With a potential "baby bust" on the horizon, key facts about fertility in the U.S. before the pandemic. Washington, DC, Pew Research Center, May 7, 2021. Available at: https://www.pewresearch.org/fact-tank/2021/05/07/with-a-potential-baby-bust-on-the-horizon-key-facts-about-fertility-in-the-u-s-before-the-pandemic. Accessed July 6, 2021.

Bennett A, Hodkinson P (eds): Ageing and Youth Cultures: Music, Style and Identity. London, Routledge, 2012

Bennett A, Taylor J: Popular music and the aesthetics of ageing. Popular Music 31(2):231–243, 2012

Billari FC, Liefbroer AC: Why still marry? The role of feelings in the persistence of marriage as an institution. Br J Sociol 67(3):516–540, 2016 27411956

Blatterer H: Adulthood: the contemporary redefinition of a social category. Sociol Res Online 12(4):1–11, 2007a

Blatterer H: Coming of Age in Times of Uncertainty. New York, Berghahn Books, 2007b

Blatterer H: The changing semantics of youth and adulthood. Cult Sociol 4(1):63–79, 2010

Borschel E, Zimmermann J, Crocetti E, et al: Me and you in a mobile world: the development of regional identity and personal relationships in young adulthood. Dev Psychol 55(5):1072–1087, 2019 30702311

Bray BC, Dziak JJ, Lanza ST: Age trends in alcohol use behavior patterns among U.S. adults ages 18–65. Drug Alcohol Depend 205:107689, 2019 31707270

Brown PT, Sheffield R: U.S. marriage rates hit new recorded low. United States Congress Joint Economic Committee, April 29, 2020. Available at: https://www.jec.senate.gov/public/index.cfm/republicans/2020/4/marriage-rate-blog-test. Accessed July 17, 2021.

Carroll JS, Willoughby B, Badger S, et al: So close, yet so far away: the impact of varying marital horizons on emerging adulthood. J Adolesc Res 22(3):219–247, 2007

Ceci L: Distribution of TikTok users in the United States in 2022, by age group. New York, Statista, February 9, 2023. Available at: https://www.statista.com/statistics/1095186/tiktok-us-users-age. Accessed May 16, 2023.

Chused JF: Neutrality in the analysis of action-prone adolescents. J Am Psychoanal Assoc 38(3):679–704, 1990 2229881

Cilluffo A, Cohn D: 6 demographic trends shaping the U.S. and the world in 2019. Washington, DC, Pew Research Center, April 11, 2019. Available at: https://www.pewresearch.org/fact-tank/2019/04/11/6-demographic-trends-shaping-the-u-s-and-the-world-in-2019. Accessed June 21, 2021.

Colarusso CA: The development of time sense in young adulthood. Psychoanal Study Child 46:125–144, 1991 1788372

Corbett F, Spinello E: Connectivism and leadership: harnessing a learning theory for the digital age to redefine leadership in the twenty-first century. Heliyon 6(1):e03250, 2020 31993523

Creamer J, Shrider E, Edwards A: More young adults lived with their parents in 2019: estimated 17.8% of adults ages 25 to 34 lived in their parents' household last year. Suitland, MD, U.S. Census Bureau, September 15, 2020. Available at: https://www.census.gov/library/stories/2020/09/more-young-adults-lived-with-their-parents-in-2019.html. Accessed June 3, 2021.

Curtin SC, Sutton PD: Marriage rates in the United States, 1900–2018. Atlanta, GA, Centers for Disease Control and Prevention, April 2020. Available at: https://www.cdc.gov/nchs/data/hestat/marriage_rate_2018/marriage_rate_2018.htm. Accessed July 14, 2021.

Dennison RP: Transition to adulthood, in The Wiley Blackwell Encyclopedia of Family Studies. Edited by Shehan CL. Oxford, UK, Wiley-Blackwell, 2016, pp 235–255

Desilver D: Increase in living with parents driven by those ages 25-34, non-college grads. Washington, DC, Pew Research Center, June 8, 2016. Available at: https://www.pewresearch.org/fact-tank/2016/06/08/increase-in-living-with-parents-driven-by-those-ages-25-34-non-college-grads. Accessed June 3, 2021.

Dougherty I, Clarke A: Wired for innovation: valuing the unique innovation abilities of emerging adults. Emerg Adulthood 6(5):358–365, 2018

Duell N, Steinberg L, Chein J, et al: Interaction of reward seeking and self-regulation in the prediction of risk taking: a cross-national test of the dual systems model. Dev Psychol 52(10):1593–1605, 2016 27598251

Duell N, Steinberg L, Icenogle G, et al: Age patterns in risk taking across the world. J Youth Adolesc 47(5):1052–1072, 2018 29047004

Emery LR: Why getting married in your 30s is the new normal. Brides.com, January 15, 2021. Available at: https://www.brides.com/why-getting-married-in-your-30s-is-the-new-normal-4768894. Accessed July 20, 2021.

Erikson EH: Ego development and historical change: clinical notes. Psychoanal Study Child 2:359–396, 1946 20293640

Erikson EH: Childhood and Society. New York, WW Norton, 1950a

Erikson EH: Growth and crises of the "healthy personality," in Symposium on the Healthy Personality. Edited by Senn MJE. New York, Josiah Macy Jr Foundation, 1950b, pp 91–146

Erikson EH: The problem of ego identity. J Am Psychoanal Assoc 4(1):56–121, 1956 13286157

Erikson EH: Identity: Youth and Crisis. New York, WW Norton, 1968

Erikson EH: Identity and the life cycle: selected papers [monograph]. Psychol Issues 1:1–171, 1979

Fogarty M: "Each one teach one": B-boying and ageing, in Ageing and Youth Cultures: Music, Style and Identity. Edited by Bennett A, Hodkinson P. London, Routledge, 2012, pp 53–65

Forde NJ, Ronan L, Zwiers MP, et al: Healthy cortical development through adolescence and early adulthood. Brain Struct Funct 222(8):3653–3663, 2017 28417232

Fry R, Passel JS, Cohn D: A majority of young adults in the U.S. live with their parents for the first time since the Great Depression. Washington, DC, Pew Research Center, September 4, 2020. Available at: https://www.pewresearch.org/fact-tank/2020/09/04/a-majority-of-young-adults-in-the-u-s-live-with-their-parents-for-the-first-time-since-the-great-depression. Accessed June 15, 2021.

Gilmore K: Is emerging adulthood a new developmental phase? J Am Psychoanal Assoc 67(4):625–653, 2019 31604388

Gilmore KJ, Meersand P: Normal Child and Adolescent Development: A Psychodynamic Primer. Washington, DC, American Psychiatric Publishing, 2014

Goldhaber MH: The attention economy and the net. First Monday 2(4), 1997. Available at: https://firstmonday.org/ojs/index.php/fm/article/view/519. Accessed November 30, 2022.

Gorlitz K, Tamm M: Parenthood, risk attitudes and risky behavior. J Econ Psychol 79:1–20, 2020

Goulding C, Shankar A, Elliot R: Working weeks, rave weekends: identity fragmentation and the emergence of new communities. Consumption, Markets and Culture 5(4):261–284, 2002

Graf N: Key findings on marriage and cohabitation in the U.S. Pew Research Center. Washington, DC, Pew Research Center, November 6, 2019. Available at: https://www.pewresearch.org/fact-tank/2019/11/06/key-findings-on-marriage-and-cohabitation-in-the-u-s. Accessed June 30, 2021.

Gunsberg L: Separation and divorce: reverberations throughout the life span. Psychoanal Study Child 72(1):40–50, 2019

Gurrentz B: For young adults, cohabitation is up, marriage is down: living with an unmarried partner now common for young adults. Suitland, MD, U.S. Census Bureau, November 15, 2018. Available at: https://www.census.gov/library/stories/2018/11/cohabitation-is-up-marriage-is-down-for-young-adults.html. Accessed June 30, 2021.

Gurrentz B, Mayol-Garcia Y: Love and loss among older adults: marriage, divorce, widowhood remain prevalent among older populations. Suitland, MD, U.S. Census Bureau, April 22, 2021. Available at: https://www.census.gov/library/

stories/2021/04/love-and-loss-among-older-adults.html. Accessed November 29, 2021.

Hakim C: Economies of desire: sexuality and the sex industry in the 21st century. Economic Affairs 35(3):329–348, 2015a

Hakim C: The male sexual deficit: a social fact of the 21st century. Int Sociol 30(3):314–335, 2015b

Hall GS: Adolescence in literature, biography, and history, in Adolescence: Its Psychology and Its Relations to Physiology, Anthropology, Sociology, Sex, Crime, Religion and Education, Vol 1. New York, D Appleton, 1904, pp 513–589

Heldman C, Wade L: Hook-up culture: setting a new research agenda. Sex Res Social Policy 7(4):323–333, 2010

Heller Z: Down with love. The New Yorker 98(8):54–58, 2022. Available at: https://www.newyorker.com/magazine/2022/04/11/how-everyone-got-so-lonely-laura-kipnis-noreena-hertz. Accessed April 11, 2022.

Hill JM, Bosick SJ: "Boomeranging" and delinquent behavior in emerging adulthood: a person-centered approach to studying role change. Emerg Adulthood 5(6):417–430, 2017

Hoffman L: From "making out" to "making love": sexual passions in late adolescence and emerging adulthood. J Am Psychoanal Assoc 68(5):995–1006, 2020

Hunter JD: Wither adulthood? Hedgehog Review, Spring 2009. Available at: https://hedgehogreview.com/issues/youth-culture/articles/wither-adulthood. Accessed November 30, 2022.

Jones JM: U.S. church membership falls below majority for first time. Gallup: Politics, March 29, 2021. Available at: https://news.gallup.com/poll/341963/church-membership-falls-below-majority-first-time.aspx. Accessed July 14, 2021.

Khan S, Greene J, Mellins CA, et al: The social organization of sexual assault. Annu Rev Criminol 3:139–163, 2020

Kiersz A: This chart shows the exact age when you're most likely to get married. Business Insider, February 12, 2020. Available at: https://www.businessinsider.com/average-marriage-age-united-states-2019-2. Accessed November 10, 2021.

Kins E, Beyers W: Failure to launch, failure to achieve criteria for adulthood? J Adolesc Res 25(5):743–777, 2010

Kitchener C: What's causing the sex recession? The Atlantic, November 14, 2018. Available at: https://www.theatlantic.com/membership/archive/2018/11/whats-causing-the-sex-recession/575890. Accessed November 29, 2022.

Krahn HJ, Howard AL, Galambos NL: Exploring or floundering? The meaning of employment and educational fluctuations in emerging adulthood. Youth Soc 47(2):245–266, 2015

Kuperberg A: Premarital cohabitation and direct marriage in the United States: 1956–2015. Marriage Fam Rev 55(3):447–475, 2019

Lament C: The impact of divorce on children: the view from the perch of adulthood. Psychoanal Study Child 72(1):16–23, 2019

Lei L, South SJ: Racial and ethnic differences in leaving and returning to the parental home: the role of life course transitions, socioeconomic resources, and family connectivity. Demogr Res 34:109–142, 2016 27110219

Leonhardt ND, Willoughby BJ, Carroll JS, et al: "We want to be married on our own terms": non-university emerging adults' marital beliefs and differences between men and women. J Fam Stud 28(2):1–23, 2020

Licoppe C, Rivière CA, Morel J: Grindr casual hook-ups as interactional achievements. New Media and Society 18(11):2540–2558, 2016

Lindell AK, Campione-Barr N, Killoren SE: Implications of parent-child relationships for emerging adults' subjective feelings about adulthood. J Fam Psychol 31(7):810–820, 2017 28517943

Little S: Women, ageing and hip hop: discourses and imageries of aging femininity. Fem Media Stud 18(1):34–46, 2018

Livesey CM, Rostain AL: Involving parents/family in treatment during the transition from late adolescence to young adulthood: rationale, strategies, ethics, and legal issues. Child Adolesc Psychiatr Clin N Am 26(2):199–216, 2017 28314451

Lowe K, Arnett JJ: Failure to grow up, failure to pay? Parents' views of conflict over money with their emerging adults. J Fam Issues 41(3):359–382, 2020

Maida AS: U.S. millennials and the hook-up culture: an online descriptive survey of hook-up attitudes, beliefs, and experiences. School of Education Doctoral Paper 403, St. John Fischer University, Rochester, NY, 2018

Mehta CM, Arnett JJ, Palmer CG, et al: Established adulthood: a new conception of ages 30 to 45. Am Psychol 75(4):431–444, 2020 32378940

Mendle J, Turkheimer E, Emery RE: Detrimental psychological outcomes associated with early pubertal timing in adolescent girls. Dev Rev 27(2):151–171, 2007 20740062

Michael R: Adulthood, in The Course of Life: Psychoanalytic Contributions Towards Understanding Personality Development, Vol III: Adulthood and the Aging Process. Edited by Greenspan SI, Pollock GH. Madison, CT, International Universities Press, 1980, pp 25–34

Monto MA, Carey AG: A new standard of sexual behavior? Are claims associated with the "hookup culture" supported by general social survey data? J Sex Res 51(6):605–615, 2014 24750070

Nathanson H: What it feels like to turn 30: four women on the "big" milestone. Elle Magazine, May 1, 2020

Nelson LJ, Padilla-Walker LM, Carroll JS, et al: "If you want me to treat you like an adult, start acting like one!" Comparing the criteria that emerging adults and their parents have for adulthood. J Fam Psychol 21(4):665–674, 2007 18179338

Nievera R: The hook up hangover: the decline in traditional dating beyond the college campus—before formal commitment. Master's Thesis 1466, Loyola University, Chicago, IL, 2013. Available at: https://ecommons.luc.edu/luc_theses/1466. Accessed November 29, 2022.

Obschonka M, Hakkarainen K, Lonka K, et al: Entrepreneurship as a twenty-first century skill: entrepreneurial alertness and intention in the transition to adulthood. Small Business Economics 48:487–501, 2017

Omelchenko E, Nartova N, Krupets Y: Escaping youth: construction of age by two cohorts of chronologically young Russian women. Young 26(1):34–50, 2018

Parker K, Igielnik R, Kochhar R: Unemployed Americans are feeling the emotional strain of job loss; most have considered changing occupations. Washington, DC, Pew Research Center, February 10, 2021. Available at: https:// www.pewresearch.org/fact-tank/2021/02/10/unemployed-americans-are-feeling-the-emotional-strain-of-job-loss-most-have-considered-changing-occupations. Accessed September 3, 2021.

Rea JK, Serido J, Borden LM, et al: Who says "I do"? Financial resources and values on relationship choices of emerging adults. J Finan Couns Plan 31(1):28–41, 2020

Reeves RV, Krause E: Report: Cohabiting parents differ from married ones in three big ways. New York, The Brookings Institution, April 5, 2017. Available at: https://www.brookings.edu/research/cohabiting-parents-differ-from-married-ones-in-three-big-ways. Accessed October 17, 2021.

Rindfuss RR, VandenHeuvel A: Cohabitation: a precursor to marriage or an alternative to being single? Popul Dev Rev 16(4):703–726, 1990

Rotz D: Why have divorce rates fallen? The role of women's age at marriage. J Hum Res 51(4):961–1002, 2016

Roupa M, Kusendová D: Emerging adulthood and later parenthood. Acta Geographica Universitatis Comenianae 61(1):3–26, 2017

Savickas ML: Career adaptability: an integrative construct for life-span, life-space theory. Career Dev Q 45(3):247–259, 1997

Shimkowski JR, Punyanunt-Carter N, Colwell MJ, et al: Perceptions of divorce, closeness, marital attitudes, romantic beliefs, and religiosity among emergent adults from divorced and nondivorced families. J Divorce Remarriage 59(3):222–236, 2018

Shulman S, Barr T, Livneh Y, et al: Career pursuit pathways among emerging adult men and women: psychosocial correlates and precursors. Int J Behav Dev 39(1):9–19, 2015

Siemens G: Connectivism: a learning theory for the digital age. Washington, DC, Siemens, 2004. Available at: https://jotamac.typepad.com/jotamacs_weblog/files/Connectivism.pdf. Accessed November 29, 2022.

South AL: Perceptions of romantic relationships in adult children of divorce. J Divorce Remarriage 54(2):126–141, 2013

Spear LP: Adolescents and alcohol. Curr Dir Psychol Sci 22(2):152–157, 2013 25309054

Steinberg L: A social neuroscience perspective on adolescent risk-taking. Dev Rev 28(1):78–106, 2008 18509515

Steinberg L: Age of Opportunity: Lessons From the New Science of Adolescence. New York, Houghton Mifflin Harcourt, 2014

Stice E, Presnell K, Bearman SK: Relation of early menarche to depression, eating disorders, substance abuse, and comorbid psychopathology among adolescent girls. Dev Psychol 37(5):608–619, 2001 11552757

Stone L: The rise of childless America. Charlottesville, VA, Institute for Family Studies, June 4, 2020. Available at: https://ifstudies.org/blog/the-rise-of-childless-america. Accessed July 22, 2021.

Strohschein L: Parental divorce and child mental health trajectories. J Marriage Fam 67(5):1286–1300, 2005

Sugarman A: The impact of internet pornography on male adolescent mental organization. Psychoanal Study Child 74(1):174–190, 2021

Sumner CC: Adult children of divorce: awareness and intervention. J Divorce Remarriage 54(4):271–281, 2013

Tanner JL: Recentering during emerging adulthood: a critical turning point in life span human development, in Emerging Adults in America: Coming of Age in the 21st Century. Edited by Arnett JJ, Tanner JL. Washington, DC, American Psychological Association, 2006, pp 21–55

Tapscott D: Grown Up Digital: How the Net Generation Is Changing Your World. New York, McGraw Hill, 2009, p 114

Taylor J: Performances of post-youth sexual identities in queer scenes, in Ageing and Youth Cultures: Music, Style and Identity. Edited by Bennett A, Hodkinson P. London, Routledge, 2012, pp 24–36

Taylor P: The well-being of young adults in the "Next America." Am J Orthopsychiatry 85(5S):S4–S13, 2015 26460714

Taylor P: The Next America: Boomers, Millennials, and the Looming Generational Showdown. New York, PublicAffairs, 2016

Theobald D, Farrington DP, Piquero AR: The impact of changes in family situations on persistence and desistance from crime, in The Oxford Handbook of Developmental and Life-Course Criminology. Edited by Farrington DP, Kazemian L, Piquero AR. New York, Oxford University Press, 2018, pp 475–494

Torkelson J: A queer vision of emerging adulthood: seeing sexuality in the transition to adulthood. Sex Res Social Policy 9(2):132–142, 2012

Tosi M: Boomerang kids and parents' well-being: adaptation, stressors, and social norms. Eur Sociol Rev 36(3):460–473, 2020

U.S. Census Bureau: Number, timing and duration of marriages and divorces. Suitland, MD, U.S. Census Bureau, April 22, 2021. Available at: https://www.census.gov/newsroom/press-releases/2021/marriages-and-divorces.html. Accessed November 23, 2022.

Ventriglio A, Bhugra D: Sexuality in the 21st century: sexual fluidity. East Asian Arch Psychiatry 29(1):30–34, 2019 31237255

Whitton SW, Rhoades GK, Stanley SM, et al: Effects of parental divorce on marital commitment and confidence. J Fam Psychol 22(5):789–793, 2008 18855515

Wilkinson and Finkbeiner Family Law Attorneys: Divorce statistics: over 115 studies, facts and rates for 2022. San Diego, CA, Wiksinson and Finbeiner, 2022. Available at: https://www.wf-lawyers.com/divorce-statistics-and-facts. Accessed May 16, 2023.

Willoughby BJ, James SL: The Marriage Paradox: Why Emerging Adults Love Marriage Yet Push It Aside. New York, Oxford University Press, 2017

Willoughby BJ, Olson CD, Carroll JS, et al: Sooner or later? The marital horizons of parents and their emerging adult children. J Soc Pers Relat 29:967–981, 2012

Willoughby BJ, Hall SS, Goff S: Marriage matters but how much? Marital centrality among young adults. J Psychol 149(8):796–817, 2015 25494858

Wooden A: Why are we having less sex today than ever before? Johns Hopkins News-Letter, February 14, 2019. Available at: https://www.jhunewsletter.com/article/2019/02/why-are-we-having-less-sex-today-than-ever-before. Accessed November 29, 2022.

Wyn J: A sociology of youth: defining the field. J Sociol (Melb) 20:1440783320936739, 2020a

Wyn J: Conclusion, in Youth and the New Adulthood: Generations of Change. Edited by Wyn J, Cahill H, Woodman D, et al (Perspectives on Children and Young People, Vol 8; Wyn J, Cahill H, Cuervo H, series eds). New York, Springer, 2020b, pp 151–160

Zoutewelle-Terovan M, Van Der Geest V, Liefbroer A, et al: Criminality and family formation: effects of marriage and parenthood on criminal behavior for men and women. Crime Delinq 60(8):1209–1234, 2012

PART III

Developmental Tasks and the Role of the Peer Group in Emerging Adulthood

5

Identity in Emerging Adulthood

The concept of identity is most closely associated with the seminal work of Erik Erikson, who used the term *identity* to represent an individual's experience of "persistent sameness within oneself (selfsameness) and a persistent sharing of some kind of essential character with others" (Erikson 1956, p. 57). Within his theory, identity functions at the interface of the mind and the social environment; it is marked by the sense of oneself as a familiar, cohesive individual who is simultaneously recognized by others. As a psychoanalytic and psychosocial thinker, Erikson viewed this construct as encompassing not just conscious facets of the self (social roles, values, attitudes) but also unconscious parts of personality (self- and other representations, modes of defense, patterns of relatedness) that powerfully shape intrapsychic and social experience. Although Erikson formulated identity as a lifelong psychological and sociocultural process, he proposed late adolescence as a period of heightened significance. During this developmental phase, the parent-based identifications of childhood no longer suffice as the basis for self-definition; the young person begins to strive for a separate, autonomous self, which results in a normative identity crisis. The identity crisis of the late teens is distinct from *identity diffusion* (described more fully in the section "Identity Pathology and the Concept of Identity Diffusion"), which refers to a pathological state of incoherence characterized by inconsistent and often distorted views of self and others (Ensink et al. 2015; Erikson 1956, 1968).

Driven by a sense of urgency to establish a unique, individualized identity, the late adolescent embarks on a process of active exploration, trying on various versions of the self and seeking feedback from the social environment. Ideally, such experimentation is facilitated by a psychosocial moratorium, a period when major life decisions and binding commitments are postponed, which allows the young person to engage freely in self-discovery (Erikson 1956, 1968). Ultimately, identity formation reflects a synthesis of childhood, adolescent, more recent, and ongoing identifications and self-experiences; this process draws together one's diverse self- and other representations, social roles, values, and goals into a coherent whole. In Erikson's view, the young adult's identity formation stabilizes the sense of self as a separate and cohesive person, setting the stage for subsequent psychological health. Importantly, identity provides a solid foundation from which to enter into intimate relationships without fear of losing one's individuality. Similarly, it facilitates the capacity to accommodate diverse events and social demands (managing conflicts in the workplace, becoming a parent, taking on a new professional position, dealing with illness in oneself and family members) without losing internal sameness and constancy. These dual, interrelated functions—stabilizing the sense of self and simultaneously facilitating a flexible adjustment to and integration of novel roles and experiences—mark identity formation as both a key developmental task and an ongoing, open-ended process of the human life span.

The following description of Ariana, an American student introduced in Chapter 3 ("Late Adolescence") as she headed off to her first year in college, captures a typical picture of late adolescent identity exploration across several realms, including social roles, sexuality, ethnicity and family history, and values and personal goals.

Case Vignette: Ariana

Ariana completed her first year of college with a new but well-established group of friends, primarily from her performing arts courses. She was thrilled to have secured a small but important role in her school's upcoming musical production, scheduled for the following autumn; everyone was excited about what appeared to be the gradual receding of the SARS-CoV-2 disease (COVID-19) pandemic, which meant that the performances could likely be done in person. At the same time, Ariana had felt deeply influenced by a couple of classes in sociology that had introduced her to theories about gender and racial/ethnic inequities. In particular, a charismatic young teaching assistant had inspired her, challenging many of her previously unquestioned assumptions and opening up her awareness of her own ethnicity. This young man drew on his experiences as a person of color growing up in a small Southern town; he depicted a childhood completely different from anything Ariana had ever imagined. Some of his stories resonated with long-forgotten narratives told by her mother and grandmother, who had emigrated to the United States from South America in the 1970s, initially encountering suspicion and anti-immigrant attitudes in their new community. However, they had always emphasized the value of assimilating into the mainstream culture, learning English as quickly as possible, extinguishing their accents as much as they could, and adopting the holidays and customs of the Irish and Italian neighborhood in which they lived.

Although she had never paid much attention to these family conversations, Ariana felt an uptick of interest in her mother's stories and in her country of origin and felt some regret and even mild anger that she had not been more deeply educated in the customs and mores of that culture. Certainly, she spoke Spanish with her older relatives, who had never quite mastered English, but English had always been the dominant language at home among her, her mother, and her American-born father. Ariana wondered if she should enroll in some advanced Spanish grammar classes or delve into Spanish literature; she glanced briefly at the course offerings for the next semester.

More urgently, Ariana wondered if she should shift altogether her current academic direction, which was headed toward majoring in the performing arts, in favor of a more rigorous-seeming academic pathway that might lead her toward making a greater impact on the world around her: law, social work, some sort of public advocacy? She raised these concerns with her theater friends, some of whom had taken the same sociology class; they questioned if the arts were not perhaps just as critical to social change, citing examples of songs, performance art, writings, or other creative products that had shone a light on contemporary issues. Still, privately, Ariana was not convinced; she knew she did not have to decide right away and resolved to take a few more classes in sociology and political science before formally declaring her choice of major. In addition, she had plans to travel after college and to acquaint herself with other parts of the world that were different from her limited upbringing. One of her political science professors had mentioned her experiences in the Peace Corps, and Ariana had briefly done some internet research on that before concluding that such a lengthy stay in another part of the world might prove daunting. She felt bad about giving in to her anxieties but assuaged her tensions by reminding herself that she had time before making any long-term commitments. The young teaching assistant had encouraged Ariana to read certain books, which she eagerly procured before returning home for the summer. In addition, she was planning to interview her mother and grandmother about their immigration experiences; this would ensure her continuing connection to the teaching assistant for the following year, because he was running a research project on oral storytelling.

Ariana's romantic life had also become far more varied than in high school, where she had dated primarily two boys, each for a few months. Ariana had been slightly disappointed by her initial sexual encounters, mostly conducted hastily when parents were not at home; she attributed this to both her and her boyfriends' lack of experience. Her high school friends' enthusiastic accounts of their own hookups had made it hard for her to confide her feelings of disillusionment; she knew that she was relatively shy and inhibited about such matters and that her peers found it strange that she had been with only a couple of boys. Once at college, she was determined to present herself as less naive and more confident. There were limited partying options during COVID-19, and classes were mostly remote, but many of her new friends were making contacts by socializing in the dorms or via dating apps. Her roommate helped her select an app and set up a profile. Ariana soon connected not only with a young man at a neighboring college who had come to visit one of her friends but also with a couple of women she had matched with on the app. She was not sure if she was really bisexual, despite having recently come out to her high school friends as such, or whether she was just enjoying experimenting. However, she did not feel concerned about labeling herself in a permanent way; certainly, she had been pleased and felt validated by the positive, affirming responses of her old friends to her social media postings that depicted herself in a romantic pose with an attractive young woman.

At the moment, packing up her room as the first year drew to a close, Ariana's main concern centered on the return home. She felt like a different person at school and was filled with a sense that she would lose that new self when she walked back into her parents' house. They hardly knew her at this point. She was also aware that as much as she missed them, she felt conflicted about the prospect of seeing her old friends; she was most afraid that her recently acquired sense of social confidence and sexual desirability would not be sustainable in an old environment, where her former chums might still consider themselves more worldly and experienced even after being informed about her recent sexual liaisons.

A year into college, Ariana has accrued an array of novel experiences and relationships; her exposure to new individuals and viewpoints interfaces with her natural curiosity and thoughtful nature, her wish to transform the sense of herself as overly cautious and somewhat inhibited, and her growing desire to make her mark in the world. Unexpectedly, her encounter with an engaging young teaching assistant ignites new interest in her own family history—for the first time, she questions her mother's insistence on cultural assimilation and ponders the meaning of her own ethnic heritage. It is not yet clear whether these interests will become integral to Ariana's sense of self or whether they are tied primarily to her idealization of the aspiring teacher.

Ariana tests out newfound social concerns and sexual behaviors by presenting them to her old high school friends as well as to her newer associates; she is eager for their responses, reflects on their comments, and considers the fit with her own genuine feelings. At times, she attempts to integrate potential goals and ideals with her own natural temperament and tendencies, such as when she realizes that she is frightened by the idea of a Peace Corps–like commitment. She derives excitement and pleasure from various domains of exploration, most notably sexuality, but does not feel any desire to focus on one individual or to establish a specific sexual preference. Like many emerging adults, Ariana is focused primarily on self-discovery, on the sense of the many available possibilities, and on her own potentials.

At the same time, the shifts in her sense of herself feel tenuous enough that she does not feel certain she can sustain them when she reenters her old, familiar childhood environment; she dreads the return to her childhood room, to her parents' affectionate but infantilizing behaviors, and even to her old friends' perception of her as their shy, sexually inhibited pal. Her knowledge that social media will keep her connected to her new friends, a few scheduled reunions with them over the summer, and her plan for reengagement with the inspiring teaching assistant all help her face the long upcoming weeks of summer.

In Video 5, a 29-year-old recruiting and human resources manager with a congenital disorder has recently married and is embarking on a career path that she has pursued for several years. She reflects on the unique ways in which her physical challenges have shaped her sense of self, relationships, and professional choices.

 Video 5: Integrating the identity process with a chronic medical condition

---

Post-Erikson Identity Theory

Psychodynamic Theories

Erikson's original work on identity gave rise to an expansive literature with various definitions of this complex concept. Most writers theorize identity as synonymous with a sense of personal cohesion, encompassing at least some of the following facets of personality: ways of being with others; habitual modes for managing affective arousal; and emotional commitments to a set of core beliefs, attitudes, and roles within the social environment (Abend 1974; Auberbach and Diamond 2017; Jørgensen 2010; Kernberg 2006). Like Erikson, most theorists view late adolescence and the early 20s as high season for identity exploration and for the gradual formation and stabilization of key aspects of self-definition. However, beyond these basic commonalities, definitions tend to differ depending on the theoretical orientation of the writer and the intended uses of the term (e.g., research vs. clinical applications); in addition, there is no unified position on the degree to which key aspects of identity may remain in flux beyond the initial period of exploration.

Within psychodynamic theories, identity is seen as comprising not just aspects of conscious mental life but also the underlying conflicts, defenses, feelings, and fantasies about self and others that powerfully affect an individual's social and cultural experience; these deeply embedded facets of identity, which may elude self-reports or other empirical tools, include mechanisms for managing guilt and anxiety, characteristic relational patterns, and wishes and fears that tend to arise in the context of intimate connections (Jørgensen 2010; Schechter et al. 2018). Identity is conceptualized as integrating multiple mental systems, including key components of an individual's ego strengths, interpersonal capacities, and superego functioning.

Despite Erikson's training as a psychoanalyst, this community deemed his conceptualizations as insufficiently intrapsychic and overly sociological (Abend 1974; Wallerstein 1998); certainly, Erikson himself credited his study of social anthropology and education for leading him to formulations about identity, but he viewed such cross-fertilization with psychoanalytic concepts as highly productive (Erikson 1956). Within the field of psychoanalysis, notions of self- and other representations eclipsed the construct of identity; efforts to differentiate between the two proposed self- and self-with-other awareness as arising during earlier, embodied, core subjective and intersubjective experiences (affective mutuality, agency, self-regulation), whereas identity is hypothesized to involve more mature social-cognitive awareness and higher-level processes, such as language and reflection (Gerson 2014; Stern 1985). Often, however, psychodynamic writers use the terms *self* and *identity* interchangeably, without specifying distinctions.

Although Erikson's overall body of work was not given prominence within mainstream psychoanalytic writings, the notion of identity as an integrative, stabilizing component of personality nonetheless retained great significance within theories about character formation and character pathology. Traditional psychoanalytic writers described identity formation as a key developmental task of the late teens and as a cornerstone of personality cohesion; however, unlike Erikson, who emphasized identity as a fluid and lifelong process, these thinkers tended toward a view of identity solidification during the late adolescent phase (Blos 1968; Ritvo 1971). Personality theorists posited coherent aspects of identity—stable representations of self and other, reliable mechanisms for maintaining emotional equilibrium—as foundational for favorable adult functioning, allowing the individual to handle shifting interpersonal situations and emotionally arousing events without loss of internal consistency (Ensink et al. 2015; Kernberg 2006). At the end of this chapter in the section "Identity Pathology and the Concept of Identity Diffusion" and in Chapter 7 ("Psychopathology and

Emerging Adulthood"), we discuss more thoroughly the concept of identity diffusion and the vulnerabilities that arise when fundamental aspects of the self-concept lack coherence and continuity.

Empirical Studies

Although Erikson's writings were not immediately integrated into broader psychoanalytic theorizing, his basic ideas soon became central to a substantial empirical literature on identity development. Within this body of work, identity is conceptualized as a unified self-concept that arises from the gradual integration of personal qualities (abilities, preferences, needs) with availabilities in the social environment; the process of identity development comprises a continual interplay among young people's behavioral experimentation with novel roles, the evoked responses of the social surround, and their subsequent reflection and reconsideration (Marcia 1966; Meeus et al. 2010). Different identity domains (social roles, relationships, affiliations with groups or values) are not necessarily processed in tandem and may undergo exploration at varying points in time. The meaning that an individual attributes to particular identity categories determines whether sexuality and gender, career, race/ethnicity, religion, or multiple other roles and aspects of culture will be prioritized (Mayseless and Keren 2014). Ultimately, the identity formation process integrates these various domains into a cohesive sense of self.

Empirical writers tend to focus on aspects of identity that can be operationalized and measured, often via self-reports; for example, individuals might endorse a particular level of commitment to a specified value or role (Castillo et al. 2020; Meeus et al. 2010). Along these lines, identity status research assesses the extent to which subjects endorse active engagement with identity domains and then applies classifications such as moratorium (active exploration), achievement (commitment to a particular identity domain, following a period of active investigation), or foreclosure (commitment without prior exploration). Analysis of these categories indicates that identity formation is a gradual, multifaceted process in which young people transition between states of exploration, reconsideration, and commitment while traversing major arenas of love and sexuality, work, friendship, and personal values (Arnett and Tanner 2006; Erikson 1968; Marcia 1966; Meeus et al. 2010; Schwartz et al. 2013). Such studies further support the notion of an identity process in which the individual repeatedly tries on various roles and behaviors, displays them and receives feedback within the social environment, and reflects on the fit of the new identity domain with evolving visions of the self.

From a different vantage point, narrative identity studies emphasize the young person's experience of key chronological questions about the self, such as "Where is my life going?" and "How did I come to be who I am?" Within this body of work, the late adolescent and emerging adult's enhanced capacity to grasp causal coherence (i.e., to reflect on ways in which the past affects one's current and future self) marks a new level of autobiographical continuity; these writers view personal memories and individual history as integral to a cohesive and coherent sense of self (Lilgendahl and McLean 2020; McAdams and McLean 1985; Pasupathi and Hoyt 2009).

Although empirical studies shed light on the identity-searching process and its contents, they also suggest that pathways of self-definition and discovery are nonlinear, unpredictable, and lacking in clear end points. Some writers propose a progressive developmental trajectory, beginning in the late teens, toward a steadily increasing number of identity commitments that ultimately define the self. Others note considerable variation in these patterns, with ongoing subtle but meaningful shifts in the ways people think and feel about their chosen paths, even after major identity roles are embraced; these writers note that many individuals, well into their 20s, demonstrate substantial flux within major identity arenas (Carlsson et al. 2015; Mackey et al. 2001; Meeus et al. 2010). For example, although some young people embark early on a highly defined path of preprofessional development (e.g., engineering, medicine), such commitments may yield a sense of efficacy and stability that contributes to fuller exploration in other nonwork arenas (Huff et al. 2019). More typical career trajectories often include changes of jobs and location, periods of unemployment, and retrainings that do not necessarily resolve in the later 20s. Similarly, in the arena of intimate relationships, although many emerging adults gradually move from superficial bonds toward deeper and more committed ones, the 20s are often characterized by casual connections, hookups, and more transient cohabitations (Shulman and Connolly 2013). These suggestions of ongoing identity exploration and reconfiguration, which extend well into the third decade of life, are consistent with current conceptualizations of the identity process and with the effect of emerging adulthood research on contemporary developmental thinking.

In Video 6, a 27-year-old multimedia artist and dog walker reflects on the ways in which she has synthesized her diverse creative interests and career opportunities with the pragmatic needs of day-to-day life. She recognizes the role that her racial and cultural identities played in her childhood and adolescent experience.

 Video 6: Late emerging adult grapples with responsibilities while exploring different roles

Contemporary Identity Theory

Research on Emerging Adulthood

Emerging adulthood research has reshaped identity conceptualizations, demonstrating that the active period of self-discovery continues well beyond the late teens. Indeed, identity exploration marks the preeminent task of the decade-long emerging adulthood phase and weaves together the five main defining characteristics of this cohort: an investment in role exploration, a focus on the self, a sense of instability, a belief in multiple possibilities, and a sense of a period between adolescence and adulthood (Arnett 2004; Schwartz et al. 2013). The lengthy duration of this developmental phase, along with a deferment of customary roles and commitments (e.g., becoming a spouse or parent); a loss of traditional jobs and pathways toward financial stability; and the greater possibilities for diverse roles, relationships, and careers within contemporary culture, is conducive to extensive experimentation across a broad range of identity domains (Arnett 2004; Gilmore 2019; Schwartz et al. 2013).

The emerging adult's turn toward self-exploration is simultaneously fueled by internal maturations that facilitate interaction with new people, novel ideas, and experiences beyond the family; these include an increased desire and capacity for autonomy, expanded abilities for self-reflection, and greater awareness of others' needs and subjectivities (Besser and Blatt 2007; Stambler 2017). Fantasy and daydreams alone no longer suffice: the young person feels growing pressure to engage with the outside world, establish a meaningful place vis-à-vis others and society, experience life firsthand, and test personal powers and competence (Eichler 2011; Meeus et al. 2010). Ideally, the emerging adult's improved self-reliance and increasing desire for independence dovetails with an environment that provides opportunities for exploring and working out identity issues. Colleges, with their innumerable academic and social offerings, represent an ideal moratorium wherein the student gains exposure to new experiences, ideas, and relationships that need not lead to immediate life-defining decisions (Schwartz 2016). However, any setting that provides novel roles and perspectives and a chance to experiment with social affiliations that are distinct from those of childhood can function as an environment conducive to the young person's self-discovery.

Studies on Social and Cultural Identity

A growing body of work seeks to elucidate the powerful role of deeply embedded culture-laden perspectives and social attitudes in the process of identity exploration and formation as well as in existing theories and clinical assumptions; an example of such often unquestioned beliefs includes American-reared individuals' tendency to place high value on familiar notions of independence and individualism rather than on family and collectivist-oriented viewpoints. Such underlying value systems not only affect the expectations for young people coming of age within a particular society but also influence researchers' and clinicians' ways of thinking about key developmental tasks.

Studies on social identity examine the meanings, feelings, and behaviors that individuals associate with membership in particular groups as well as the ways in which the sense of belonging is explored and maintained; such groups may be defined by characteristics of religion, ethnicity, gender, sexuality, and so forth (Rogers et al. 2015; Umaña-Taylor et al. 2014). Burgeoning contemporary research on the development of minority identities, discussed in the following sections of this chapter, reflects a confluence of recent trends; in the United States, these include an overall increase in population diversity, larger numbers of biracial and multiracial births, growth in immigration from Asia and Latin America, an overall resurgence of identity groups, and the gain in prominence of social movements such as Black Lives Matter (Eschbach 1993; Jones and Bullock 2012; Lee and Bean 2007; Neblett et al. 2019). Minority identity studies demonstrate that hostile interpersonal encounters (e.g., microaggressions) as well as experiences of more pervasive racist systems (such as diminished access to services and opportunities) have negative effects on emerging adults; they contribute to overall psychological distress and the internalization of unfavorable stereotypes, eroding the young individual's personal sense of worth (Jones 2000; White 2002; Willis et al. 2021).

Research on intersectionality provides a framework for assessing the ways in which systems of power and privilege intertwine and affect individuals who identify with multiple marginalized groups, such as LGBTQ+ youths of color (Sattler and Zeyen 2021). When the negotiation of minority identity is further complicated by immigration, in particular if dislocation occurs in the context of fleeing trauma and violence, the young person faces a unique set of vulnerabilities, including the internalization of anti-immigration sentiment, the loss of cultural continuity, sudden changes in mores and behaviors, intense feelings of marginalization, and the pressures of assimilating into the dominant culture (Akhtar 1995; Boulanger 2004; Eng and Han 2000; Tummala-Narra 2014).

Like other aspects of self-definition, minority identities attain special significance during the emerging adulthood phase; although parents may be the major determinants of how children and young adolescents view ethnicity, race, and gender, emerging adults begin to negotiate these domains by and for themselves, seeking their own meanings and avenues for exploration and self-expression (Padilla et al. 2021). The enhanced social-cognitive awareness of this developmental phase fuels a sense of sharing history and experience with specifically defined groups; at the same time, the young person's gains in independence mean that hateful attitudes and behaviors are experienced more directly, without the protection and mediation of the family (Levy-Warren 2017; Song 2019; Umaña-Taylor et al. 2014; Wantchekon et al. 2021; Wilkinson and Dunlop 2020; Willis et al. 2021). Emerging adults who are negotiating nonconforming gender and sexual identities may encounter a somewhat different experience, because these fundamental aspects of the self are frequently not shared with family members and may not be supported by them; meaningful connections with and positive feedback from peers and groups assume greater urgency. Psychosocial moratorium settings, such as college, serve important functions in facilitating identity exploration and mediating internalized negative attitudes toward the self; ideally, such environments provide the young person with access to open conversations and encouraging communities, offer friends and mentors, and increase the salience of group affiliation (Blake 2019; Sellers et al. 2003; Umaña-Taylor et al. 2014; Wantchekon et al. 2021).

Racial/Ethnic Identity

We begin this section by acknowledging our lack of lived experience in the development of racial/ethnic identity. To address this deficiency, we enlisted the counsel of William Cross, Ph.D., a renowned Black identity theorist of the conversion school, whose extensive work from the 1970s onward on the evolution of Black identity represents an approach that has influenced many generations of writers and theorists. In addition, we explored critical race theory perspectives and psychoanalytic contributions to racial/ethnic identity development and consulted our own clinical experience. We base the following discussion on our perspective as developmental psychoanalysts, hoping to bring contemporary insights and modifications into conceptualizations of human development in which race has traditionally been ignored (Stoute 2021), even invisible. Racial/ethnic identity development in emerging adulthood is almost inevitably a crucial component of overall identity formation.

The constructs of race and ethnicity are problematic in terms of their specificity and meaning—influenced by "ideology, political climate, and adherence to old paradigms...as much as by advances in science" (Cokley 2007, p. 224). Although the dispute over their overlap and distinctions is not the focus here, we use the proposal of Cross and Cross (2008) (also quoted by Umaña-Taylor et al. 2014) that, on the level of individual psychological experience, racial/ethnic identity encompasses the person's racial/ethnic–cultural identity amalgam arising from the interface of psyche and culture (Stoute 2021). Race is socially constructed and, in the United States, frequently complicated by intersectionality (i.e., the coincidence of identity components each with its own history of oppression, particular vulnerabilities, and sources of rage that can fragment group affiliations). As we see in the vignette later in this section about Molly, intersectionality in a biracial individual can pose a unique challenge to the formation of a coherent identity.

Critical race theory focuses on the basic assumptions that perpetuate pervasive racism; it makes abundantly clear that the multidetermined nature of racist thinking in U.S. culture is structurally determined, that is, so deeply embedded in the social system that the system is ill-equipped to redress the wrongs in U.S. history (Delgado and Stefancic 2017). Kanwal (2021) and Stoute (2021) independently suggested that this same problem makes psychoanalysts ill-equipped to see, much less to address therapeutically, the degree to which the field has evolved because of blindness to many issues. Its blind spots, as related to the neglect of race, ethnicity, class, culture, sexuality, and gender in much of psychoanalytic thinking, interfere with our capacity to see these problems in proper perspective. In contrast to these blind spots, the field of psychoanalysis has had experience with preconceived prejudices that problematize or perpetuate biased sociopolitical attitudes (exemplified by the fight over whether homosexuality is a psychopathological disorder). However, there is a growing effort to recalibrate our developmental thinking in order to face squarely these central components of identity, to see the effect of cultural bias and so-called medical expertise, and to apply the open mind of the psychoanalyst to the complexity of identity and mental development.

Racial/ethnic identity is a core aspect of identity that develops from birth; infants are born into a social world with which they immediately interact (Weil 1970), develop attachments, and embark on a lifelong process of mutual influence. Just as there is no nonverbal phase of infancy (Vivona 2012), there is no nonracial phase of development (Rogers et al. 2020); infants attend to faces and distinguish features that convey strangeness or familiarity. Racial/ethnic priming begins in the first year of life (Williams et al. 2020): after birth, infants' multipotential receptivity to socialization gradually narrows so that by 9 months they are focused primarily on the familiar. In combination with the processes of attachment and developmental anxieties of stranger anxiety and separation anxiety, these tendencies result in preferences for certain facial configurations. This is a process that is preconscious and, of course, individualized on the basis of the diversity of the infant's interpersonal surround. It does not become a conceptual distinction until much later when the recognition of "people like me" takes on meaning and significance (Williams et al. 2020).

Early preparation primes children for encounters in other contexts; it becomes relevant and meaningful when, over time, children begin to have experiences in the larger society. How this evolves is as complex as most aspects of development and includes the important amplification and diversification due to intersectionality (when other group memberships associated with other forms of bias shape the individual identity; Gillborn 2015). As the birthrate of multiracial infants skyrockets (Livingston 2017), intersectionality must be considered a complication for a growing percentage of the population. Intersectionality is an implicit feature of nonlinear dynamic systems developmental theory: individual development is the product of the confluence of constitutional, familial, cultural, interpersonal, intrapsychic, and random factors, and these factors in interaction contribute to the gradual and unique construction of identity. Contemporary use of the term *intersectionality* focuses on the intersection of identities that incur bias and discrimination, but there are intersections that can bring in a privileged component, such as high socioeconomic status or nonminority parentage.

Especially relevant to our topic is the priming achieved by lifelong racial socialization that shapes adolescent and later emerging adult identity exploration. For minority children, a range of influences, including parenting, random events, traumatic moments, constant correction of linguistic patterns, pressure to code-switch from grade school onward (i.e., a method whereby minority youths shift the way they talk, act, and interact depending on what world they are in; see further discussion later in this section), and attitudes in their communities, can make their developing racial/ethnic identity more or less salient at a given moment. The effect of such events on children is shaped by their socioemotional attunement and cognitive capacities; these moments can remain in the mind, to be continuously reinterpreted by the evolving mental organizations and experiences of childhood, adolescence, and emerging adulthood. Although highly homogeneous cultures or sharply boundaried, thoroughly segregated cultures can create the illusion of color blindness, minority children inevitably come into contact with the dominant culture or the world at large. With contemporary access to the internet and digital exposure to vastly different societies across the globe, cultural differences come into focus, and, sooner or later, the young person recognizes racial disparities and bias woven into every society. Depending on the type of community, such confrontations may come earlier in childhood as part of daily life, may coincide with the beginning of formal schooling, may be delayed until high school graduation or a first job, or may be precipitated by what Cross (1971) called "an encounter." An *encounter* is an event that occurs in adolescence or more typically young

adulthood that shatters the individual's naive acceptance of cultural stereotypes; for Cross himself, it was the murder of Martin Luther King Jr. Most
observers suggest that the process of racial awareness proceeds unevenly
and with varying degrees of salience, but emerging adult identity tasks and
accomplishments inevitably hasten the realization of the meaning of being
nonwhite in U.S. society.

The cognitive capacities that emerge in adolescence and develop in
emerging adulthood shift the childhood experience of family socialization
from unreflective receptivity to a more active questioning posture, greater
openness to peer group influence, and a dawning realization of one's place
in society (Douglass and Umaña-Taylor 2016). Sensitivity and a deeper
comprehension of public regard are in full development during emerging
adulthood; an expanding awareness of social forces, bias, racial/ethnic barriers, and alternative worlds facilitates the capacity for *double consciousness*—
the "sense of always looking at oneself through the eyes of others" (Du Bois
1903/2007, p. 8). Such awareness can accumulate gradually or be abruptly
awakened by the encounter that delivers a shock to racial/ethnic identity
development. The notion of *private regard*—individuals' own feelings about
their racial/ethnic group—is clearly not a simple achievement because
racial/ethnic identity must be continuously remodeled. But for emerging
adults, there are new, invaluable sources of self-esteem regulation; a supportive and assertive peer group may provide feedback radically different
from both childhood sources and society. Private regard is elaborated in the
context of the emerging adult's relative autonomy from childhood parental
influence, from nonfamilial childhood identifiers, and from racial/ethnic
stereotyping. For example, the vignette about Deshawn in Chapter 6 ("Youth
Culture"), whose racial/ethnic identity development before college was
limited by his mother's anxiety and prohibitions, illustrates the enormous
value he drew from greater access to his peers, both in sports and ultimately
in college, where he developed his political beliefs and his confidence in
himself as a Black man.

However, embarking on a college career as a minority youth and/or an
individual of lower socioeconomic status can be equally fraught with potentially undermining experiences: microaggressions, including microinsults,
microinvalidations, and microassaults, can destabilize racial/ethnic identity,
creating a sense of exclusion from full participation (Gray et al. 2018). These
conditions require *identity work*, more or less continuously, in order to with-
stand insults and restore equilibrium. Racial/ethnic identity differences are
pervasive and unacknowledged: examples include prior access to better college preparation, familiarity with the world through travel, and possession
of more advanced technology and devices; moreover, the less affluent students often must take campus jobs, which adds to their feeling of diminished

status. Identity work as lived and experienced relies on a few techniques, including buffering, code-switching, and bridging (Cross et al. 2017).

Code-switching, a term from linguistics that concerns circumstantial shifts in linguistic code, is used more broadly to refer to any context-related transformations in communication and expression (Cross et al. 2017; Whiting 2020). Code-switching is a method whereby minority youths shift the way they talk, act, and interact depending on what world they are in—the white world or their own world. It is a controversial method, viewed as both imperative in order to get ahead in the white world and racist, because little effort is made in that world to promote diversity and tolerate a range of linguistic codes (Whiting 2020). In a Pew Research Center study, 48% of Black college graduates described the need to code-switch to deal with interactions with other races. This kind of identity shifting is viewed by the people using this method as a way to fit in and be less threatening (Steele 2010) and more adaptable to the white world; it is also described as exhausting and obstructive to being oneself. This is a different kind of double awareness, in which one persona is replaced by another as the young person moves from, for example, an interview for a job in corporate finance to a pickup game of basketball on campus or hanging out with friends. It is not language alone, of course, but hairstyle, attire, leisure activities, music, and the deliberate effort to avoid stereotyping. Today this is described as essential in some settings but arduous; it is experienced as an unavoidable response to systemic racism in U.S. society that begs for other solutions.

Many disadvantaged emerging adult groups are keenly aware of context in terms of modulating their presentation; their demeanor and standards of comportment depend on the people around them and their goals in the interaction. For emerging adults in the active process of differentiating from family, the peer group and youth culture are invaluable supports; many describe feeling more at home, more open, and more "themselves" with their peer group around them. There is often shared understanding of the need for code-switching and compensatory efforts at self-affirmation (Steele 2021).

The identity challenges of multiracial individuals (whose numbers are growing at a rate three times as fast as the population as a whole; Parker et al. 2015) are complex; bristle with intersectionality; and often create fundamental dilemmas in terms of self-location in society, access and connection to heritage, fluidity and confusion in identity, and racial identity invalidation (Franco et al. 2016; Lusk et al. 2010). First there is the problem of self-designation as biracial, monoracial, or shifting. Social class is strongly associated with the choice of nonminority or biracial identity (Townsend et al. 2012), but physical appearance also is a determinant. Racial invalidation typically happens in the school setting, extending from grade school through college, when peer questioning or doubting ("You aren't Black enough!")

can affect self-esteem and sense of belonging. Despite school being a setting for invalidation, many of the experiences of emerging adulthood can help to consolidate self-experience and group affiliation.

In the following vignette, a biracial emerging adult had a relatively unusual experience in which racial identifications were not promoted or even acknowledged. Instead, affluence and circumstances allowed her to be shielded from the realities of American society during a period of racial turmoil. Within her family, her unmistakably Black appearance was not recognized as a potential source of pride; instead, there was an emphasis on dressing her in expensive outfits and accessories. Behind all of these issues was deep shame about her white father's criminal activities.

Case Vignette: Molly

Molly was a 22-year-old biracial woman in the fashion production business. Her mother was a Black Muslim woman who had immigrated from an East African country in young adulthood. Molly's white father, a high-level, highly paid contractor, was regularly employed by the U.S. Department of Defense to build technical plants in the Southwest where the family lived. Molly was raised with her two brothers in an affluent enclave with few other people of color in her school or neighborhood. Molly remembered her childhood as protected and sunny, defined by her affluence; her access to fine things; and her well-regarded and successful father, who had considerable status in the area. As she got older, her relationship with her mother grew tense. Molly was irritated by her mother's religious and traditional attitudes about the "girl's role" in family life and the need for faultless propriety outside the home. Her mother's prohibition of miniskirts as "slutty" was a particular point of resentment. However, despite her hovering overprotectiveness, Molly's mother was oblivious to Molly's "work-arounds." Despite the reality that she and her brothers stuck out in school and the neighborhood because they were biracial and looked Black, Molly denied having any experiences that confronted her with her difference or that reflected bias or bigotry.

This childhood idyll suddenly imploded and calamity struck, plunging the family's finances, social status, and lifestyle into chaos: their home was invaded by federal agents seeking evidence that Molly's father had been fraudulently overcharging the federal government for the work he provided. Her father had always been a casual gambler, but now it became clear that he was in serious debt. In order to pay his gambling debts and maintain the family's lifestyle, he had resorted to padding contracts. The family was suddenly confronted with the truth about a man who had always been revered. A frightening financial collapse quickly ensued. By the time Molly was 11, her father was in custody, and her remaining family members (her mother and two brothers) were homeless, moving from relative to relative while the father awaited trial. Molly suffered enormous shame about this experience, which received considerable local publicity; she refused contact with her father while he served his sentence and after his release.

Molly moved in with her godparents, whom she called her parents, who rescued her at age 12 from this deteriorated home life. The godparents, a white, affluent Chicago-based couple with no children of their own, had always been involved with Molly, visiting monthly and treating her to shopping sprees in fancy stores, cultivating her manners and comportment, and instilling the importance of "dressing for the occasion" and the value of gracious gift-giving and other such social graces. They enrolled her in a small private girls' school in Chicago where there were only a few other girls of color from similarly affluent families. This experience was followed by college at a small liberal arts school nearby, chosen to allow her to easily spend weekends at home. Just to be sure of frequent contact and oversight, her godparents bought a little "lake house" even closer to the school so that Molly could be with them whenever she needed.

Difficulties emerged during college: Molly was drawn to excessive use of drugs, primarily marijuana; she hung out with girls with similar predilections, and she repeatedly broke promises to her godparents by keeping weed in the lake house, inviting friends over to stay when her godparents were in Chicago, and covering up such transgressions with transparent lies that inevitably came to light. Molly and her godmother frequently fought about both her lying and her failure to execute basic errands or chores. The conflicts around her drug use became the greatest source of strife. Finally, her godparents insisted that she regularly attend an outpatient emerging adult drug rehabilitation program, called the Lakeside Institute, which served a mostly affluent but diverse group of young people. Molly's reluctant participation there gradually shifted to resignation to her fate and then to growing engagement with counselors and new friends.

The program seemed to initiate the emergence of racial identity awareness in Molly. Molly mentioned in a group discussion that despite having spent her teenage years in Chicago, she had virtually no close contact with other Black people her age. Indeed, the program staff was astonished by her lack of race consciousness; she never talked about encounters with racism and was uninformed about the police shootings of Black people. This was all the more noteworthy because so many events highlighting systemic racism had occurred in recent years: the Charlottesville Unite the Right march, the growing number of shootings of unarmed Black people, the killing of George Floyd, and the Black Lives Matter movement. Molly's obliviousness first emerged when she told her group about an experience in a bar where she was surrounded by a group of young white men who flirted with her and insisted she play pool with them; she was curious about the "PB" on their baseball caps but, when told, did not know who the Proud Boys were. The group was astonished not only by her lack of awareness but also by her lack of proper vigilance around a group of men who might be harboring violent intentions toward her. The question of how either set of parents had advised their children about being Black in America came under discussion. Molly said that she had not had such conversations with any parent (she had reluctantly told her life story to the group in a state of acute anxiety when her father received early release from jail). In another group meeting, intended as a gripe session titled "My mother annoys me," Molly complained about her godmother's attitude toward her hair, which was shoulder length, coily, and a little wild; both godparents were always pressuring her to straighten it or at least pull it back so she would look "right" in her designer clothes.

Molly's counselor was increasingly concerned about Molly's problems with her identity, which felt fragile in many ways; it frequently seemed that Molly's attitudes, thoughts, and feelings were lifted out of whole cloth from her parents' pronouncements and that her access to her inner life was limited. The family's emphasis on appearance achieved by "costumes" stood in stark contrast to their lack of recognition of Molly's unmistakable Blackness and their failure to facilitate her racial/ethnic identity. There was no recognition of her unique African heritage and how it affected her identity in contrast to an African American heritage; there was also no discussion of how that difference did not usually affect the attitudes of others.

The counselor, an opera buff, knew that Molly's family had exposed her to a lot of "high-brow" culture, so when *Iolanta*, the opera by Tchaikovsky, was performed at the local opera house, she arranged an outing with Molly and two other young people in the program with an interest in classical music and opera, who fortuitously had some degree of social consciousness. The story of Iolanta concerns a blind princess whose father, the king, is so distraught that she might discover that she is different from others that he places her with caregivers in an isolated location designed to be "blindness blind." He orders that she must not realize her difference from the people around her: there can be no references to vision, to personal appearance, or to the appearance of the natural world. Moreover, the king refuses help from a healer who insists Iolanta can be treated only if she knows that she cannot see. The counselor tried to use this story as a talking point about racial awareness, how its absence over the course of development creates a kind of blindness to the self and to external reality that leads to a lack of recognition of racism in the environment and in interpersonal relationships. Molly listened and wanted to hear more about this; she was urged to join a discussion group about race and started to talk, rather pedantically, to her brothers about the risks of being young Black men in U.S. society.

Molly is an extreme example of someone in whom the pervasive denial of racial difference seems to erase any effect of early priming by her primary caregiver, leaving her without a racial/ethnic identity and without stable identifications on which to build her identity. Her childhood affinity for her white father, whose presence was of course another source of priming, was crushed by the events of her early adolescence. Her godparents increasingly represented idealized and aspirational models, unfortunately complicated by their not really being her blood relations. The inordinate focus on clothing and on being dressed for the occasion created a conviction that the right outfit was the best protection for her intense anxiety about who she was and how she would be received. Interestingly, she was impervious to events in her adolescence and emerging adulthood that might have served as pivotal encounters to awaken her to racial realities.

This vignette also highlights the complexity created by the intersectionality of identity components and the contribution that double consciousness can make to identity stabilization and cohesion, for better or for worse.

The salience of racial/ethnic identity in mental life, which, according to Cross (2020), can vary greatly in the mind, is inevitably affected by the surrounding culture and how the individual is reflected in the eyes of others. Molly's racial/ethnic identity and its reflection in her interpersonal world was, like Princess Iolanta's, constructed, deliberately or inadvertently, to deny the existence of an identity element that was nonetheless evident to anyone who met her.

Identities of Gender and Sexuality

Exploring and integrating gender and sexual identities into an overall self-concept marks a major task of emerging adulthood. Compared with previous generations, a longer duration of premarital life, along with changes in societal attitudes, facilitates greater opportunities for contemporary young people's experimentation and self-discovery in the domains of gender identity and sexual attraction, fantasy, behavior, and romantic feelings (Arnett 2004). Despite the potential for increased freedom, however, young people who are negotiating minority sexual and gender identities face unique social and psychological challenges. Indeed, a widespread body of research suggests that LGBTQ+ youths experience elevated rates of psychological conditions due to ongoing societal stigmas, negative interpersonal encounters, and the general distress of the identity process; the latter includes coming out to family, friends, and others and risking experiencing unsupportive or downright hostile reactions (Camp et al. 2022; Ehrensaft 2011; Sattler and Zeyen 2021). Unlike racial/ethnic identities, which are often shared by parents and siblings, LGBTQ+ identities frequently differ from those of family members; furthermore, developing nonconforming identities in these arenas may conflict with family and community religious beliefs, leading to substantial internal conflict and negative feelings about the self (Mallory et al. 2021; Parmenter et al. 2020).

Contemporary gender and sexuality studies, in contrast to older work within this field, attempt to encompass the complexity of potential identity domains. Such efforts include marking significant differences in the experience of monosexual (lesbian, gay) compared with plurisexual (e.g., bisexual, pansexual) individuals as well as between cis, nonbinary, and transgender people; moreover, more recent research acknowledges that single-label sexual orientations or gender categories may not be relevant for many LGBTQ+ emerging adults (Paz Galupo et al. 2015). Prior research models of coming out, which tended to emphasize the experience of gay white males, have required substantial revision. These frameworks tended to propose an invariant sequence: gaining an awareness of same-sex affinity in late childhood, initiating same-sex behaviors in early adolescence, self-identifying as gay during middle adolescence, disclosing to others during late adolescence, and then establishing romantic relationships between ages 18 and 20 years (Bishop et al. 2020; Dubé and Savin-Williams 1999). More recent research recognizes that gender and sexual self-disclosures now tend to occur at younger ages; in addition, these writings emphasize that sexual minority identity, like identity in general, attains particular importance during emerging adulthood but represents a continuous and ongoing process, subject to varied and individual pathways as well as to multiple individual, family, and sociocultural systems (Bishop et al. 2020; Dubé and Savin-Williams 1999). Although many young people have identified patterns of sexual attraction by late adolescence, key developments in the arenas of gender identity and sexual preference may continue, with potential for shifts over the life span as the person acquires awareness and experience (Morgan 2012).

Coming out to others about gender and sexual identity is a complex and often prolonged process that potentially enhances self-esteem and facilitates feeling known and accepted; expressing true, fundamental aspects of identity within relationships and the larger social environment is integral to a sense of coherence and consistency between inner self and outer self (Galatzer-Levy and Cohler 2002). Self-disclosure and self-expression in the face of others' positive reception and validation, joining in LGBTQ+ activities, and affiliating with supportive communities are known to be correlated with self-acceptance and positive self-regard (Camp et al. 2022). Despite the importance and potential benefits of the coming out process, negative reactions from others or the young person's own internal conflicts can create significant distress. Minority gender and sexual identities may be incompatible with other important self-domains, such as religious belief systems; some young people may negotiate these conflicts by muting the salience of one identity arena in order to avoid what feels like unresolvable aspects of the self, ultimately denying faith or suppressing sexual orientation (Parmenter et al. 2021). Emerging adults who are exploring a range of intersecting minority identities, racial/ethnic identity as well as LGBTQ+, may also experience marginalization by one of these communities; for example, a particular ethnic group may evince negative attitudes toward certain gender or sexual behaviors, or a gender community may harbor racist views (Mallory et al. 2021; Parmenter et al. 2021; Scroggs et al. 2020).

Role of Digital Media in Emerging Adulthood Identity Exploration

The use of digital media is ubiquitous among the emerging adult population; indeed, it is estimated that more than 90% of this cohort own a smartphone, and most visit social networking sites multiple times per day, often negotiating two or more sites simultaneously (Coyne et al. 2013; Perrin and Anderson 2019; Pew Research Center 2021; Stockdale and Coyne 2020; Vanucci et al. 2018). For many of these digital natives, independent and unstructured media use—without parental oversight—is relatively novel. Their internet practices reflect a significant facet of autonomy and self-management; the urge to be included in group chats and social media posts, the fear of missing out, and the absorption in digital sites must be integrated into the demands of work and education as well as balanced with exercise, other recreations, and nonvirtual social activities. In addition, using media responsibly and managing others' digital aggression (e.g., cyberbullying) are other developmental challenges that must be navigated in the absence of adult supervision.

Emerging adults recruit digital media for diverse purposes, including being entertained and gaining knowledge about wide-ranging topics. Social platforms, which allow users to share and interact around updates and other posts, including photographs and videos, serve as major forums in which young individuals manage all aspects of friendship and romantic life. These sites (e.g., Facebook, Twitter, Snapchat, Instagram, TikTok, dating apps) facilitate making new contacts, establishing hookups and meetups, communicating and receiving social news, presenting real and more idealized aspects of the self, and sustaining connections with existing friends and acquaintances. Young people with specific cultural interests that might not be shared by their nonvirtual age-mates (e.g., comics, television series, video games) can identify like-minded peers via online groups, such as fandom communities; the latter enable a potential for self-expression, discussion, and information-sharing in a safe, accepting setting (McInroy and Craig 2020).

Although emerging adults recruit media for their own uses, digital platforms simultaneously impact them, shaping their self and social experience. The potential impacts of technology range from positive (expanding one's base of knowledge, achieving new perspectives, meeting new friends, and consolidating relationships) to more problematic (becoming overly absorbed in online endeavors, obsessing over the number of "likes" and the quality of others' comments, deriving idealized standards with which to compare one's body and social life). Some studies suggest that underlying motivations operating outside conscious awareness, as well as the engaging quality of technology and the perceived power of online responses, can create and exacerbate emerging adults' vulnerabilities (Coyne et al. 2013). Desires for social connection and belonging represent major purposes of using digital media, but the young person's needs to relieve boredom, assuage loneliness, and seek stimulation are concomitant motivations; in addition, using digital media may serve as a method of coping with age-salient pressures and as a potential route of escape from social and emotional pain (Arnett 1995; Biondo 2018; Coyne et al. 2013; Lemma 2010). For the most part, these affective-based purposes reflect normative developmental needs and stressors, such as the college student's struggle to manage lonely feelings and fears of not making friends during a first semester away from home or the older emerging adult's desire for relief from the anxieties of a first full-time job or from the pressures of consequential decisions in the arenas of relationships and occupation. However, emotional vulnerability can contribute to an overreliance on the escapist potential of the digital world, anxious ruminations about others' responses to personal postings, and an excessive need for validation of online self-presentations, ultimately absorbing inordinate amounts of time and energy and negatively affecting academic and work performance, self-esteem, and identity cohesion (Yang et al. 2017).

As emerging adults' unrestricted, unsupervised access to and use of digital platforms have skyrocketed, problems associated with cyberaggression also have trended upward; indeed, college students' newfound freedom from parental oversight and their attendant high use of online platforms do not correlate with greater knowledge about internet safety (Alipan et al. 2018). Cyberbullying involves the use of text, group chat, or other social media outlets for the purpose of intentionally embarrassing, excluding, or otherwise harming others; deliberately revealing sensitive, private information, also known as doxing, is another form of harassment that seeks to expose and humiliate the targeted individual (Hinduja and Patchin 2010; Khan et al. 2020). Theories about the nature of online aggression include the notion that cybercommunications feel more anonymous or less based in reality to the sender, which creates a false sense of reduced consequences and erodes normal levels of self-control and empathy (Khan et al. 2020).

To date, research on cyberaggression has focused primarily on middle and high school students. However, the need for further examination of this problem among emerging adult populations is apparent: several studies found that between 10% and 30% of undergraduates report at least one occurrence in which they were targeted by intentionally harmful messaging (Feinstein et al. 2014; Hinduja and Patchin 2010; Varghese and Pistole 2017). Repeated cybervictimization is associated with a range of adverse psychological effects, including higher levels of overall distress, ruminative and depressive thinking, elevated mood symptoms, a decline in self-esteem and self-confidence, worsening academic engagement and performance, and a significant increase in suicide attempts (Alipan et al. 2018; Feinstein et al. 2014; Hinduja and Patchin 2010). Compared with nonvirtual bullying, the potential for a targeted individual to feel exposed and rejected before large numbers of peers is clearly increased. Emerging adults' methods of coping with acts of cyberaggression include the following: technologically based responses involve blocking the offender, deleting one's accounts, or reporting the abuse to online authorities; social and emotional coping strategies encompass seeking interpersonal support or engaging in an array of avoidant behaviors that range from attempts at ignoring or minimizing the situation to more potentially destructive actions such as drinking or engaging in self-harm (Alipan et al. 2018).

At the same time, these technological platforms serve positive functions as major modes for identity exploration across several domains. Emerging adults use digital media to gain experience with diverse social and political views that might not otherwise be available in their immediate surroundings as well as to acquire knowledge about social roles and relationships (Arnett 1995; Coyne et al. 2013). They use social platforms to present and experiment with multiple aspects of the self, including real, false, and idealized versions, before a potentially large audience; trying on such diverse identities and receiving feedback form a crucial part of the identity exploration process for contemporary youths, despite the potential risks of receiving scant or negative responses (Michikyan 2020). Many emerging adults recruit these sites to express and experiment with roles and ideas they might feel reluctant to expose directly to others, fearing criticism or rejection (Michikyan 2020; Tosun 2021). Social networking platforms represent a particularly vital resource for those who are exploring sexual and gender minority identities; as mentioned in the preceding section, these emerging adults may not receive support from or share identities with their families or childhood friends. They turn to digital environments as safe spaces for making self-presentations, gaining information about how peers are negotiating similar aspects of the self, and receiving supportive feedback on their own struggles and solutions (Parmenter et al. 2021).

Identity Pathology and the Concept of Identity Diffusion

Erikson (1956) described identity diffusion in contrast to the normative, transient identity crisis of adolescence; the latter marks a necessary developmental upheaval that fuels the young person's turn toward autonomy and self-discovery, whereas the former involves a loss of self-definition that leads to feelings of emptiness and isolation. Indeed, identity diffusion impedes forward development, causing regression to the earlier identifications of childhood or manifesting as fear and avoidance in key realms of young adult life, such as making decisions about one's future, achieving physical and emotional intimacy with others, tolerating competition, and managing complex social situations.

Contemporary personality disorder studies conceptualize identity as a multifaceted construct that accounts for a sense of personal cohesion and constancy. Within this body of research, identity encompasses the following components: stable self- and other representations; feelings of integration and continuity over time and in different contexts; an ongoing sense of affiliation with certain social groups; an established set of norms and values; and deep emotional commitments to relationships, roles, and personal goals (Jørgensen 2010). Disturbances in these aspects of identity, pathognomonic of identity diffusion, are associated with borderline personality disorder, a condition known to be correlated with complex biological, developmental, and environmental risk factors, which may include temperamental tendencies toward aggression, deficits in cognitive and behavioral controls, insecure attachment, a personal history of trauma, and having a parent with borderline personality disorder (Ensink et al. 2015; Jørgensen 2010; Kernberg 2006).

During emerging adulthood, identity pathology often takes the following forms: a painful lack of a sense of personal coherence; poorly regulated emotional reactions; a tendency to seek action-oriented outlets for strong feelings, including risky and self-injurious behaviors; vague viewpoints or conformist overidentifications with particular persons and groups; difficulty undertaking a search for personal authenticity; and trouble making age-appropriate commitments to goals, values, and relationships (Ammaniti et al. 2015; Wilkinson-Ryan and Westen 2000). Distorted beliefs and fantasies about the self, along with poorly modulated affects, can propel the emerging adult toward postponing or prematurely foreclosing on identity commitments. Self-distortions, in combination with overreactivity and impulsivity, impede the gradual process of trying on roles; receiving and integrating others' feedback; and balancing choices with increasing knowledge of personal needs, talents, and strengths (Schechter et al. 2018).

Kernberg (1974) suggested that identity diffusion tends to coexist with the young person's relative lack of capacity for guilt and concern, difficulty achieving deep understanding of others, paucity of long-lasting relationships, and failure to acquire an expanding and deepening set of personal values. Close relationships are difficult to sustain because a fragile sense of inner coherence is often maintained by using others for evacuating non-integrated aspects of the self (Jørgensen 2010). Personal narrative and autobiographical cohesion are also affected: disturbances in the sense of self make it hard for the young person to integrate the past with current events, to see connections between previous and here-and-now experience, and to achieve a sense of continuity over time; as a result, personal narratives may have a fragmented, disjointed quality (Lind et al. 2019; Sajjadi et al. 2022).

As developmental writers and clinicians, we are cautious in applying the concept of identity diffusion, as well as the diagnosis of borderline personality disorder, to the emerging adult population. Certainly, we would agree that painful feelings of self-incoherence, diminished capacities for guilt and empathy, deficits in emotional self-regulation, and distorted self-beliefs represent serious vulnerabilities and risk factors during the identity process, a cornerstone of emerging adult development and of forward developmental progression. However, when appraising identity diffusion, we find it important to keep in mind that late adolescents and 20-somethings are frequently in a state of flux; instability, uncertainty, and confusion, along with seemingly superficial and transient attachments to roles and systems of belief, may be highly visible in major realms of selfhood, including gender identifications, sexual preferences, and personal values. The same holds true in the arena of relationships: this age group is often still in conflict with and struggling to achieve a sense of autonomy vis-à-vis their family members and actively experimenting with social-gender-sexual roles and types of romantic connections. Friendships sometimes offer a clearer forum for determining the quality of and capacity for enduring connections; even here, however, there is often a desire to redefine and reinvent the self via establishing new friends and group affiliations and loosening former ties. Emotional and behavioral self-regulation, and realistic appraisals of risky behavior, continue to mature throughout the third decade of life. In Chapter 6, we discuss more fully our developmental perspective on the psychopathology of emerging adulthood.

Conclusion

The construct of identity draws heavily from Erik Erikson's original formulations, in which he used the term *identity* to represent a sense of personal coherence and sameness, particularly in relationship to others. Within his theory, identity is a lifelong psychosocial process that achieves prominence during the early years of emerging adulthood; ideally, a psychosocial moratorium (such as a college experience) provides a time and setting in which the young person can explore different identity domains, engaging in self-discovery and self-definition without the need for immediate commitments. Identity serves to integrate diverse conscious and unconscious aspects of the self (mental representations of oneself and others, social roles, attitudes, and beliefs). Achieving a relatively stable identity facilitates the young individual's capacity to retain a sense of cohesion, separateness, and individuality during emotional upheavals, unsettling events, and intimate connections to others.

Contemporary research has expanded our understanding of the duration and breadth of the identity process and highlighted the powerful effect of cultural and societal attitudes and behaviors on the developing sense of self. Emerging adulthood research shows that the late teens through the late 20s are an extended time of active exploration and flux involving an array of identity domains, including gender and sexuality, friendships and romantic relationships, values, and professional goals; indeed, individuals who are coming of age in the twenty-first century do not necessarily seek to define themselves through assuming traditional roles or occupations. Young people who are exploring minority identities (race and ethnicity, gender and sexuality, and the intersection of these) face additional pressures and obstacles from deeply embedded systems of power and privilege, negative attitudes, interpersonal aggressions, and conflicts with family.

KEY POINTS

- Identity research reveals that young people explore and experiment within several domains, engaging in a gradual process in which they try on various identities; seek feedback from the social surround; and then reflect on the fit between self and particular roles, relationships, interests, and values.

- Contemporary studies on racial/ethnic identity explore the powerful effect of deeply embedded social hierarchies and attitudes, as well as interpersonal instances of prejudice and microaggression, on the emerging adult's sense of self and level of psychological stress.

- Negotiating minority identities in the domain of gender and sexuality involves a unique set of pressures. These may include having a fundamental identity that is different from members of one's family; engaging in the process of coming out in the face of uncertain responses; and dealing with widespread societal stigmas and prejudices.

- Digital technology represents an essential forum for contemporary identity exploration. Potential benefits include easy access to novel information and points of view and the ability to identify supportive peers and communities. However, more vulnerable emerging adults may become preoccupied with others' responses to social media postings or develop highly unrealistic standards and images for themselves.

- Contemporary writing on personality disorders suggests that a stable identity forms a crucial component of healthy adult functioning. Identity components include stable representations of self and others; a sense of personal cohesion in different situations; and affective investment in relationships, goals, ideals, and interests. Identity diffusion is characterized by a painful lack of self-coherence, poor emotional self-regulation, and difficulty achieving stable relationships.

References

Abend SM: Problems of identity: theoretical and clinical applications. Psychoanal Q 43(4):606–637, 1974 4431852

Akhtar S: A third individuation: immigration, identity, and the psychoanalytic process. J Am Psychoanal Assoc 43(4):1051–1084, 1995 8926325

Alipan A, Skues JL, Theiler S: "They will find another way to hurt you": emerging adults' perceptions of coping with cyberbullying. Emerg Adulthood 9(1):22–34, 2018

Ammaniti M, Fontana A, Nicolais G: Borderline personality disorder in adolescence through the lens of the Interview of Personality Organization Processes in Adolescence (IPOP-A): clinical uses and implications. J Infant Child Adolesc Psychother 14(1):82–97, 2015

Arnett JJ: Adolescents' use of media for self-socialization. J Youth Adolesc 24:519–533, 1995

Arnett JJ: Emerging Adulthood: The Winding Road From the Late Teens Through the Twenties. New York, Oxford University Press, 2004

Arnett JJ, Tanner JL (eds): Emerging Adults in America: Coming of Age in the 21st Century. Washington, DC, American Psychological Association, 2006

Auberbach JS, Diamond D: Mental representations in the work of Sydney Blatt. J Am Psychoanal Assoc 65(3):509–523, 2017

Besser A, Blatt SJ: Identity consolidation and internalizing and externalizing problem behaviors in early adolescence. Psychoanal Psychol 24(1):126–149, 2007

Biondo D: The digital world and developmental pain. Italian Psychoanalytic Annual 12:129–144, 2018

Bishop MD, Fish JN, Hammack PL, et al: Sexual identity development milestones in three generations of sexual minority people: a national probability sample. Dev Psychol 56(11):2177–2193, 2020 32833471

Blake MK: Self and group racial/ethnic identification among emerging adults. Emerg Adulthood 7(2):138–149, 2019

Blos P: Character formation in adolescence. Psychoanal Study Child 23:245–263, 1968 5759022

Boulanger G: Lot's wife, Cary Grant, and the American dream: psychoanalysis with immigrants. Contemp Psychoanal 40(3):353–372, 2004

Camp J, Vitoratou S, Rimes KA: The self-acceptance of sexuality inventory (SASI): development and validation. Psychol Sex Orientat Gend Divers 9(1):92–109, 2022

Carlsson J, Wängqvist M, Frisén A: Identity development in the late twenties: a never ending story. Dev Psychol 51(3):334–345, 2015

Castillo K, Reynolds JD, Lee M, et al: Black-Asian American identity: an exploratory study on how internalized oppression impacts identity development. Asian Am J Psychol 11(4):233–245, 2020

Cokley K: Critical issues in the measurement of ethnic and racial identity: a referendum on the state of the field. J Couns Psychol 54(3):224–234, 2007

Coyne SM, Padilla-Walker LM, Howard E: Emerging in a digital world: a decade review of media use, effects, and gratifications in emerging adulthood. Emerg Adulthood 1(2):125–137, 2013

Cross WE Jr: The negro-to-black conversion experience. Black World 20(9):13–27, 1971

Cross WE Jr: Reflections on the lifespan model for ERI development. Res Hum Dev 17(2–3):177–185, 2020

Cross WE, Cross TB: Theory, research, and models, in Handbook of Race, Racism, and the Developing Child. Edited by Quintana SM, McKown C. Hoboken, NJ, Wiley, 2008, pp 154–181

Cross WE Jr, Seaton E, Yip T, et al: Identity work: enactment of racial-ethnic identity in everyday life. Identity 17(1):1–12, 2017

Delgado R, Stefancic J: Preface to the third edition, in Critical Race Theory: An Introduction, 3rd Edition. New York, New York University Press, 2017, pp xix–xxi

Douglass S, Umaña-Taylor AJ: Time-varying effects of family ethnic socialization on ethnic-racial identity development among Latino adolescents. Dev Psychol 52(11):1904–1912, 2016 27709995

Dubé EM, Savin-Williams RC: Sexual identity development among ethnic sexual-minority male youths. Dev Psychol 35(6):1389–1398, 1999 10563729

Du Bois WEB: The souls of black folk, in Three Negro Classics (1903). Edited by Franklin JH. Chicago, IL, AC McClurg, 1965, pp 207–389

Du Bois WEB: Of our spiritual strivings, in The Souls of Black Folk (1903). Edited by Edwards BH. Oxford, UK, Oxford University Press, 2007, pp 7–14

Ehrensaft D: Boys will be girls, girls will be boys: children affect parents as parents affect children in gender nonconformity. Psychoanal Psychol 28(4):528–548, 2011

Eichler RJ: The university as a (potentially) facilitating environment. Contemp Psychoanal 47(3):289–316, 2011

Eng DL, Han S: A dialogue on racial melancholia. Psychoanal Dialogues 10(4):667–700, 2000

Ensink K, Biberdzic M, Normandin L, et al: A developmental psychopathology and neurobiological model of borderline personality disorder in adolescence. J Infant Child Adolesc Psychother 14(1):46–69, 2015

Erikson EH: The problem of ego identity. J Am Psychoanal Assoc 4(1):56–121, 1956 13286157

Erikson EH: Identity: Youth and Crisis. New York, WW Norton, 1968

Eschbach K: Changing identification among American Indians and Alaska Natives. Demography 30(4):635–652, 1993 8262285

Feinstein BA, Bhatia V, Davila J: Rumination mediates the association between cyber-victimization and depressive symptoms. J Interpers Violence 29(9):1732–1746, 2014 24346650

Franco MG, Katz R, O'Brien KM: Forbidden identities: a qualitative examination of racial identity invalidation for black/white biracial individuals. Int J Intercult Relat 50:96–109, 2016

Galatzer-Levy R, Cohler BJ: Making a gay identity: coming out, social context and psychodynamics. Annual of Psychoanalysis 30:255–286, 2002

Gerson MJ: Reconsidering self and identity through a dialogue between neuroscience and psychoanalytic theory. Psychoanal Dialogues 24(2):210–226, 2014

Gillborn D: Intersectionality, critical race theory, and the primacy of racism: race, class, gender, and disability in education. Qualitative Inquiry 21(3):277–287, 2015

Gilmore K: Is emerging adulthood a new developmental phase? J Am Psychoanal Assoc 67(4):625–653, 2019 31604388

Gray B, Johnson T, Kish-Gephart J, et al: Identity work by first-generation college students to counteract class-based microaggressions. Organization Studies 39(9):1227–1250, 2018

Hinduja S, Patchin JW: Bullying, cyberbullying, and suicide. Arch Suicide Res 14(3):206–221, 2010 20658375

Huff JL, Smith JA, Oakes WC: Identity in engineering adulthood: an interpretive phenomenological analysis of early career engineers in the United States as they transition to the workplace. Emerg Adulthood 7(6):451–467, 2019

Jones CP: Levels of racism: a theoretic framework and a gardener's tale. Am J Public Health 90(8):1212–1215, 2000 10936998

Jones NA, Bullock J: The Two or More Races Population: 2010. Suitland, MD, U.S. Census Bureau, 2012

Jørgensen CR: Invited essay: identity and borderline personality disorder. J Pers Disord 24(3):344–364, 2010 20545499

Kanwal GS: More than simply human: intersectionality in psychoanalytic theory, practice, and establishment. Contemp Psychoanal 57(2):270–305, 2021

Kernberg OF: Mature love: prerequisites and characteristics. J Am Psychoanal Assoc 22(4):743–768, 1974 4423688

Kernberg OF: Identity: recent findings and clinical implications. Psychoanal Q 75(4):969–1004, 2006 17094369

Khan F, Limbana T, Tehrim Z, et al: Traits, trends, and trajectory of tween and teen cyberbullies. Cureus 12(8):e9738, 2020 32821629

Lee J, Bean FD: Reinventing the color line: immigration and America's new racial/ethnic divide. Social Forces 86(2):561–586, 2007

Lemma A: An order of pure decision: growing up in a virtual world and the adolescent's experience of being-in-a-body. J Am Psychoanal Assoc 58(4):691–714, 2010 21115753

Levy-Warren MH: Growing up with hatred: a psychoanalytic developmental perspective. J Infant Child Adolesc Psychother 16(3):209–218, 2017

Lilgendahl JP, McLean KC: Narrative identity processes and patterns of adjustment across the transition to college: a developmentally contextualized approach. J Pers Soc Psychol 119(4):960–977, 2020 31829656

Lind M, Vanwoerden S, Penner F, et al: Inpatient adolescents with borderline personality disorder features: identity diffusion and narrative incoherence. Pers Disord 10(4):389–393, 2019 31033329

Livingston G: The rise of multiracial and multiethnic babies in the U.S. Washington, DC, Pew Research Center, June 6, 2017. Available at: https://www.pewresearch.org/fact-tank/2017/06/06/the-rise-of-multiracial-and-multiethnic-babies-in-the-u-s. Accessed December 30, 2021.

Lusk EM, Taylor MJ, Nanney JT, et al: Biracial identity and its relation to self-esteem and depression in mixed black/white biracial individuals. J Ethn Cult Divers Soc Work 19(2):109–126, 2010

Mackey K, Arnold ML, Pratt MW: Adolescents' stories of decision making in more or less authoritative families: representing the voices of parents in narrative. J Adolesc Res 16(3):243–268, 2001

Mallory AB, Pollitt AM, Bishop MD, et al: Changes in disclosure stress and depression symptoms in a sample of lesbian, gay, and bisexual youth. Dev Psychol 57(4):570–583, 2021 34711995

Marcia JE: Development and validation of ego-identity status. J Pers Soc Psychol 3(5):551–558, 1966 5939604

Mayseless O, Keren E: Finding a meaningful life as a developmental task in emerging adulthood: the domains of love and work across cultures. Emerg Adulthood 2(1):63–73, 2014

McAdams DP, McLean KC: Narrative identity. Curr Dir Psychol Sci 22(3):233–238, 1985

McInroy LB, Craig SL: "It's like a safe haven fantasy world": online fandom communities and the identity development activities of sexual and gender minority youth. Psychology of Popular Media 9(2):236–246, 2020

Meeus W, van de Schoot R, Keijsers L, et al: On the progression and stability of adolescent identity formation: a five-wave longitudinal study in early-to-middle and middle-to-late adolescence. Child Dev 81(5):1565–1581, 2010 20840241

Michikyan M: Linking online self-presentation to identity coherence, identity confusion, and social anxiety in emerging adulthood. Br J Dev Psychol 38(4):543–565, 2020 32686856

Morgan EM: Contemporary issues in sexual orientation and identity development in emerging adulthood. Emerg Adulthood 1(1):52–66, 2012

Neblett EW, Roth WD, Syed M: Ethnic and racial identity development from an interdisciplinary perspective: introduction to the special issue. Emerg Adulthood 7(2):79–84, 2019

Padilla J, Vazquez EJ, Updegraff KA, et al: Mexican-origin youth's ethnic-racial identity development: the role of siblings. Dev Psychol 57(2):302–308, 2021 33346675

Parker K, Horowitz JM, Morin R, et al: Multiracial in America: proud, diverse and growing in numbers. Washington, DC, Pew Research Center, June 11, 2015. Available at: https://www.pewresearch.org/social-trends/2015/06/11/multiracial-in-america. Accessed January 2, 2022.

Parmenter JG, Galliher RV, Yaugher AC, et al: Intersectionality and identity configurations: a qualitative study exploring sexual identity development among emerging adults within the United States. Emerg Adulthood 8(10):1–14, 2020

Parmenter JG, Galliher RV, Maughan ADA: LGBTQ+ emerging adults perceptions of discrimination and exclusion within the LGBTQ+ community. Psychol Sex 12(4):289–304, 2021

Pasupathi M, Hoyt T: The development of narrative identity in late adolescence and emergent adulthood: the continued importance of listeners. Dev Psychol 45(2):558–574, 2009 19271839

Paz Galupo M, Mitchell RC, Davis KS: Sexual minority self-identification: multiple identities and complexity. Psychol Sex Orientat Gend Divers 2(4):355–364, 2015

Perrin A, Anderson M: Share of U.S. adults using social media, including Facebook, is mostly unchanged since 2018. Washington, DC, Pew Research Center, April 10, 2019. Available at: https://www.pewresearch.org/fact-tank/2019/04/10/share-of-u-s-adults-using-social-media-including-facebook-is-mostly-unchanged-since-2018. Accessed November 30, 2022.

Pew Research Center: Mobile fact sheet. Washington, DC, Pew Research Center, April 7, 2021. Available at: https://www.pewresearch.org/internet/fact-sheet/mobile. Accessed November 30, 2022.

Ritvo S: Late adolescence: developmental and clinical considerations. Psychoanal Study Child 26:241–263, 1971 5163228

Rogers LO, Scott MA, Way N: Race and gender identity among black adolescent males: an intersectionality perspective. Child Dev 86(2):407–424, 2015 25363136

Rogers LO, Kiang L, White L, et al: Persistent concerns: questions for research on ethnic-racial identity development. Res Hum Dev 17(2–3):130–153, 2020

Sajjadi SF, Gross J, Sellbom M, et al: Narrative identity in borderline personality disorder. Pers Disord 13(1):12–23, 2022

Sattler FA, Zeyen J: Intersecting identities, minority stress, and mental health problems in different sexual and ethnic groups. Stigma Health 6(4):457–466, 2021

Schechter M, Herbstman B, Ronningstam E, et al: Emerging adults, identity development, and suicidality: implications for psychoanalytic psychotherapy. Psychoanal Study Child 71(1):20–39, 2018

Schwartz SJ: Turning point for a turning point: advancing emerging adulthood theory and research. Emerg Adulthood 4(5):307–317, 2016

Schwartz SJ, Zamboanga BL, Luyckx K, et al: Identity in emerging adulthood: reviewing the field and looking forward. Emerg Adulthood 1(2):96–113, 2013

Scroggs B, Love HA, Torgerson C: Covid-19 and LGBTQ emerging adults: risks in the face of social distancing. Emerg Adulthood 9(5):639–644, 2020

Sellers RM, Caldwell CH, Schmeelk-Cone KH, et al: Racial identity, racial discrimination, perceived stress, and psychological distress among African American young adults. J Health Soc Behav 44(3):302–317, 2003 14582310

Shulman S, Connolly J: The challenge of romantic relationships in emerging adulthood: reconceptualization of the field. Emerg Adulthood 1(1):27–39, 2013

Song M: Learning from your children: multiracial parents' identifications and reflections on their own racial socialization. Emerg Adulthood 7(2):119–127, 2019

Stambler MJL: One hundred years of adolescence and its prehistory from cave to computer. Psychoanal Study Child 70(1):22–39, 2017

Steele CM: Whistling Vivaldi: How Stereotypes Affect Us and What We Can Do. New York, WW Norton, 2010

Steele CM: A new approach to schooling in a diverse society: a research fable. J Soc Issues 77(3):911–916, 2021

Stern DN: The Interpersonal World of the Infant: A View From Psychoanalysis and Developmental Psychology. New York, Basic Books, 1985

Stockdale LA, Coyne SM: Bored and online: reasons for using social media, problematic social networking site use, and behavioral outcomes across the transition from adolescence to emerging adulthood. J Adolesc 79:173–183, 2020 31978836

Stoute BJ: Black rage: the psychic adaptation to the trauma of oppression. J Am Psychoanal Assoc 69(2):259–290, 2021 34039068

Tosun LP: Motives for Facebook use and expressing "true self" on the internet. Comput Human Behav 28(4):1510–1517, 2021

Townsend SS, Fryberg SA, Wilkins CL, et al: Being mixed: who claims a biracial identity? Cultur Divers Ethnic Minor Psychol 18(1):91–96, 2012 22250901

Tummala-Narra P: Cultural identity in the context of trauma and immigration from a psychoanalytic perspective. Psychoanal Psychol 31(3):396–409, 2014

Umaña-Taylor AJ, QuintanaSM, LeeRM, et al: Ethnic and racial identity during adolescence and into young adulthood: an integrated conceptualization. Child Dev 85(1):21–39, 2014 24490890

Vanucci A, Ohannessian CM, Gagnon S: Use of multiple social media platforms in relation to psychological functioning in emerging adults. Emerg Adulthood 7(6):501–506, 2018

Varghese ME, Pistole MC: College student cyberbullying: self-esteem, depression, loneliness and attachment. J Coll Couns 20(1):7–21, 2017

Vivona JM: Is there a nonverbal period of development? J Am Psychoanal Assoc 60(2):231–265, 2012 22467444

Wallerstein RS: Erikson's concept of ego identity reconsidered. J Am Psychoanal Assoc 46(1):229–247, 1998 9565906

Wantchekon KA, Umaña-Taylor AJ, Sladek MR, et al: Adolescents' ethnic-racial centrality moderates effect of school-based intervention on ethnic-racial identity exploration. Dev Psychol 57(3):432–442, 2021 33570985

Weil AP: The basic core. Psychoanal Study Child 25(1):442–460, 1970 5532125

White KP: Surviving hating and being hated: some personal thoughts about racism from a psychoanalytic perspective. Contemp Psychoanal 38(3):401–422, 2002

Whiting K: Code-switching: 4 forum voices on what it is—and why we need to talk about it. Geneva, Switzerland, World Economic Forum, November 10, 2020. Available at: https://www.weforum.org/agenda/2020/11/code-switching-systemic-racism-work. Accessed January 10, 2022.

Wilkinson DE, Dunlop WL: Ethnic-racial life scripts: relations with ethnic-racial identity and psychological health. Emerg Adulthood 10(2):402–419, 2020

Wilkinson-Ryan T, Westen D: Identity disturbance in borderline personality disorder: an empirical investigation. Am J Psychiatry 157(4):528–541, 2000 10739411

Williams CD, Byrd CM, Quintana SM, et al: A lifespan model of ethnic-racial identity. Res Hum Dev 17(2–3):99–129, 2020

Willis HA, Sosoo EE, Bernard DL, et al: The associations between internalized racism, racial identity, and psychological distress. Emerg Adulthood 9(4):384–400, 2021

Yang C, Holden SM, Carter MDK: Emerging adults' social media self-presentation and identity development at college transition: mindfulness as a moderator. J Appl Dev Psychol 52:212–221, 2017

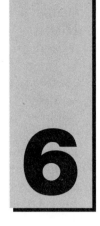

Youth Culture

And these children that you spit on
As they try to change their worlds
They're immune to your consultations
They're quite aware of what they're going through

Ch-ch-ch-ch-Changes
(Turn and face the stranger)
Ch-ch-Changes
Don't tell them to grow up and out of it
Ch-ch-ch-ch-Changes
(Turn and face the stranger)
Ch-ch-Changes
Where's your shame?
You've left us up to our necks in it

"Changes," David Bowie (1971)

I gave 'em chance and chance and chance again
I even done told them please
I find it crazy the police'll shoot you and know that you dead
But still tell you to freeze
Fucked up, I seen what I seen
I guess that mean hold him down if he say he can't breathe

It's too many mothers that's grieving
They killing us for no reason
Been going on for too long to get even

It's bigger than black and white
It's a problem with the whole way of life
It can't change overnight
But we gotta start somewhere
Might as well gon' 'head start here
We done had a hell of a year
I'ma make it count while I'm here
God is the only man I fear

"The Bigger Picture," Lil Baby (2020)

What Is Youth Culture?

Youth culture is a phenomenon that arose in the early twentieth century and blossomed in postwar society. The myriad forms of coexisting and sequential youth cultures, despite the bad reputation of many of them, all contribute to the developmental process by shepherding late adolescents into adulthood. As young people move away from their childhood homes, their selected cultures provide a bridge populated by like-minded peers whose acceptance and affirmation are critical supports to evolving autonomy vis-à-vis the family and to the search for self-determined identity. Each culture contains variations on the common features of music, art forms, social consciousness, group ethos, group activities, clothing and jewelry, and substances to abuse, and each accumulates a specific vernacular. Each appeals to a specific cohort whose affinities align with its offerings. Frequently, one or all of these components include an element of protest or resistance to the adult world, from the established conventions of ambition, morality, and lifestyle—sometimes rejected outright and sometimes caricatured—to the insufficiently examined flaws in the fabric of society, such as systemic racism, the economic divide, or the destruction of the environment.

Although seen prior to World War II (as in the flapper movement), youth culture emerged full force in postwar society. Theories offered to explain this emergence differ depending on the sector of society examined. For example, the flowering of youth cultures has been linked to greater economic security, the advent of age-segregated and compulsory schooling (until age 16 or 18 depending on the state), greater opportunities for the pursuit of leisure activities, increased disposable income, and the recognition of adolescence as a developmental entity (Parsons 1942). From a radically different perspective, the blossoming of youth culture has been understood as a response to the failures of the social order: youth cultures chronicle the experience of immigration, the impoverishment of inner-city populations dominated by Black and brown people, and the widening gap between the affluent mainstream and marginalized youths. These two formulations encompass the main historical trends in the scholarly approach to youth culture, traditionally the purview of sociologists. Talcott Parsons (1942) focused his studies on the youth culture of the white mainstream population in suburban high schools and colleges. Even in the culture arising in this relatively affluent, elite youth cohort, he described a unifying note of resistance to the social order and adult expectations: youth culture was a "culture of irresponsibility" (Galland 2003, p. 163). Parsons (1942, p. 607) viewed youth culture as first and foremost a reaction to conventional adult values; it rejected adult responsibility, including social and career roles, elevating instead the pursuit of enjoyment, sports, and attractiveness. Boys were "swell guys," and girls were admired as they approximated the ideal of the "glamour girl." Parsons noted that youth culture facilitated the transition from dependency on parents to autonomy, via dependency on the peer group (Fasick 1984). In contemporary society, Greek culture represents an updated version of this type of youth culture.

A different, class-based perspective arose from two centers of scholarly inquiry—one at the University of Chicago in Chicago, Illinois, and the other at the Centre for Contemporary Cultural Studies in Birmingham, United Kingdom. The Chicago school was especially focused on the effect of urbanization on delinquency, describing the social ecology of youth culture in its relation to deviance from the culture at large, represented by the development of gangs and criminal activities. The historical de-emphasis on class and urban youths was further challenged by the groundbreaking theory of youth culture that emerged from the Centre for Contemporary Cultural Studies beginning in the 1950s with the rise in juvenile delinquency in Britain. That approach, which informs many thinkers today, was influenced by neo-Marxist theory and cultural studies; it saw youth culture as not merely displaced and coded expressions of the parent culture but also the opportunity for attempts at solving participants' larger, problematic societal experience of class, racism, homophobia, and exclusion (Lave et al. 1992). It challenged the idea of youth culture as classless and elevated social class as the main driver in the creation of cultures that appear in any given epoch. It also underscored the meaningful commentary on society contained in youth culture.

Although the sociological debate is beyond the scope of this book, it seems clear to us that youth cultures must be contextualized in the larger culture, the historical epoch, and the circumstances in which they develop. Whether youth culture represents neotribalism, subcultures, or simply "scenes" (Hodkinson 2007), issues of class, income level, and, especially in the United States, race are intrinsic to the nature of youth cultures today. And despite changing styles and forms, youth cultures cannot be dismissed as evanescent, superficial, or frivolous or, alternatively, criminal, violent, and aggrieved, because reverberations run deep and often linger in the adulthood of the participants. Many of the causes embraced by a given culture spread to different age groups and spawn new editions of youth culture. In a world dominated by digital communication, the globalization of youth cultures and trends ensures that there is cross-fertilization among them and that they likely carry seeds of other cultures in their own. A broader notion of youth culture, that is, one not mainly assigned a deviant tendency, extends the peer culture concept to become more inclusive; to transcend geography and language; and to identify with belief systems, music, activities, online activities, substances, and fashion from around the world. It also promotes international and intergenerational participation, such that many youth cultures increasingly include (or tolerate) participants well beyond age 30. This is nowhere better exemplified than by the rise of hip-hop culture from an impoverished enclave in the South Bronx, New York, to a dominant force in global networking containing a clear message of social unrest and resistance and of defiance of so-called cultural values, contributing to identity formation, and ultimately creating a "transnational cultural product" (Silva et al. 2016, p. 134).

It is noteworthy that from its introduction, youth culture was said to address the needs of an "in-between" phase of development (Moore 2015), corresponding to emerging adulthood, because of the loss of structured paths to adulthood and the age segregation created by extended schooling. Youth culture has thus been linked to the circumstances of twentieth- and twenty-first-century youths as they negotiate the unregulated transition between childhood and adulthood. In agreement with Arnett's observations, youth culture scholars emphasize that this transition is increasingly elongated and fluid, as the formerly static and circumscribed aspects of developmental progression and identity have loosened in contemporary society (Hodkinson 2007). From this perspective, youth culture can be understood to provide roles and rituals (in the broadest sense) no longer present in conventional society because of the breakdown of traditional pathways to adulthood that formerly guided youths (Ciocan 2015); the diminished importance of social positions and roles; and the delay or decline in engagement with hallowed institutions such as religion, marriage, and parenthood. With increasing urbanization, immigration, and inequality regarding race and class, the more explicit elements of defiance and anti-authoritarianism have entered into some movements.

Many of the themes that occupy a given youth culture reflect the cohort's particular position in and struggle with the culture at large. As the sociologist Mike Brake (1985) suggested in addressing subcultures in general, these "arise as attempts to resolve collectively experienced problems resulting from contradictions in the social structure, and...generate a form of collective identity from which an individual identity can be achieved outside that ascribed by class, education and occupation" (p. ix). (It should be noted that some contemporary activist groups can facilitate individual identity by the opposite means—that is, by strengthening ties to just those ascribed signifiers.) This is an aspect of youth culture that serves a crucial role in identity formation in emerging adulthood, because it supports self-determination and self-definition within the group ethos, in defiance of roles assigned by society. The older generation may view the sorority girl or the surfer as an example of unthinking identification with a peer group, but to the youths involved, their participation is an escape from cultural pigeonholing into membership in a rich and exciting world full of like-minded youths.

As noted earlier, youth cultures are typically distinguished by their favored clothes, popular music, sports, vocabulary, communication preferences, preferred substances, gender expression, social consciousness, and sexual mores; the defining feature can be one or many of these elements. Whereas some cultures—for example, those in elite surroundings like college campuses—seem primarily focused on pleasure, clothing, shared musical or video game tastes, drug consumption, or consumption of material goods, others encompass a specific opposition to or deviation from the larger cultural milieu and participate prominently in political movements such as the civil rights, gay rights, antiwar, gun control, anti–climate change, or Black Lives Matter (BLM) movements. Of course, no singular youth culture draws the entire generation into its practices, even if in retrospect the youths of an era may be referenced by a singular moniker, such as "hippies." Not all young people of the late 1960s and 1970s were hippies, civil rights activists, and antiwar activists who wore beads and bell-bottom jeans; smoked pot; believed in free love; and listened to Joan Baez, Bob Dylan, or, from a different tradition, David Bowie and the Rolling Stones. Within any given generation are many groups that embrace very different sensibilities, styles, and agendas.

In other words, the relation of youth cultures to the parent culture is complex, varied, and widely distributed, as attested to by the co-occurrence of what seem like vastly different youth cultures within a larger cultural milieu: for example, from the 1970s through the 1990s, while hip-hop culture was forming and gaining momentum, other musical genres, such as rock and roll, soul, disco, heavy metal, and house music, each with more or less its own culture, had their own trajectories. Especially today with the vast reach of digital and social media, there is a mingling and integration of components of different youth cultures in addition to their co-optation by the surrounding milieu and by the marketplace. The rise of various youth cultures, their scaffolding and means of dissemination, and their transitions are closely connected to contemporaneous new media (beginning with the radio and onward to the digital age). This ensures that movements, initially consigned to isolated neighborhoods, can gain momentum from elsewhere, gathering musical resources, dance styles, fashion, acolytes, and shared sensibility; thus, hip-hop is a cultural product developed over decades of social transformation, migration, formation of inner cities, and frequently political outrage among Black artists (Ogbar 2018). By the twenty-first century, it had achieved domination in terms of both its scope and influence and its market share; more than 30% of all on-demand audio and video streams in the United States in 2020 were of tracks recorded by rhythm and blues and hip-hop artists (Ingham 2021). As hip-hop culture demonstrates, the interface between youth culture and mainstream culture is bidirectional (Best and Lynn 2016), as when commercialization and commodification of youth cultural artifacts cash in on the trends.

The relationship of youth culture to the market and to technology is deep and troubled; determining who is actually driving various components, like new equipment, drug paraphernalia, and fashion, is often impossible. This has led to grave warnings about the nature of the intimate connections among what youths consume, the medium by which their consumption is shaped, and how they identify themselves (Best and Lynn 2016). It is true that advances in technology tend to be greeted by an outcry regarding their seductions, as well as their moral dangers for young people, beginning with television and extending to contemporary incarnations such as TikTok, YouTube, and Instagram. The marketplace has been accused of aggressively co-opting the creative energy of youth cultures, often without seriously engaging with the sensibility of the innovators (Sola-Santiago 2017). Given the rapid transformation in the past three decades to an information and technological society associated with the emergence of the internet, smartphones, and social networking sites, youth culture is increasingly shaped by the extended reach of commerce. Communication through digital media and social networking sites is sponsored by advertising; similarly, charismatic leaders, artists, and spokespeople are elevated to prominence by commercial backers.

Twenty-first-century youth culture is thus a complex cocreation of technology, evolving art forms, consumerism, targeted marketing and youth trends, Western values, and the young people who influence and are influenced by it. Although commercial interests have a huge and pervasive presence in the digital world of young people, there has also been the opportunity for youths to turn into *prosumers*, both by creating digital content of their own and by asserting their preferences in product development.

The importance of access to devices and broadband capacity has been augmented exponentially by the SARS-CoV-2 disease (COVID-19) pandemic, which took people off campuses and off the street, out of work, and into their parental homes. However, even before this forced reliance on social networking, access to the internet was a key facilitator of youth culture. We continue to highlight the interface of the digital world with youth culture as this chapter progresses. But first, we delve into the considerable interface of youth culture and the mind, which is bidirectional—both mutually enhancing and potentially at cross-purposes—and illustrate these dynamics through a small sampling of youth cultures.

The Relationship of Youth Culture to Mental Development in Adolescence and Emerging Adulthood

All youth cultures can be understood as providing support in the quest of young people in transition to define themselves, to establish their relationship to the existing order, and to create a sense of kinship with a community of peers (Moore 2015). In this way, youth culture provides an invaluable resource in shoring up psychic boundaries, individuating from the family of origin, developing meaningful identity components, providing a new sense of belonging and community, and promoting the inexhaustible creative capacity of this age group (Dougherty and Clarke 2018). Because participation in youth cultural activities does not necessarily encompass daily life, it can strain emerging adults' capacity to regulate their impulses, to manage their states of mind and shift their orientations between the values of the clan and those of the larger culture, and essentially to meet the challenge of achieving ego integration and identity formation in two cultural planes simultaneously.

Certainly, some aspects of all youth cultures can exacerbate the differences between the states of mind and self-representations in the culture and those in the real world. The darker side is a given youth culture's potential to promote and facilitate drug use; applaud risky activities, including life-threatening extreme sports and other dangerous and criminal behavior; and in some cases, such as with cults, insist on full submission of the individual will, moral reasoning, and personal standards to the cult leader. But most youth cultures, at least at entry, seem to fulfill the emerging adult's drive to achieve the psychological function of autonomy and self-actualization, of "making your own decisions, of controlling your own life, or deciding with whom to associate, of deciding which actions to pursue, and of deciding which and whose ends to advance" (Olivier 2006, p. 102).

The degree to which a youth culture encompasses a full-service identity that can travel between youth cultural activities and real life, with an income and future potential, varies considerably by individual and by culture. When this occurs—for example, when a popular musician develops a makeup brand or when an elite snowboarder gets prestigious endorsements—the person achieves a kind of legitimate adulthood recognized by peers, followers, and the larger society. That is, the completeness of their cultural world, culminating in financial success, is established by this sturdy, commercial bridge between the cultures that elevates the youth culture persona to a version of adulthood on a par with the parent generation's version. In Video 7, a 30-year-old parkour expert has transformed a passion into a key identity feature and a profession.

 Video 7: Passion for an athletic activity becomes a life's work

The Importance of Action

Despite the evidence against universal "storm and stress" (Hollenstein and Lougheed 2013), the adolescent process involves some degree of upheaval, as rapid physical, hormonal, and brain maturation poses new challenges intrapsychically and interpersonally. Many developmental pressures and conflicts throughout adolescence and emerging adulthood are managed through *action* (Chused 1990); action is required to test new capabilities and to assert autonomy, to pursue intense feelings and sensations, and to enjoy the higher levels of reward stimulation occurring in the adolescent brain. The development of physical strength and adult sexual capacity forces a reconfiguration of the parent-child relationship; the former reliance on parental guidance and support now poses potential threats for the young person beset by sexual feelings, aggressive impulses, and regressive urges, any of which, if expressed toward family members, may illicit punishment, guilt, or fear of reprisal. The struggle to differentiate the superego from its roots in parental dos and don'ts and the associated need to detach from oedipal objects, related to the heightened threat of sexual and aggressive feelings, often leave the adolescent feeling lonely and abandoned.

   Action is essential to creating physical distance from parents, to rebelling, and to finding a new community to guide behavior and new objects of desire to deflect sexual drive from within the family and seek satisfaction elsewhere. At the same time, action serves the growing pressure to achieve self-definition—part of the ongoing effort to establish an individuated and autonomous identity. In this context, the peer group is essential. Connecting and belonging to a peer group can provide a strong source of family-like community, shared values and tastes, and codes for behavior and beliefs, not to mention peer facilitation of excitement and fun. Sensation- and novelty-seeking, associated with the characteristic spike in risk behaviors, relies on the peer group for support, encouragement, and actualization. This confluence of factors augments the importance of the peer group and the opportunities it offers for sexual exploration, new standards of behavior and self-assessment, greater willingness to experiment and take risks, and new supports for identity development. When a peer group rises to the level of peer culture, the implication is that the focus is no longer simply on the network of local individuals and the complexity of their relationships. The group ethos, via its underlying assumptions and shared predilections, connects or expands to larger groups that further elaborate the meaning of membership. Membership can then confer a more enduring identity.

Action, Risk Behaviors, and the Peer Group

The statistically demonstrable predilection for risk behavior in late adolescence and emerging adulthood is developmental, that is, it is a typical outcome of the constellation of brain and physical growth, sexual development, and socioemotional transformations that occur in this decade (Oosterhoff and Wray-Lake 2020). Proneness to risk-taking creates the substrate for a range of actions, including political activity as well as the more typically cited transgressive behavior—that is, binge drinking and the use of other illicit substances, casual sexual encounters without protection or unwanted sexual encounters achieved by doping, reckless driving, extreme sports, reckless illegal takeover and use of spaces, cyberbullying, and certain forms of group-condoned criminal activity. All of these are important manifestations of this action orientation. The strong connections between an inclination toward risk and the peer group that begin in puberty and extend to the end of emerging adulthood are supported by empirical research (Gardner and Steinberg 2005; Jeon and Goodson 2015; Keyzers et al. 2020; Lamblin et al. 2017). With involvement in certain youth cultures, the invitation to engage in risk behaviors, which is heightened by the crucial facilitating presence of peers and the frequent presence of alcohol (Sherman et al. 2019) or other substances, becomes integrated into activities that are intrinsic to belonging: rave parties, the occupation of vacant spaces, graffiti wars, skateboarding in construction sites, drug trafficking, drug use, various sexual practices, and public demonstrations (including some demonstrations that entail violence or invite violent suppression). A range of these activities can lead to arrest, and although some are in direct defiance of legal strictures, others may be only dimly recognized by participants as potentially consequential. Many provide context for further reckless behavior without contemplation. The excitement of painting graffiti on a tall building with friends is multiplied when police helicopters are circling above, further enhancing the addictive pleasures of risk.

The role of peers in the persistence of risk behaviors has been examined by many researchers. Assessments of the efficacy of educational programs for reducing risk behaviors consistently document their limitations (Steinberg 2008; Sunstein 2008); the conclusion is that it "is not what they know, but what they do" (Sunstein 2008, p. 147). Rational discussions and warnings of consequences are simply not deterrents when everyone is having fun taking drugs and dancing in abandoned warehouses. We review theories about brain development relevant to persistent risk behavior shortly, but in regard to the relationship between risk behavior and youth culture, it is noteworthy that many prominent thinkers and researchers repeatedly return to the importance of the peer group in exacerbating developmental trends and quieting internal prohibitions.

Risky behavior as a developmental entity has been addressed by many different disciplines, each from their vantage point. Neuroendocrinologists, neurogeneticists, psychiatrists, developmental scientists, sociologists, psychoanalysts, and many other specialists offer insights for understanding this adolescent and emerging adult phenomenon (Dahl 2004); it is clear that there is no simple linear causality, no bedrock etiology for a phenomenon that unfortunately can exact a high price in terms of accidental death, initiation and perpetuation of substance abuse, criminal behavior, suicide, arrest, and incarceration.

The prominence of the theory of raging hormones in adolescent risk behavior has declined from its status in the 1990s (Pharo et al. 2011), but pubertal hormones remain implicated in every aspect of the dramatic changes of puberty and adolescence. They are essential for physical development, including changes in the face, skin, body hair, and other secondary sex characteristics; musculoskeletal size and overall maturation; growth of sexual and reproductive organs; and burgeoning socioemotional interest in sex. Gonadal hormones play an important role in the two active periods of brain sculpting in human development—the perinatal period and the pubertal period. Current research supports the idea that these are not discrete events but rather two peaks in ongoing brain remodeling: the first is mostly organizational, and the second is activational for the circuits established in the earlier period (Schulz and Sisk 2016); the contemporary view is that an organizational component in the pubertal period is also present (Vijayakumar et al. 2018). The second wave is part of the complex cascade that produces new connectivity in brain circuitry, neurogenesis, programmed cell death, pruning and dendrification, sexual differentiation, and so on (Schulz and Sisk 2016). This second wave of structural brain transformation in adolescence is globally correlated with various behaviors associated with puberty and adolescence, but clear correspondences with typical adolescent behavior, such as moodiness and depression, self-related preoccupations, and rapid fluctuations in self-esteem, have not been established; the most consequential factor correlated with these behaviors, as well as with aggression and predilection to delinquency, is pubertal timing (Buchanan et al. 1992; Mrug et al. 2014). In summary, contemporary viewpoints note the temporal correspondence between puberty and changes in brain systems that pertain to risk and other typical adolescent behavior, but there is little empirical evidence of the effect of pubertal hormones directly on these systems (Vetter-O'Hagen and Spear 2012).

Developmental neuroscientist Laurence Steinberg (2008) proposed that the dramatic upsurge in risky behavior reflects variable rates of development in different brain systems. The dual brain systems model delineates two circuits whose development is unsynchronized and thus creates the potential for risk behavior (Steinberg 2010). The first, the socioemotional system (the dopaminergic system with nodes in the amygdala, nucleus accumbens, orbitofrontal cortex, medial prefrontal cortex, and superior temporal sulcus), which governs both reward-seeking and sensitivity to reward, develops early. The second, the cognitive control system, which governs self-regulation, is, in contrast, slow to develop and not complete until the mid- to late 20s. (This fact fundamentally challenges the potential of cognitive approaches aimed at younger children to successfully reduce risk in adolescence, such as "Just Say No" [Landmark Recovery 2018], Project Charlie [McGurk and Hurry 1995], D.A.R.E. [Drug Abuse Resistance Education; https://dare.org/about], and Scared Straight [Hale 2010]; indeed, many studies suggest that such programs may even be harmful.) In other words, reward-seeking is unchecked by simultaneous cognitive input promoting delayed gratification, future thinking (Bromberg et al. 2015), and higher executive function. The presence of peers is a consistent enhancing condition for the responsiveness of the socioemotional system (Chein et al. 2011). Interestingly, the movement away from the larger peer group into couples that occurs as emerging adults move into their mid- to late 20s is temporally correlated with the shift in balance between the two systems. The timing of these events provides support for the expectation that marriage and family tend to curb risk behaviors. However, this expectation is under renewed scrutiny.

Reward-seeking has been described as "one of a suite of developmental domains...linked to puberty-specific maturational changes" (Dahl 2004, quoted in Steinberg 2010, p. 217). Reward-seeking and risk-taking have evolutionary advantages for all mammals, because venturing outside of familiar territory prevents inbreeding. The emerging adult period shows the full flowering of these behaviors, evidenced not only by peak alcohol consumption and peak binge drinking (Patrick et al. 2019) but also by other aspects of risk-taking that have come to be viewed as habit-forming, like the adrenaline rush that makes thrill seekers adrenaline junkies. Many participants claim that they are seeking flow and state alteration. Another important question is whether these behaviors reliably decline as age 30 is approached.

The varying perspectives on the socio-, neuro-, biopsychological risk-seeking of this age group all acknowledge that *context* is an important component that modulates the effect of hormones or uneven brain development on the saliency of reward. The presence of peers is a consistent source of reward enhancement and a stimulus for upping the ante. Youth cultures provide a circle of peers who reward the behaviors that identify participants as members, some of which may border on recklessness, substance abuse, and a range of other impulsive actions. This is one important reason that youth cultures foment action—acts of courage and daring, acts of cruelty, acts of self-destructiveness, and so on.

For example, risk-taking associated with protests, demonstrations, and political positions is certainly facilitated by peer recruitment and peer affirmation, often through social media (Bisafar et al. 2020). Recruiters adept at social media can mobilize youths to convene for demonstrations or draw them into dangerous affiliations, such as terrorist groups. One researcher (DiGrazia 2014) examined readiness to engage in "conventional" and "unconventional" activities and noted that the groups differed by virtue of their position in society and their conformity to mainstream values; typically, youths from higher socioeconomic classes, on the pathway to achieving conventional adulthood (e.g., marriage, a stable job), gravitate toward the conventional, less risky activities. The degree of disadvantage, investment in the cause, and peer encouragement become key factors in determining a willingness to overstep boundaries or to violate the law. No doubt there is excitement associated with such activities, in addition to fervent political belief; enthusiasm among peers consolidates affiliations. These factors promote the identity function of youth cultures described in the following subsection.

Development of Identity

Youth cultures offer the in-between emerging adult a community, providing outlets for physical feats, sexual activity, and other sources of sensation; a shared interest in specific risk-taking behaviors; shared beliefs in self-determined moral positions; and an acclaimed sense of identity. The identity support fills or expands the space formerly occupied by familial identifiers, including genetic, ethnic, racial, religious, political, and moral elements that define the family at large, as well as intrafamilial identifiers, such as the role assigned in the sibling cohort, the descriptors, the critiques, and myriad other features that descend on a child beginning at birth. Some emerging adults jump into a formed culture on the basis of their predilections, friends, and crushes, whereas others develop their peer culture by chance, from being recruited on social media, or from scratch. In a remarkable global example, Greta Thunberg's first steps into activism were initiated by her personal response to learning of climate change as a grade school student; she borrowed from the example of the March for Our Lives activists (a self-generated movement secondary to the school shooting in Parkland, Florida) by conducting school strikes and went on to galvanize youth climate activists everywhere. Today, the youth consciousness regarding climate in addition to issues such as race, gun control, gay rights, and women's rights contradicts turn-of-the-century critiques leveled at youths for their complacency (McNulty 2019) and has become part of the sensibility of a broad swath of youth cultures. As has often been the case, protests define generations and promote identity development, in addition to fostering superego autonomy. Cause-focused groups are a particular type of youth culture that tends to welcome like-minded adults: the quarrel is with the larger culture's failure to redress wrongs, especially those affecting the current and future lives of youths.

In the following vignette, a young man of color was greatly disadvantaged in developing a peer group that supported racial identity by the effect of trauma on his nuclear family. His mother had been widowed with two young children at age 28; her effort to earn a living and protect her family resulted in the widespread prohibition of any contact with or connection to the neighborhood. After an isolated childhood, Deshawn finally experienced a glimmer of belonging when he became a valued player on his high school sports team. In college, his participation in the sports culture was modulated by his growing engagement with political activism, which became his most committed group experience, especially as youth presence in the BLM movement began to mushroom following the events of the summer of 2020. Although the BLM movement extends across generations, the role of late adolescents and young adults is considerable, much as it is in environmental activism and was in the civil rights and antiwar movements of the past.

Case Vignette: Deshawn

Deshawn was the older child and only son of two Caribbean immigrants; his mother was a nursing assistant at a local teaching hospital, and his father had been an orderly in the affiliated Veterans Health Administration hospital. When Deshawn was 4, his father, then only 24, died of a gunshot to the head, apparently in the context of a drug deal. Deshawn remembered very little about him, especially as his mother discouraged his questions, removed any memorabilia, and refused contact with paternal family members. She made clear her determination to help her children become achievers in the mainstream. She was intent on improving the family's prospects single-handedly by moving up in the ranks of nursing, eventually obtaining a bachelor of science degree in nursing in night school while she continued working her daytime job. Deshawn was often left alone with his sister, who was 2 years younger, with only a neighbor's telephone number ("just in case") while his mother pursued her degree. He remembered long evenings with his sister in their tiny apartment, hearing gunshots and feeling terrified, because the neighborhood was plagued by gun violence and the drug trade. He felt responsible for shielding his little sister and therefore obligated to present himself as calm and adult, trying to manage mounting anxiety without adult presence or guidance.

Deshawn worked hard and excelled at school. He socialized very little, except in the context of team sports. His height, athleticism, and good grades led to his recruitment by the basketball team of the local magnet high school; there he was able to develop friendships with other conscientious, ambitious athletes, many of whom had shared some of his exposure to neighborhood violence. As he approached his final year of high school, his mother received her degree and decided to move to a different state for a good nursing position. She planned to take Deshawn's little sister but offered him the choice of staying put for his last year of high school. He was determined to stay, hoping to further augment his recruitment potential for college: he was finally to be captain of his state-champion basketball team and would have more time to consolidate his reputation with his coach and teachers, who in turn would support his applications. His mother made loose arrangements for Deshawn's care during his final year of high school, asking parents of his friends and his coach's family to take turns housing him in order to provide him with a semblance of stability. Deshawn was abashed at his enforced dependency on these relationships. He was determined to contribute to the families that kept him for months at a time by doing chores and running errands, despite the protests of the family members. He dreaded appearing needy or pitiful. In their homes, he comported himself as a courteous and serious young man who rarely opened up to the adults and who never spoke of the real cause of his father's death.

As a result of contemporaneous events of that particular time, there were many conversations in these families of color about their growing sense of impotent outrage around gun violence, first in regard to shootings related to crime and drug dealing and then in regard to gun violence inflicted on young Black men by the police. However, Deshawn was mindful of his mother's admonition to steer clear of conflict and "just get ahead"; such lifelong instruction had curtailed his interest in and exploration of political movements. The pressure of her conventional ambitions and her wish that he "stay out of trouble and fit in" exerted an inhibiting power over his mental life and his freedom of expression. At the same time, his unresolved mourning of his father was an unprocessed trauma that frightened him (was he going to be like his father, involved in the drug world and dead at 24?) and fueled his suppressed anger over the loss of his father and his own subsequent "imprisonment" by his strict but absent mother, who now had completely abandoned him.

Born the year of the Columbine school massacre (1999), Deshawn knew that gun concerns were not confined to the inner city. He was impressed with the action taken by the Parkland, Florida, students, especially Emma Gonzalez and her famous speech "We Call B.S."; he attended and watched firsthand as inner-city victims of gun violence found a place in the March for Our Lives protest in Washington, D.C., organized in the wake of the Parkland massacre. He realized that he was looking for an avenue to vent his anger and frustration, but because he was afraid his mother would disown him completely if he became active in BLM protests, he instead engaged in actions around gun control and participated in organizing efforts to form coalitions with local chapters. His athletic talent and hard work resulted in a full scholarship to the large university in the city where his mother now resided; much to her chagrin, he brought the same interest and activism to that scene as well. In addition to being relieved to be once again in the same geographic area as his family, Deshawn felt buoyed by the peer group he found at college, whose members were multiracial and all interested in political activism in addition to rap music, video-gaming, and style statements. His group engaged in deep conversations about the BLM movement, and he increasingly identified with participation in that movement. He did not yet share this interest with his mother.

At one BLM demonstration, Deshawn met a young woman, Aniyah, from a different college within his university, whose more assertive politics he both feared and admired. His tentative approach to getting to know her was warmly welcomed, because she had noticed him too. Their similar experiences growing up in an inner city created a feeling of safety in their relationship, and he began to seek her company regularly. Their intimacy grew and finally led him to discuss his father's murder for the first time. She expressed sympathy and, perhaps most important to him, a sustained curiosity about his father and paternal family, and she encouraged him to pursue his occasional research into the many unknowns about this aspect of his life. Although Deshawn knew that she was "wilder" than he was—more sexual, more willing to experiment with substances—he was confident that she had a level-headed sensibility in terms of her political views and that she would be able to help him manage both the disclosure to his mother of his commitment to BLM and the fallout. This proved a sustained challenge in which Aniyah's already established warm connection to his mother plus her evident intelligence and ambition were invaluable. The couple continued to participate in BLM protests; Deshawn's interest and evolving leadership abilities led him to seek organizational and recruitment roles.

Deshawn's development was deeply shaped by the violent death of his father and the experienced loss of his mother. As is often said about parental death in childhood, the loss of the surviving parent, as a result of depression, remarriage, the economic demands of raising the family, or any of many other reasons, further complicates the trauma. Deshawn's mother was absent from the home because of her desperate desire to improve her family's circumstances. The same rationalization led her to deny him access to or knowledge of his father, the paternal family, and cultural history and thus left him with a gaping hole in his mental construction of his father. Deshawn had no mental scaffolding for identity development related to a sense of his father's character, cultural heritage, and family. He did not even know if his father had been an innocent bystander or a hardened gang member, which severely challenged another important pillar of development in terms of identifications, values, and ideals: was he the offspring of a criminal or a good man? His mother's severe admonitions and real restrictions on his freedom to engage with his peer group became an oppressive inhibition, limiting his access to shared thoughts and feelings about race and inner-city experience. Over time, his engagement with activism provided support for the development of his own set of values. Deshawn's participation in the world of college basketball and the culture of activism on campus and beyond served many aspects of his development in late adolescence and emerging adulthood in addition to identity formation: it provided him with a pathway to individuation and autonomy, superego modulation, a sense of belonging, and peer relationships. In this case, his youthful participation seemed to pave the way for an adult role in his organization; if he was recruited into the National Basketball Association, all the better.

Presumably, the importance of the identity function of youth cultures declines with passage through the 20s. The activities, styles, music, drugs, and other signifiers certainly may diminish in aging emerging adults, as these persons consolidate identities by virtue of evolving careers, marriage, and adult responsibility and affiliations. But, as discussed in Chapter 4, "What Is Distinct About the Second Part of Emerging Adulthood?," the contemporary version of adulthood may depend less on the classic adult markers and more on other identifications and capacities, such as adaptability, flexibility, entrepreneurship, and autonomous decision-making (Arnett 2000). The requirements for fluency, adaptability, and creativity in technology thoroughly differentiated the emerging adults at the turn of the twenty-first century from their parents; today's differentiation is less marked, because the parent generation is now able to speak the language and even provide mentorship. The developmental outcomes of the passage to adulthood are far more complex and original than those defined by adult markers.

Elements of youth culture, from preferred music to political leanings, from preferred recreational drug use to massive group activities, may be sustained deep into adulthood. Evidence of brain maturation, a decline in sensation-seeking, and an action orientation should coincide in the mid-20s as age 30 is approached. In many ways, the classic adulthood of the late twentieth century is "obsolete" (Hunter 2009, p. 27) and without intrinsic social status; some features may eventually appear without the same significance. Even the five features in Arnett's original report persist, reflecting a fundamental change in visions of adulthood; Arnett and Mitra (2020) published a report of a national survey that showed that more than half of the respondents in age groups up to 60 endorsed the continued experience of four out of five features of emerging adulthood (excluding feeling in-between), which suggests that the stereotype of the stable settled adult is shifting to an ideal of openness to opportunities and to change, to living in unstable circumstances, to continuing to engage in self-focused explorations, and even to continuing to see change in their future. In Video 8, a 26-year-old former raver and ambitious pharmaceutical sales representative shows a complex amalgam of identities derived from family and heritage, a strong work ethic, and a love of rave parties.

 Video 8: The "in-between" experience of emerging adulthood

Depersonalization and Autonomy of the Superego

Any given youth culture can foster values that constitute a radical departure from the childhood version of the superego and can even delay or impede the development of enduring, stable, and ego-syntonic versions, as risky behavior is rewarded in the presence of like-minded others (Chein et al. 2011). As emerging adults grapple with individuation from their families of origin and attempt to divest themselves of parental influence, youth culture draws participants into a new orbit of practices, beliefs, values, and behaviors that may be contrary to many standards maintained by parents in early life. A given youth culture can loosen constraints on conservative, rule-following, and law-abiding aspects of parental influence; in some arenas, the new sensibility is experienced by youths as more enlightened and appropriate. This is amply demonstrated by Deshawn's development and gradual commitments.

Given the reality that emerging adults often live, at least temporarily, in their childhood homes, there is an extended opportunity for communication between generations. On the most general level of technology-speak, the passing up of technological savvy and, increasingly, the mutual education between parents and children are evolving. Specific youth cultural engagement can draw in the parent generation and prompt a shift in attitudes. Whether this is welcome, resented, or simply entertaining to the involved emerging adult varies according to the culture, the activity, and the individual. Alternatively, some parents draw their emerging adult children into their own youth culture, introducing them to extreme sports (or possibly tamer versions); explaining the values of goth culture, deejaying, and the parents' style of dancing; or initiating them into classic rock and marijuana culture. The influence can thus be bidirectional, further blurring the alleged generational divide between youth culture and serious adult life. Certainly, youth cultures draw the interest of the adults who hope to profit by them; such financial compensation from the corporate world promotes a different set of values, the potential for selling out, or the admiration of the family as the breadwinner or star.

Elements of Youth Cultures

Features of a given culture can be loosely itemized into a recognizable collection. Hip-hop has deejaying, emceeing, graffiti, dance, rap music, and streetwear. Ravers are distinguished by their underground partying; spectacular lit-up, neon wild-fit clothing; ecstasy; dance moves; and the development of several musical forms (predominantly electronic dance music but also incorporating house music, techno, and dubstep; Burch and Sachs 2021). Snowboarders have streetwear; boards; snow parks; and after-snow parties fueled by alcohol, marijuana, and prescription drugs. Less spectacular youth cultures may have fewer emblems of belonging or shared sensations, but over the past decades, some of these, such as comic book and video game fandoms, have attracted commercial interests and gained sponsorship that supports massive conventions or tournaments. For example, in the mid-twentieth century, comic book fans had little access to others with similar tastes until comic book stores became spaces where aficionados of comics, costumes, action figures, and other paraphernalia could gather in impromptu meetings. When comic-cons (comic book conventions) began to draw huge crowds eager to display their costumes and to purchase paraphernalia, this fandom catapulted to a new level. The active interface between fans and commercial interests creates prosumers whose ideas shape the marketplace and promote the community. The following elements are usually present in youth cultures of various types.

Fashion

Youth cultures are often associated with an emblematic clothing item or style that undergoes serial editions as wearers add their variations; in the digital era, the rapid dissemination of these transformations via Instagram, YouTube, and other social media ensures that new styles get noticed. Streetwear itself is a culture, a culture of innovation and collecting. Streetwear designers and its passionate collectors (known as sneakerheads [Sola-Santiago 2017] and hypebeasts [Rajendran 2012]), with inspiration from hip-hop and surfer and skateboarding cultures, have developed styling and collecting into its own culture.

The story of the streetwear movement's uneasy relationship with luxury fashion is a drama of co-optation and realignment. Some decry the relationship between the fashion industry and streetwear as superficial, an exploitative embrace of the style currently made popular by Black celebrities, victims of racism (Trayvon Martin's hoodie), and rappers; these emblems of lethal racism, power, or resistance are now fashion items, produced by an industry without any real interest in Black culture or serious integration of its own infrastructure. As stars achieve renown within their particular youth culture, they are often sponsored and engaged in designing their own fashion items. Some fashions have soared beyond the reach of the average fan by virtue of collaborations with luxury brands and endorsements or designs of celebrities. Within hip-hop, fashion can be an important tool in asserting status over other artists: in the so-called gold rush of the late twentieth century, the "spirit of competition" among artists epitomized by the extravagance of dookie chains (thick gold chains), grillz (gold mouthpieces), and door knocker earrings (Jenkins 2018, p. 45) inspired competitive excesses. Collaboration with elite jewelers and escalation of the status of gaudy and extravagant led to the immortalization of some jewelry designers in song, as in the hit song "Grillz" (Nelly et al. 2005).

While hip-hop culture has created a highly visible fashion sensibility, other youth cultures have joined by contributing recognizable and innovative fashion accoutrements. A steady stream of small businesses repeatedly seek to reassert the modest beginnings of popular fashion in the surfer and hip-hop communities; co-optation by luxury brands is a violation of the political and racial sensibilities that these clothing items represent. A simple, affordable fashion item—the oversized T-shirt or the hoodie—is the blank canvas that invites transformation and serves to broadcast the affiliation of the individual with both the genre of youth culture and the fashion item's emblematic meaning.

Streetwear has become a do-it-yourself movement, initially a reaction against luxury brands, favoring "rawness, attitude, creativity, and community" (Petty 2019). Early incarnations of streetwear were co-opted by the fashion industry to appear on runways as designer tracksuits, baseball caps, and sneakers. Subsequently, the style was reclaimed by brands that cater to young people. These brands create affordable items or outfits inspired by their wearers, often members of cultures such as hip-hop, surfing, skateboarding, and parkour, captured in photographs or videos and disseminated via Instagram and other social media. Some brands continue to form collaborations with luxury designer brands, such as Supreme and Off-White, whereas others are committed to the template of the blank T-shirt and thus the ethos and price point of streetwear: Stüssy, Kith, and many others (Meyer 2023). These brands are open to the innovation and creativity of urban, diverse, immigrant youths and remain streetwear oriented and affordable.

Sports

Extreme sports are risky, thrilling, and dominated by young people with young bodies. There are many types of extreme sports (Lockwood 2022) associated with a range of terrains, equipment, and gathering spaces and featuring different types of danger and excitement generated by the moving body. The draw for emerging adults may be related to the emphasis on extreme sensation, risk, and the competitive challenge. Some of these sports naturally develop a surrounding youth culture, often hedonistic, reckless, adamantly heterosexual, and fueled by drugs and alcohol. Moreover, participation in the surrounding lifestyle is "connected to notions of cultural commitment and authenticity, identity and belonging" (Thorpe 2012, p. 38). Two such cultures arose from the California surfing scene, both with millions of adherents, massive commercial sponsors and investors, and a place in the Olympics: snowboarding and skateboarding.

Skateboarding now has more than 11 billion participants and supports a multibillion-dollar industry that includes the production of boards, parks, fashion, and music (Montgomery 2009). Skateboarders' search for the next new location is part of the thrill, as boarders seek increasingly improbable territory to practice their skills. Long associated with risk, creativity, rebellion, and freedom from adult rules and constraints, it has also become thoroughly commercialized, institutionalized in skate parks and as a competitive sport in the Olympics. Although the field is dominated by males, female skateboarders have become increasingly active. Sadly, the debut of female skateboarders in the 2020 Olympics was canceled because of the pandemic.

Snowboarding, from a similar lineage but trailing with a mere 70 million boarders worldwide (Thorpe 2012), shares important features with skateboarding: their demographics are almost identical—mostly male, almost exclusively heterosexual, mostly middle- to upper-class, white, and suburban. Snowboarding has had a similar ascent, but unlike skateboarding, snowboarding invaded an existing turf—that is, ski resorts. In recent decades, the growing popularity of snowboarding has shifted the resort culture from an affluent, white, elitist, family-style sensibility to a "drunk and disorderly" party (Howe 1998), also white and elitist, with its own rules and values. The geographic requirement for snow and mountains draws aficionados to resorts and resort towns; these are liminal spaces removed from daily life and responsibilities and peopled by transients, all of which promote disinhibition and anonymity. Moreover, the legalization of marijuana in many ski states has cemented the central role of this drug in this culture, where it is not just an après-snow item but a vital ingredient in facing terrifying challenges and "get[ting] into the groove" (Thorpe 2012, p. 33).

Gay Youth Culture

Gay culture has a long history of political persecution, medical mislabeling, and aggressive oppression in the United States beginning in the 1950s. Steps toward community were galvanized by the Stonewall Riots in 1969. The riots led to the creation of the Pride movement, which was launched by a march marking the anniversary of Stonewall. In the ensuing years, homosexuality was officially pathologized by psychiatric, psychoanalytic, and psychological organizations and then gradually officially destigmatized. In 1979, the first National March on Washington for Lesbian and Gay Rights occurred, which led to the Democratic Party's endorsement of gay rights in its 1980 platform. Very soon afterward, AIDS was identified and mobilized the gay community to seek research, fair pharmaceutical practices, and dissemination of information about AIDS (PBS 2021). These events and many others that followed were instrumental in the progressive lifting of discriminatory laws and practices. Many of these steps arose from the hard-won official recognition of mistreatment, pathologizing, and hardship; however, they also added to the narrative of suffering and overcoming as intrinsic to growing up gay. The series of gay youth suicides in 2010 drew further attention to the plight of gay youths (Waidzunas 2012), which mobilized efforts to understand and ameliorate the suffering of young people; despite some questioning of the validity of statistics concerning gay youth suicides, the recognition of gay youths as an entity may have fostered the creation of a gay youth culture and identification with that culture (Waidzunas 2012). Similarly, beginning in 2010, the It Gets Better Project, in which adult LGBTQ+ spokespeople encouraged youths with the idea of a better future life, positioned gay youths as struggling and provided encouragement to find happiness through adaptation to heteronormative goals. Widespread objections to this skewed view of what makes for happiness led to the abandonment of that project.

The specific hurdles in the internal struggle to accept a profoundly impactful aspect of identity—that is, its relative lack of visibility, its emergence over an extended developmental arc, and the frequent lack of a ready geographically available community—can make this identificatory process challenging and lonely. Depending on their independence and mobility, many youths in nonurban settings can collect cultural capital by visiting urban areas with a gay scene, in order to elaborate an aspect of their identity that lacks the peer support of the usual youth culture (Conner and Okamura 2021). Furthermore, the potential for gay youths to come together, especially given the complexity, geographic dispersion, and diverse circumstances of the gay youth population, has been greatly enhanced by digital communication and platforms.

The internet offers many opportunities for authentic self-representation, for identity enhancement, and for bonding with peers through the circulation of imagery, videos, and written text (Lovelock 2019); these opportunities help consolidate a peer culture without borders. For example, an examination of coming out videos on YouTube (Lovelock 2019) shows how this audiovisual digital medium allows vloggers to express intensely personal feelings about the experience of growing up outside of heteronormative expectations. Although intended for public display, contemporary coming out announcements, both verbal and performative, focus on being yourself and accepting yourself, albeit in the context of potential marginalization. Such videos generate conversations, elicit support, and provide education to other young people.

The geographic isolation in adolescence of nonurban gay youths, simply in terms of access to like-minded individuals, is improved by entry into the college scene or at least temporary relocation to urban settings where gay individuals can meet at bars, connect through apps such as Grindr, unite at pride marches, and benefit from friendship and some degree of exposure to gay culture. But what is gay culture today? Because of the movement toward privileges such as marriage, the co-optation of gay style by the fashion establishment, and "gay news" by corporate operations like NBC Out, it might seem that some of the more subversive aspects of gay culture have been neutralized and normalized. However, the male gay circuit party tradition continues, persisting over objections through the COVID-19 pandemic. Circuit parties, essentially networks of events and eventually nightclubs where a type of house music called "circuit music" was played, were established in the 1980s by Black and Latino men in Detroit, Michigan, and Chicago to create opportunities for solidarity in addition to hookups, drugs, and fun. In the decades since their initiation, circuit parties seem to have become increasingly white and overrun by hypermasculine ideals of beauty and by "body fascism" that exclude those who do not conform to the cut, hypermasculine standard (Conner 2021). Apps offer access to a robust "ParTy and Play" (the capital T refers to the current street name for methamphetamine, Tina) scene in the gay community, wherein sales of drugs, hookups, and parties featuring drugs of choice, especially crystal methamphetamine and methylenedioxymethamphetamine (MDMA; ecstasy), are arranged. The platforms for these arrangements include Grindr and SCRUFF, where emojis and private codes communicate available substances and types of sex. PnP is an app developed to facilitate connections; with instant geo-location capacity, users can connect to nearby individuals or parties of choice. But, according to op-ed contributor David Halperin, gay culture is not merely style, sex, or drugs; it is a "sly and profound critique of what passes for normal" (Halperin 2012). So although the pride marches, dance parties, music fads, diva worship, and drag performances do continue, engaging in gay cultural events is a crucial form of affirmation for youths who have struggled with acceptance and are ready to embrace who they are.

Greek Life

Before considering the serious transgressions and the deleterious effect on other aspects of college life that have become associated with fraternities (and to a lesser extent, sororities), it is important to remember that these organizations remain a valued connection for college students who are members (Biddix et al. 2014). Fraternities differ from most other youth cultures (at least for now) in certain noteworthy ways: they are institutionalized organizations, with written bylaws and covenants, and they have a history in U.S. culture dating back to the eighteenth century, beginning with the founding of Phi Beta Kappa in 1776 at the College of William and Mary. Membership unlocks resources via alumni directories and services that facilitate careers and networking in general. But these organizations also share some features of other youth cultures: they provide a sense of belonging in a period of considerable turmoil as first-year college students leave home and settle into campus life; they require initiation rituals that demand submission and sometimes considerable risk; they are a fount of pleasurable activities and opportunities, often awash with alcohol; and they provide a scaffold for identity formation in a period of exploration. To the degree that there is greater access to participation regardless of race, class, or religion, they offer testing grounds for acquiring "prestige cultural capital on campus by way of leadership programs, social skill building and etiquette dinners" (Arnold and Barratt 2015, p. 189, also quoted by Bureau et al. 2021, p. 88)—the last mentioned a clear indication of the assimilative influence of Greek life.

Fraternities remain a significant part of college life, although they are increasingly criticized by former members, administrators, concerned commentators on student health, and students at large. In addition to their history of deaths by hazing, of drugging and sexual assault, of binge drinking, and of alcohol poisoning, fraternities and sororities have come under fire in the COVID-19 era for being responsible for superspreader events (Stewart 2020). Fraternities are also infamous for perpetuating racist, sexist, and elitist attitudes in their admissions practices in addition to encouraging excessive drinking and sexual aggression. Over the past century, fraternities have faithfully mirrored the history of sexism and racism in their colleges and writ large in the surrounding society (Gillon et al. 2019). Beginning in 1923, fraternities not only practiced racist exclusion in their selection process but also included a bylaw explicitly limiting membership to white men with Christian values (Harris et al. 2019). The effect has been to stimulate the creation of such organizations among women and minority students, with the sense that by doing so, the experience of exclusion, isolation, harassment, and devaluation socially and in the classroom could be alleviated. This compensation has been realized in some cases, for example, by some Black Christian Greek letter societies (see McGuire et al. 2020). However, membership often involves some form of conformity—for example, among people of color for whom participation may require disidentification with intersecting identities, such as in the case of membership in sororities in which one's nonbinary gender expression and queer sexual interests are of necessity negated (Garcia and Duran 2021).

Substances, especially but not exclusively alcohol, are a core part of Greek life. Like some extreme sports, fraternities can also promote an ambient culture of hypermasculinity, misogyny, elitism, and extreme alcohol use. Admission procedures for fraternities, called "hazings," are notorious for exposing inductees to dangerous intoxication, humiliation, abuse, and injury. Media coverage of injuries and deaths has led to the criminalization of hazing in 44 states; nonetheless, hazing continues as an important initiation experience and is generally "normalized" in college life (Allan and Madden 2008). Hazings are "1) coalitional, 2) unidirectional, 3) temporary, and 4) coercive" (Schiffer et al. 2022, p. 1); that is, they are intended to create a bond of membership, coercively inflicted on the applicant by an established member for a discrete period. They have been described as reinforcing traditional masculine norms and serve to sustain "masculine honor beliefs"—the idea that "aggression/violence is necessary and justifiable in response to provocation or in the protection of oneself or others" (Schiffer et al. 2022, p. 2). Clearly, such beliefs, subject to individual interpretation, can promote the toxic masculinity that is associated with aggression and entitlement.

Indeed, despite negative publicity and efforts to reform Greek life on campuses, there is evidence—such as continuing dating violence, cyberdating violence, and high rates of sexual assault on campus—that, like in other youth cultures, approval of risky and even criminal behavior and group promotion of hypermasculine, aggressive attitudes are part of the sensibility of many fraternities. In fact, according to a study published in 2022, one in five women experience a sexual assault in college; sorority members are three times more likely than women who are not in a sorority to experience rape (Emelianchik-Key et al. 2022).

Nevertheless, fraternities and sororities have been found to reduce loneliness in college and improve well-being on campus; in one study, such benefits exceeded those associated with participation in religious organizations (Turton et al. 2018). Moreover, the more active and committed the member, the more benefit is accrued. Interestingly, despite the connection between fraternities and abuses associated with masculinity, the protected homosocial space of fraternities can permit expression of contrasting feelings: greater warmth and intimacy among participants, more vulnerability, and sustained brotherhood. As one member of a Black Christian fraternity described it, "Brotherhood to me is like an active word. It's continuous. You continuously build brotherhood, you continuously do things for your brother" (McGuire et al. 2020, p. 596). Like many other networks, fraternities initiate lasting relationships that can be counted on throughout life.

Technology and Innovation

Although not typically conceptualized as a youth culture per se, the major innovators in the digital world form a kind of kinship and an elite social club and almost exclusively hire emerging adults (people younger than 30 who are mostly white and mostly male). These young technology innovators join techno-corporate campuses that offer high salaries and foster casual, even playful ambiances, setting the stage for camaraderie and the evolution of a culture. In fact, the inhabitants of Silicon Valley refer to it as not a place at all but "an abstraction of the tech industry itself" (Cook 2020, p. 13). LinkedIn founder Reid Hoffman offered the notion that "Silicon Valley is a mindset, not a location" (Cook 2020, p. 13). However, it is no less a location, a sphere of affluence embedded in a geographic area that is increasingly plagued by homelessness and a shrinking middle class.

It is widely understood that the ideals of the early internet innovators have been gradually eroded by commercialization and that participation in its increasingly corporate culture has the potential to corrupt. For example, the 2013 novel *The Circle* (Eggers 2013) portrays a dystopian vision of the corporate technology world wherein an emerging adult woman, age 24, becomes submerged in a dark vision of the future in the hands of a malevolent technology-world giant. She rises to prominence with her vast accumulation of likes in reviews of her customer service. She gradually endorses the intrusive and secretive management. Ironically, the corporate motto is "Secrets are lies," "Sharing is caring," and "Privacy is theft."

However, unlike the other cultures described here, entry into the corporate technology world is a domicile, job, and career, however constrained by the unacknowledged age limit of 30 (Fottrell 2017). Its requirements of work, purpose, and commitment already take it out of many youth cultures' sensibility, although the prominent presence of ideology and ethos is comparable. There are certainly commonalities with college life and even military service.

The Role of Music in Youth Culture and Development

The importance of music in mental life, particularly in adolescent and emerging adult development, has struggled to achieve the recognition it deserves within psychology (Rentfrow and McDonald 2010; for an ardent plea for such recognition, see Miranda 2013). This is despite the historical recognition within psychology, by foundational thinkers such as Maslow (1968), that its power and ability to create peak experience put music on a par with sex. The intersection of favored music with personality type, affect states, affiliations, identity, gender roles, and self-regulation is widely recognized. Youth cultures historically have had recognizable "soundtracks" (Bennett 2009) that are, if not the signature, a critical component of the ethos, recognizable to participants and profoundly evocative. Specific musical forms have been linked to youth culture since the 1950s, and the serial invention of genres over the decades is a dazzling array: rock and roll, psychedelic rock, soul, glam rock, heavy metal, grunge and punk, reggae, rap, electronic dance music, K-pop, and more. Each has extraordinary power to elicit sensory and socioemotional states that evoke group experience. Certain sounds can bring grown-ups back to their own youth (McFerran et al. 2019). Interestingly, the digital age and deejaying have scrambled these diverse forms because remixes and other do-overs blend elements of vastly different genres. According to Bennett (2009), the "eclecticism of contemporary dance music has played its own part in the breakdown of formerly more defined youth cultural affiliations and replaced these with a new individualized musical aesthetic" (p. 266).

Music genres arise organically in relation to youth cultures, fueled by the creative capacities of this age group (Dougherty and Clarke 2018) and propagated by the harnessing of digital media to disseminate and exchange music across the planet. Clearly, the nature of the youth culture colors the choice and evolution of its preferred music. Songs can carry messages, more or less explicit, that vary in focus from romance to outrage, and the music of a given culture is a link to the community. In youth cultures defined by the dedication to causes, such as the civil rights and antiwar movements, hymns of resistance and antiwar folk songs are ready examples of musical genres that carry the group's message. In fact, some commentators, following the theoretical contributions of the Centre for Contemporary Cultural Studies in the United Kingdom (Bennett 2009), have positioned youth music as the "expression of resistance to the hegemonic order of the dominant society" (p. 265). They are referring not only to songs with an explicit message but also to sounds, spectacular and memorable shows, bands, and individual artists who embody the meaning of youth movements.

Substances of Choice

Emerging adulthood is the time in the life course when drug use is highest (Arnett 2005); although Arnett concluded that this peak use is explained by his proposed five features of this age group, it remains unclear how exactly features such as identity exploration and feeling in-between contribute to substance abuse. As described earlier in the subsection "Action, Risk Behaviors, and the Peer Group," a closer correlate is the developmental upsurge in sensation-seeking, resistance to adult constraints, and drive to push boundaries. Youth cultures influence and sustain drug use, offering "taste clusters of values, styles, norms and sensibilities" (Kelly et al. 2013, p. 289) that provide context, the crucial support of the peer group, and accessibility. Some, like nightlife scenes, create opportunities for continuing access to drugs among older emerging adults, sustaining the "social organization of drug use" (Kelly et al. 2013, p. 292). They perpetuate the use of drugs such as ecstasy in rave culture or blunts (marijuana rolled in cigar leaves) in hip-hop culture. The use of prescription drugs can become integrated into other drug use, with more than 50% of participants in electronic dance music, indie rock, certain extreme sports, gay and lesbian parties, and the alternative scene acknowledging their use; different categories of medications (painkillers, stimulants, sedatives/hypnotics) vary from scene to scene.

Some risk behaviors are closely associated with intoxication; for example, some snowboarders rely on weed and prescription drugs to increase their determination to tackle the terrain, and ravers use ecstasy to create the disinhibition and flow for full participation. Substances are used to augment the experience but may simultaneously increase the risk in these and other cultures. Ongoing participation in such scenes can extend risk behavior into the 30s.

Peers and the Adult Project

In addition to the negative effects of promoting risk, substance use, antiestablishment posturing, and criminal behavior, youth cultures provide access to compatible peers who share the same passion and keep up with trends, technology, culture-specific status symbols, and collaborative planning. Such peers are much more up-to-date and knowledgeable about the latest than most older adults (Young et al. 2015). Youth cultures encompass so much diversity that it is difficult to recognize, in each one, the way in which the culture supports developmental momentum.

It is therefore worth emphasizing that there is value in membership in youth cultures; they provide safe contexts for young people who may have never encountered peers who understand them. That is, not only are peers a stimulus and an appreciative audience for risk behaviors, but they can play a more intimate role in identity development beyond the spectacular aspects of their youth culture. These peers can normalize aspects of the self that may have felt shameful or forbidden; they legitimize certain affects, like outrage and desire; and they endow identity components with names and meanings. In addition to supplying a steady stream of like-minded people, youth cultures can promote close relationships by regularly gathering these people in venues of all kinds, from skateboard parks to the forbidden underground spaces, where they share their passion and discuss life: parents, friends, romantic relationships, and useful advice. As each individual progresses through the culture, often accruing expertise and authority, questions of authenticity and trust may arise within the culture (Mason 2018). But there are also discussions about the future and models that show a range of paths forward, some conventional and some extraordinary.

Conclusion

Youth cultures are collections of scenes, tribes, or subcultures that feed the tastes and desires of late adolescents and emerging adults, inspiring devotion and full immersion. They are a source of pleasure and excitement for their participants and are usually accompanied by a sensibility and life attitudes that are distinctive and defining. Whatever their focus, they gradually take on many of the following defining preferences and accoutrements: characteristic attire, substances of choice, favored locations, musical preferences and idealized bands, political affiliations, and actions. Whether it concerns a belief in a social or environmental cause or a dedication to a band or dance party, devotees are affiliated and connected.

Youth culture facilitates several developmental tasks of emerging adulthood. Individuation from the family of origin is supported by this alternative clan, which typically offers a supportive and admiring peer group, a moral code, and an education in real life. Identity exploration is fostered, as are leadership capacities, developing relationships, innovation, creative expression, and emotional investment in a group outside the family—all these and more find expression in various youth cultures. Such cultural commitments may eventually determine what youths wear, where and with whom they hang, what music they love, what substances they favor—choices that come to be defining and often are further refined by a preference for a sport, a type of dancing, a sociopolitical cause, and so on. As participants age, the entire scene may be completely relegated to the past or continued in an attenuated version, as in the case of weekend warriors who visit their scenes on an occasional basis. The effect of a given youth culture on the young men and women who were ardent participants can include nostalgia and pleasurable recollections of their former scene; an ongoing identification with at least some of its aspects, like its music or style; or the discovery of a vocational interest that becomes a lifelong occupation. Most participants acknowledge the enduring imprint of their youth cultures and believe that they have added something indelible to the people they are today.

KEY POINTS

- Youth cultures have extended their reach into the 20s.

- At various points in the progression through emerging adulthood, youth cultures support the development of autonomy, a value system different from childhood teachings, and the sense of belonging often lost when young people step away from their families, traditional cultures, religious observance, and associated childhood identities.

- Despite the high-risk behavior and questionable codes of honor among some youth cultures, these cultures serve as supportive teams in rebellion against childhood constraints, normative traditions, ethical strictures, and adult expectations, thereby promoting identity formation.

- Some youth cultures and derivatives can lead to severe negative outcomes, such as drug addiction, incarceration, destructive aggression, injury to others, or loss of personal legitimacy.

References

Allan EJ, Madden M: Hazing in view: college students at risk: initial findings from the National Study of Student Hazing. Collingdale, PA, Diane Publishing, March 11, 2008. Available at: https://stophazing.org/wp-content/uploads/2020/12/hazing_in_view_study.pdf. Accessed December 1, 2022.

Arnett JJ: Emerging adulthood: a theory of development from the late teens through the twenties. Am Psychol 55(5):469–480, 2000 1084426

Arnett JJ: The developmental context of substance use in emerging adulthood. J Drug Issues 35(2):235–254, 2005

Arnett JJ, Mitra D: Are the features of emerging adulthood developmentally distinctive? A comparison of ages 18–60 in the United States. Emerg Adulthood 8(5):412–419, 2020

Arnold W, Barratt W: First-generation students, in Today's College Students: A Reader. Edited by Sasso P, DeVitis J. New York, Peter Lang Press, 2015, pp 183–200

Bennett A: Spectacular soundtracks: youth and music, in Handbook of Youth and Young Adulthood: New Perspectives and Agendas. Edited by Furlong A. New York, Routledge, 2009, pp 263–268

Best AL, Lynn R: Youth and consumer markets, in Routledge Handbook of Youth and Young Adulthood, 2nd Edition. Edited by Furlong A. New York, Routledge, 2016, pp 244–251

Biddix P, Matney M, Norman E, et al: The influence of fraternity and sorority involvement: a critical analysis of research (1996–2013). ASHE Higher Education Report 39(6):1–156, 2014

Bisafar FI, Welles BF, D'Ignazio C, et al: Supporting youth activists? Strategic use of social media: a qualitative investigation of design opportunities. Proc ACM Hum Comput Interact 4:1–25, 2020

Bowie D: Lyrics to "Changes." Genius. Available at: https://genius.com/David-bowie-changes-lyrics. Accessed December 1, 2022.

Brake M: Preface, in Comparative Youth Culture: The Sociology of Youth Cultures and Youth Subcultures in America, Britain and Canada. New York, Routledge, 1985, pp ix–x

Bromberg U, Wiehler A, Peters J: Episodic future thinking is related to impulsive decision making in healthy adolescents. Child Dev 86(5):1458–1468, 2015 26110500

Buchanan CM, Eccles JS, Becker JB: Are adolescents the victims of raging hormones: evidence for activational effects of hormones on moods and behavior at adolescence. Psychol Bull 111(1):62–107, 1992 1539089

Burch K, Sachs J: Raves vs. music festival: what's the difference? iHeartRaves, June 11, 2021. Available at: https://www.iheartraves.com/pages/rave-vs-music-festival. Accessed May 18, 2023.

Bureau DA, Sasso PA, Barber JP, et al: Contextualizing social class and leadership in fraternity and sorority communities. New Dir Stud Leadersh 169(169):85–92, 2021 33871946

Chein J, Albert D, O'Brien L, et al: Peers increase adolescent risk taking by enhancing activity in the brain's reward circuitry. Dev Sci 14(2):F1–F10, 2011 21499511

Chused JF: Neutrality in the analysis of action-prone adolescents. J Am Psychoanal Assoc 38(3):679–704, 1990 2229881

Ciocan TC: Ludic role of religious rituals: the use of play for religious ceremony. Dialogo 2(1):120–128, 2015

Conner CT: How the gay party scene short-circuited and became a moneymaking bonanza. The Conversation, February 12, 2021. Available at: https://theconversation.com/how-the-gay-party-scene-short-circuited-and-became-a-moneymaking-bonanza-153424. Accessed February 12, 2021.

Conner CT, Okamura D: Queer expectations: an empirical critique of rural LGBT+ narratives. Sexualities 25(8):1–18, 2021

Cook K: The Psychology of Silicon Valley: Ethical Threats and Emotional Unintelligence in the Tech Industry. Cham, Switzerland, Springer Nature, 2020

Dahl RE: Adolescent brain development: a period of vulnerabilities and opportunities. Keynote address. Ann N Y Acad Sci 1021:1–22, 2004 15251869

DiGrazia J: Individual protest participation in the United States: conventional and unconventional activism. Soc Sci Q 95(1):111–131, 2014

Dougherty I, Clarke A: Wired for innovation: valuing the unique innovation abilities of emerging adults. Emerg Adulthood 6(5):358–365, 2018

Eggers D: The Circle. New York, Knopf, 2013

Emelianchik-Key K, Byrd R, Gill CS: Dating violence and the impact of technology: examining the lived experiences of sorority members. Violence Against Women 28(1):73–92, 2022 33827394

Fasick FA: Parents, peers, youth culture and autonomy in adolescence. Adolescence 19(73):143–157, 1984

Fottrell Q: Silicon Valley has an age problem. MarketWatch, September 30, 2017. Available at: https://www.marketwatch.com/story/silicon-valley-has-an-age-problem-2017-09-26. Accessed December 1, 2021.

Galland O: Adolescence, post-adolescence, youth: revised interpretations. Rev Fr Sociol 44(5):163–188, 2003

Garcia CE, Duran A: "In my letters, but I was still by myself": highlighting the experiences of queer men of color in culturally based fraternities. J Divers High Educ 14(2):228–239, 2021

Gardner M, Steinberg L: Peer influence on risk taking, risk preference, and risky decision making in adolescence and adulthood: an experimental study. Dev Psychol 41(4):625–635, 2005 16060809

Gillon KE, Beatty CC, Salinas C Jr: Race and racism in fraternity and sorority life: a historical overview. New Directions for Student Services 2019(165):9–16, 2019

Hale J: Scared straight? Not really. PsychCentral, November 26, 2010. Available at: https://psychcentral.com/blog/scared-straight-not-really#1. Accessed December 1, 2022.

Halperin DM: Normal as folk. The New York Times, June 21, 2012. Available at: https://www.nytimes.com/2012/06/22/opinion/style-and-the-meaning-of-gay-culture.html. Accessed January 3, 2022.

Harris JC, Barone RP, Finch H: The property functions of whiteness within fraternity and sorority culture and its impact on campus. New Directions for Student Services 2019(165):17–27, 2019

Hodkinson P: Youth cultures: a critical outline of key debates, in Youth Cultures: Scenes, Subcultures and Tribes. Edited by Hodkinson P, Deicke W. New York, Routledge, 2007, pp 1–23

Hollenstein T, Lougheed JP: Beyond storm and stress: typicality, transactions, timing, and temperament to account for adolescent change. Am Psychol 68(6):444–454, 2013 23915399

Howe S: (Sick): A Cultural History of Snowboarding. New York, St Martin's Press, 1998

Hunter JD: Wither adulthood? The Hedgehog Review, Spring 2009. Available at: https://hedgehogreview.com/issues/youth-culture/articles/wither-adulthood. Accessed November 30, 2022.

Ingham T: Nearly a third of all streams in the us last year were of hip-hop and R&B artists (as rock beat pop to second most popular streaming genre). Music Business Worldwide, January 7, 2021. Available at: https://www.musicbusinessworldwide.com/nearly-a-third-of-all-streams-in-the-us-last-year-were-of-hip-hop-and-rb-music. Accessed May 8, 2021.

Jenkins TS: Bling, in St. James Encyclopedia of Hip Hop Culture. Edited by Riggs TJ. Farmington Hills, MI, St James Press, 2018, pp 44–47

Jeon KC, Goodson P: US adolescents' friendship networks and health risk behaviors: a systematic review of studies using social network analysis and add health data. PeerJ 3:e1052, 2015 26157622

Kelly BC, Wells BE, Leclair A, et al: Prescription drug misuse among young adults: looking across youth cultures. Drug Alcohol Rev 32(3):288–294, 2013 23190213

Keyzers A, Lee SK, Dworkin J: Peer pressure and substance use in emerging adulthood: a latent profile analysis. Subst Use Misuse 55(10):1716–1723, 2020 32400279

Lamblin M, Murawski C, Whittle S, et al: Social connectedness, mental health and the adolescent brain. Neurosci Biobehav Rev 80:57–68, 2017 28506925

Landmark Recovery: "Just Say No" and its effects. December 3, 2018. Available at: https://landmarkrecovery.com/just-say-no-and-its-effects. Accessed June 11, 2021.

Lave J, Duguid P, Fernandez N, et al: Coming of age in Birmingham: cultural studies and conceptions of subjectivity. Annu Rev Anthropol 21:257–282, 1992

Lil Baby: Lyrics to "The Bigger Picture." Genius. Available at: https://genius.com/Lil-baby-the-bigger-picture-lyrics. Accessed December 1, 2022.

Lockwood S: List of 100 extreme sports (ultimate list for 2022). Extreme Sports Lab, February 3, 2022. Available at: https://www.extremesportslab.com/list-of-100-extreme-sports. Accessed May 1, 2022.

Lovelock M: "My coming out story": lesbian, gay and bisexual youth identities on YouTube. Int J Cult Stud 22(1):70–85, 2019

Maslow AH: Music education and peak experience. Music Educators Journal 54(6):72–75, 163–171, 1968

Mason W: "Swagger": urban youth culture, consumption and social positioning. Sociology 52(6):1117–1133, 2018

McFerran K, Derrington P, Saarikallio S (eds): Handbook of Music, Adolescents, and Wellbeing. New York, Oxford University Press, 2019

McGuire KM, McTier TS Jr, Ikegwuonu E, et al: "Men doing life together": black Christian fraternity men's embodiments of brotherhood. Men Masc 23(3–4):579–599, 2020

McGurk H, Hurry J: Project Charlie: An Evaluation of a Life Skills Drug Education Programme for Primary Schools, Paper 1. London, Great Britain Home Office, 1995

McNulty J: Youth activism is on the rise around the globe, and adults should pay attention, says author. University of California Santa Cruz, September 17, 2019. Available at: https://news.ucsc.edu/2019/09/taft-youth.html. Accessed May 23, 2021.

Meyer M: 33 Must-know streetwear brands in 2023 (established and underground). The VOU, March 24, 2023. Available at: https://thevou.com/fashion/streetwear-brands. Accessed May 18, 2023.

Miranda D: The role of music in adolescent development: much more than the same old song. Int J Adolesc Youth 18(1):5–22, 2013

Montgomery T: The state of the skateboarding industry. Shop-Eat-Surf.com, May 12, 2009. Available at: https://web.archive.org/web/20140812232423/http://www.shop-eat-surf.com/2009/05/the-state-of-the-skateboarding-industry. Accessed April 26, 2021.

Moore R: Sociology of youth culture, in International Encyclopedia of the Social and Behavioral Sciences, 2nd Edition. Edited by Wright JD. Amsterdam, The Netherlands, Elsevier Science, 2015, pp 813–818

Mrug S, Elliott MN, Davies S, et al: Early puberty, negative peer influence, and problem behaviors in adolescent girls. Pediatrics 133(1):7–14, 2014 24324002

Nelly, Wall P, Ali & Gip: Grillz (U.S. 12-inch single vinyl disc). Universal Records, Fo' Reel Entertainment, 2005

Ogbar JOG: Introduction, in St. James Encyclopedia of Hip Hop Culture. Edited by Riggs TJ. Farmington Hills, MI, St James Press, 2018, pp xi–xvi

Olivier S: Moral dilemmas of participation in dangerous leisure activities. Leisure Studies 25(1):95–109, 2006

Oosterhoff B, Wray-Lake L: Risky politics? Associations between adolescent risk preference and political engagement. Child Dev 91(4):e743–e761, 2020

Parsons T: Age and sex in the social structure of the United States. Am Sociol Rev 7(5):604–616, 1942

Patrick ME, Terry-McElrath YM, Lanza ST, et al: Shifting age of peak binge drinking prevalence: historical changes in normative trajectories among young adults aged 18 to 30. Alcohol Clin Exp Res 43(2):287–298, 2019 30645773

PBS: American Experience: milestones in the American gay rights movement. 2021. Available at: https://www.pbs.org/wgbh/americanexperience/features/stonewall-milestones-american-gay-rights-movement. Accessed December 24, 2021.

Petty F: How streetwear became a uniform for progressive youth culture around the world. i-D, March 14, 2019 (originally published in i-D's The Homegrown Issue, No 355, Spring 2019). Available at: https://i-d.vice.com/en/article/7xnj9x/how-streetwear-became-a-uniform-for-progressive-youth-culture-around-the-world. Accessed January 10, 2022.

Pharo H, Sim C, Graham M, et al: Risky business: executive function, personality, and reckless behavior during adolescence and emerging adulthood. Behav Neurosci 125(6):970–978, 2011 22004262

Rajendran M: The development of streetwear and the role of New York City, London, and Supreme NY. Theses and dissertations, Paper 924, Ryerson University, Toronto, ON, Canada, 2012

Rentfrow PJ, McDonald JA: Preference, personality, and emotion, in Handbook of Music and Emotion: Theory, Research, Applications. Edited by Juslin PN, Sloboda JA. New York, Oxford University Press, 2010, pp 669–695

Schiffer AA, Romo-Figueroa J, Lawless TJ, et al: Group bonding or hazing? The effects of masculine honor beliefs on perceptions of undergraduate hazing. Pers Individ Dif 186:1–10, 2022

Schulz KM, Sisk CL: The organizing actions of adolescent gonadal steroid hormones on brain and behavioral development. Neurosci Biobehav Rev 70:148–158, 2016 27497718

Sherman LE, Rosenbaum GM, Smith AR, et al: The interactive effects of peers and alcohol on functional brain connectivity in young adults. Neuroimage 197:264–272, 2019 30978496

Silva J, Silva S, Quinn J: Using hip hop culture and code switching as a way to connect, engage and empower youth, in The Young Are Making Their World: Essays on the Power of Youth Culture. Edited by Kiuchi Y, Villarruel FA. Jefferson, NC, McFarland, 2016, pp 133–156

Sola-Santiago F: Mask on: how fashion erased the politics of streetwear in 2017. CUNY Academic Works, 2017. Available at: https://academicworks.cuny.edu/gj_etds/219. Accessed December 1, 2022.

Steinberg L: A social neuroscience perspective on adolescent risk-taking. Dev Rev 28(1):78–106, 2008 18509515

Steinberg L: A dual systems model of adolescent risk-taking. Dev Psychobiol 52(3):216–224, 2010 20213754

Stewart M: The "Abolish Greek Life" movement calls for an end to toxic fraternity, sorority culture. Insight Into Diversity, September 15, 2020. Available at: https://www.insightintodiversity.com/the-abolish-greek-life-movement-calls-for-an-end-to-toxic-fraternity-sorority-culture. Accessed October 15, 2021.

Sunstein CR: Adolescent risk-taking and social meaning: a commentary. Dev Rev 28(1):145–152, 2008

Thorpe H: "Sex, drugs and snowboarding": (il)legitimate definitions of taste and lifestyle in a physical youth culture. Leisure Studies 31(1):33–51, 2012

Turton GM, Nauta MM, Wesselmann ED, et al: The associations of Greek and religious organization participation with college students' social well-being and purpose. J Psychol 152(4):179–198, 2018 29522382

Vetter-O'Hagen CS, Spear LP: Hormonal and physical markers of puberty and their relationship to adolescent-typical novelty-directed behavior. Dev Psychobiol 54(5):523–535, 2012 21953609

Vijayakumar N, Op de Macks Z, Shirtcliff EA, et al: Puberty and the human brain: insights into adolescent development. Neurosci Biobehav Rev 92:417–436, 2018 29972766

Waidzunas T: Young, gay, and suicidal: dynamic nominalism and the process of defining a social problem with statistics. Science, Technology, and Human Values 37(2):199–225, 2012

Young RA, Marshall SK, Wilson LJ, et al: Transition to adulthood as a peer project. Emerg Adulthood 3(3):166–178, 2015

PART IV
Mental Health in Emerging Adulthood

7

Psychopathology and Emerging Adulthood

Emerging adulthood marks a period of enormous psychological growth as well as peak vulnerability to mental health problems. This phase coincides with the first episodes of serious illnesses, such as bipolar and psychotic spectrum conditions, as well as with initial diagnoses of personality disorders; moreover, it encompasses the years when preexisting, subthreshold levels of depression, anxiety, or substance abuse trend toward increased severity (Burt and Paysnick 2012; Powers and Casey 2015; Reed-Fitzke et al. 2021). Indeed, overall rates of psychiatric disorders among those ages 18–29 years are significantly elevated: in the United States, for example, the 12-month prevalence of anxiety, depression, and substance abuse within this cohort is estimated at around 40%, higher than for any other age group (Arnett et al. 2014).

These uniquely high rates of psychopathology reflect the interface of a young person's neurobiology, heredity, and psychosocial history with the novel pressures and challenges of emerging adult life. For many in their late teens and 20s, the emerging adulthood phase facilitates a sense of freedom and a process of self-discovery, along with the satisfaction and confidence that accompany making one's own decisions, finding new social connections, and exploring identities that were perhaps not validated within the family system. However, more vulnerable young people, newly immersed in a less structured and less parent-directed lifestyle, may struggle during this prolonged phase of instability and flux, buffeted by upheavals in living situations, shifting social roles, and potentially risky situations. The prospect of self-exploration and the sense of future possibilities may promote anxiety and uncertainty rather than optimism, along with feelings of inadequacy in the face of novel challenges (Schulenberg and Zarrett 2006; Werner et al. 2020). Importantly, adaptation to this phase, whether favorable or more problematic, serves as a springboard for the young person's subsequent transition into adulthood and sets the stage for future personal habits, emotional and behavioral regulation, occupational functioning, and capacities for caring and caregiving relationships.

Successful adjustment to the developmental tasks and challenges of emerging adulthood requires the strengthening and cohesion of a wide range of cognitive, emotional, relational, and autonomous superego capacities, including planning and organizing personal behavior, modulating affective reactions, deferring gratification, balancing self-interest with others' needs, and maintaining stable self-esteem in the face of conflict and uncertainty. Ongoing maturation of these foundational abilities requires experience out in the world and sufficient energy, optimism, and motivation to engage in the following: managing the routines of everyday life; attaining increasingly realistic appraisals of self and others; preserving rational judgments in the face of emotionally laden situations; conducting diverse relationships and handling interpersonal dilemmas with friends, sexual partners, coworkers, bosses, and mentors; deepening romantic connections; and envisioning and planning for future goals (Burt and Paysnick 2012; Conley et al. 2014; Eichler 2011; Ritvo 1971). When emerging adults are subject to internal and external emotional pressures (distress over personal circumstances, affective instability, excessive anxiety), immersion in and adaptation to social, academic, and occupational life are impeded, which potentially increases their susceptibility to maladaptive defensive patterns (e.g., avoidance), reliance on substances, and other risks (such as self-harm). A few examples of vulnerable individuals include the 18-year-old college student whose debilitating anxiety makes it impossible to respond to social overtures, which leads to increasingly avoidant and isolating behaviors; the overreactive, easily frustrated young employee who enters into frequent conflicts with coworkers and supervisors; and the 20-something with a history of alcohol use whose binge drinking and subsequent out-of-control behavior have begun to create problems with friends, have led to a few encounters with the legal system, and have started to interfere with next-day functioning in graduate school and on the job.

The ongoing process of identity exploration creates its own set of unique developmental challenges; as diverse roles, values, and interests are pursued, experienced, and reconsidered, normative levels of identity distress often lead to worries and preoccupations over decisions and commitments (Palmeroni et al. 2020). Tolerating the vagaries of identity exploration requires flexible responsiveness, a stable and essentially positive self-concept, and a hopeful outlook as the emerging adult encounters novelty, ambiguity, and inevitable frustration. Young people who are actively processing minority identities in the arenas of gender, sexuality, race, and ethnicity often experience heightened levels of stress; additional pressures may arise externally (embedded systems of power and discrimination, harassment by others) as well as internally (painful expectations of rejection and prejudice, hypervigilance in the face of uncertain social reactions) as societal messages and interpersonal encounters interface with the individual's evolving feelings and beliefs about the self (Borgogna et al. 2019; Meyer 2003).

The phase-defining in-between status of emerging adults (Arnett 2000) applies not only to their perceived position between adolescence and adulthood but also to their relationship with mental health services. These young individuals have transitioned out of regular pediatric medical care (which was frequently arranged by their parents) and now make their own decisions about seeking professional help. However, many lack access to treatment as well as the motivation, insight, and experience to know when therapeutic services are needed. Because mood and other disorders may emerge for the first time during this developmental period, emerging adults are often just figuring out what their symptoms mean (e.g., realizing that one is not just sad but sinking into a depressive episode) and how to attend to changes in their outlook and behavior. As a result, despite exceedingly high levels of psychiatric problems, emerging adults are less likely than either younger or older cohorts to receive treatment; in addition, treatment retention and outcomes are often poor, partly because of providers' lack of understanding of the unique developmental needs of this age group (Adams et al. 2014; Arnett et al. 2014; Goodman et al. 2016). In Chapter 8 ("Therapeutic Modalities in the Treatment of Emerging Adults"), we discuss in greater detail the various psychotherapeutic approaches to working with emerging adults.

It is important to note that much of the available data on the mental health needs and treatment-seeking behaviors of the emerging adulthood cohort are based on studies of college populations, who are relatively easy for researchers to find, gather information from, and administer measures to in large numbers. This means that far less is known about the large percentage of emerging adults who never attend or soon leave postsecondary school and also that the trends for older 20-somethings are not well represented by the research.

Developmental Framework for the Psychopathology of Emerging Adulthood

Our approach to the disorders of this age group draws from contemporary psychoanalytic developmental theory as well as from the field of developmental psychopathology. These dual perspectives share the following central principles:

- An emphasis on integrating information from neighboring fields in order to understand the emergence or intensification of symptoms and disorders rather than relying solely on a biological, behavioral, social, or psychodynamic model.
- A focus on the ways in which particular age groups tend to organize their experience, make meaning of events and interactions, and develop patterns of defense and adaptation in the face of novel stressors and transitions. When the young person is functioning well, such patterns promote flexible negotiation of developmentally salient issues. For emerging adults, positive adaptations facilitate autonomous functioning, engagement in identity explorations, and deepening intimate relationships.
- A broad perspective that positions psychopathology in a developmental context in which evolving ego capacities, individual strengths and vulnerabilities, and age-salient demands are seen as intertwined with multiple other systems (such as parent-child bonds, community environments, larger social systems of power and privilege). As psychodynamic clinicians, we are particularly alert to the young person's ego and superego functions, relational patterns, and unconscious fantasies about the self and others. The interactions among these multiple systems of personality, environment, and development create nonlinear pathways and sometimes unpredictable outcomes.
- A complex view of *developmental cascades*, or longitudinal pathways, through which earlier experiences and resolutions—whether adaptive or more problematic—potentially spill over into subsequent phases. Although early relational experience, in particular the parent-infant bond, powerfully affects the evolving personality, we see all phases of development—including emerging adulthood itself—as making a unique contribution to both current and subsequent mental health functioning (Carlson et al. 2009; Cicchetti and Rogosch 2002; Gilmore and Meersand 2014; Malone et al. 2018).

This developmental framework allows us to achieve a broad view of emerging adulthood psychopathology that encompasses cases in which long-standing vulnerabilities are newly amplified (e.g., someone with a history of early separation anxiety and latency-age school phobias who experiences intense anxiety during the transition to college) as well as cases that involve the unexpected emergence of new symptoms and problems in the context of novel challenges (e.g., a previously well-functioning 20-something who struggles with feelings of isolation, loneliness, and ultimately clinical depression after graduating college, moving to a new city, and beginning a first full-time job). In addition, these principles support a complex view of earlier experience as shaping but not necessarily predicting later health or pathology. Although early relational trauma, such as maltreatment, is uniquely disruptive to childhood psychological health, such potentially derailing adversities may be moderated during subsequent periods of development; positive proximal influences and opportunities, and the emergence of new skills and capacities, can serve to recalibrate risk and promote favorable outcomes (Carlson et al. 2009; Negriff 2021). Connection with peers, the support of mentoring figures, perceived success and mastery, and personal resiliency factors—such as reflective capacities, which help the individual gain perspective and regulate intense emotions—all contribute to psychological well-being and the mitigation of negative experience (Borelli et al. 2015; Manago et al. 2012; Smith et al. 2022). Increasingly, mental illnesses and their etiologies are conceptualized within frameworks that emphasize multidetermined risk factors; multiple and nonlinear pathways toward both psychopathology and health; and complicated interactions among an individual's qualities, unique life experiences, and gene expression. For example, when applied to the most severe forms of psychopathology, such as schizophrenia, the developmental approach looks at the way in which genetics, prenatal and natal factors, the social environment, adolescent and young adult drug use, and the toll of exposure to trauma or ongoing high levels of stress may affect the emergence and course of illness (Hastings et al. 2020; Leebens and Williamson 2017; Marenco and Weinberger 2000).

Although the emerging adult period exposes the young individual to unfamiliar pressures, it also offers unique prospects for experiencing the self in new ways and reworking earlier conflicts, potentially transforming prior modes of relating and defense. Such opportunities may include developing connections with teachers and friends that elicit different aspects of self- and self-with-other experience; embodying and receiving validation for roles that are key to personal identity; discovering and pursuing interests that align with personal strengths and talents and contribute to a sense of purpose and meaning; or developing reciprocal, intimate relationships with loving and supportive feelings that expand one's capacity for empathy, sense of connection, and overall contentment.

The following vignette illustrates a developmental pathway in which a young woman's long-standing mood vulnerabilities and mild social inhibitions are moderated by positive, affirming college experiences. Novel interpersonal and intellectual opportunities, in combination with her own motivation and existing ego strengths, help open up new adaptations to personal difficulties.

Case Vignette: Sarah

As a young child, Sarah had occasionally severe separation anxiety; her refusal to go on school trips or attend drop-off events (including playdates at the homes of familiar families) and her mounting nighttime fears led her parents to seek twice-per-week play therapy for her at age 7. Her mother, who had her own lengthy history of anxiety, with prominent psychosomatic symptoms, frequently worried aloud about both her own and Sarah's health, sleep, and eating. The combination of professional support, the parents' commitment to understanding Sarah's needs, and Sarah's essentially solid developmental capacities contributed to favorable progression: by age 9, Sarah was happily attending playdates without distress, participating in group activities, and sleeping through the night in her own room. She performed well academically and got along with her classmates. Sarah's parents noticed that she still requested not to enroll in more than one after-school class per week, needed reassurance before sleepovers at others' homes, occasionally asked to leave parties after a couple of hours, and tended toward seeking the company of only one or two friends, but these preferences seemed manageable and consistent with their understanding of Sarah's naturally shy and anxious temperament.

Following her mother's brief hospitalization for pneumonia when Sarah was 11, Sarah's symptoms reemerged in the form of school refusal and mounting catastrophic thinking whenever her parents' whereabouts were unknown. Her teachers were surprised by the resistance to school, because Sarah was an excellent student who seemed to enjoy engaging in structured tasks and acquiring new skills; at the same time, they recognized that she depended primarily on one or two classmates for socialization and sometimes needed encouragement to participate in class discussions. A 6-month course of renewed therapy (with the same social worker she had seen from ages 7 to 9), coordination with the counselor at school, and parent work restored normal school attendance and helped Sarah avoid tearful reactions and repetitive calls to her mother if she arrived home from work events later than expected. Some mild anxiety symptoms continued (she needed extra parent phone calls during sleepaway camp and sometimes called home from a sleepover with friends), but Sarah and her family enjoyed a relatively calm period of academic and social engagement for the duration of the late elementary and middle school years.

Another intensification of anxiety began during high school, at age 15, as Sarah grew increasingly preoccupied with her school performance and her popularity, despite doing well in her classes and possessing a solid if small circle of friends. This coincided with a period of low mood that appeared to follow her best friend's move to another town; although it was still possible to visit, they were no longer in the same school, and this was an interruption to Sarah's beloved routines, which involved meeting in the morning before school, eating lunch together, and often taking the same bus home. Irritability with her parents and a slight withdrawal from social activities, as well as problems with sleep and concentration, were the major manifestations of what her mother increasingly recognized as a depressive episode. Sarah reluctantly agreed to return to her therapist, who recommended referral to a colleague for a medication evaluation. After a few months of talk therapy and antidepressant treatment, her depressive and anxiety symptoms gradually decreased, but Sarah remained somewhat less engaged in extracurricular endeavors. As the time for college applications approached, her parents anxiously consulted Sarah's therapist, wondering if their daughter was just not ready to leave home: should they investigate gap-year options or encourage her to enroll only in local schools? However, Sarah herself did not want to wait or live at home when most of her friends were attending out-of-town schools. Ultimately, the family settled on a small liberal arts school located about a 3-hour drive from home. Sarah agreed to continue her medication and to see her psychiatrist during trips home, to have online sessions with her therapist, and to reach out to her college's student mental health service if necessary.

Initially, when she arrived on campus, Sarah called home almost every day; she liked her roommate and her classes but had trouble sleeping and felt anxious and homesick much of the time. Concerned about appearing clingy or needy in the eyes of her roommate, she ended up eating many meals alone and feeling sad and isolated. She was in frequent contact with her best friends from high school, both of whom were attending other schools and appeared to be having easier transitions than she was; their social media postings reflected what looked like parties and various outings with new people, which caused Sarah to feel even more alone. Her parents, worried about her mood, pushed for her to establish in-person therapy with Student Health. Sarah was reluctant to seek a new relationship but increased the regularity of her online sessions, which helped her verbalize her ruminations and revisit some of the strategies she had used in the past.

Sarah pushed herself to make a few attempts at friendly behaviors, such as leaving the door to her dorm room ajar, sitting in the common area at the end of the hallway, and making at least one comment to people sitting next to her in class. A classmate responded by inviting Sarah to grab coffee, and they started spending some time together after lectures; one Friday evening, she and this new friend had fun creating a profile for Sarah on a dating website that many of the students were using. In addition, Sarah's roommate, a quiet and studious but social young woman who knew several of the people at school and had already joined a few clubs, occasionally invited Sarah to meals with her friends; ultimately, one of these friends convinced Sarah to join the campus's environmental awareness group.

Near the end of the first year, Sarah was thrilled to be asked by her favorite sociology professor to serve as a research assistant; she enjoyed in particular the planning meetings, held at a campus café, where her professor and five other students brainstormed about current findings and the next year's projects and talked about a range of topics, both personal and political. These students formed a small, tight-knit group and soon began meeting on their own, with plans to continue when the fall semester started. In addition, Sarah began to feel that her diverse academic and social interests were coming together; she and the professor had met separately to talk about ways in which she could integrate studies on social groups and environmental issues; she registered for a couple of relevant classes for the following year and began to envision an independent study project. She was nervous but excited about the possibility of studying abroad during junior year, perhaps selecting a program that one of the five older students had suggested, which would allow her to see how another country addressed climate concerns; this student, who would be entering his senior year in the fall, felt like both a friend and a somewhat older mentor. By the time the summer arrived, Sarah had secured a part-time job at home but also had multiple visits planned with her new friends.

Despite an array of ego strengths and interpersonal capacities, this young woman's long-standing struggles with anxiety—along with a period of depression in adolescence—mark vulnerabilities that could potentially interfere with her adjustment to college life: she has significant homesickness, feels nervous about making friends, worries about being perceived by her roommate as clingy, and is certain that her high school companions are enjoying greater levels of social success. In childhood, Sarah's separation fears, which are inevitably interwoven with her mother's own deep-seated separation anxieties, curtailed her full immersion in age-appropriate social interactions, such as playdates and sleepovers; negative and missed social experience contributes to Sarah never fully mastering the stress of novel social situations or group gatherings, and she tends increasingly toward avoidance in order to eschew inner tensions. At the same time, protective factors include her supportive family, a therapist, and helpful educators who are all happy to work together to soften her social fears and resolve a transient period of school refusal. In combination with Sarah's internal capacities and motivations for social connection and academic achievement, these resources ultimately yield a successful adaptation to the demands of the grade school years. Nonetheless, her inherent strengths and learned strategies do not inoculate Sarah from a typical course of worsening anxiety and depression during adolescence, exacerbated by the loss of a friendship on which she depends heavily.

Sarah's initial college adjustment is slow; she leans on behavioral coping mechanisms that she has used before to deal with social avoidance and anxiety—using problem-solving measures, taking small steps, reframing the way she is thinking about a seemingly overwhelming situation. Her affinity for academics brings positive recognition but also ushers her into a small social circle that is ideally suited to her temperament; in addition, the serendipitous presence of a roommate who is kind, studious, and more outgoing than Sarah and who is happy to share her circle of friends provides a foundation of social experience and leads to a couple of independent friendships. These peer bonds, along with a set of intellectual and extracurricular interests (sociology, environmental awareness), provide a framework for Sarah's second year on campus; she completes her first year looking ahead with significantly greater confidence and sense of belonging.

Anxiety and Depression

The prevalence of anxiety and depression, sometimes referred to as *internalizing disorders*, is strikingly high in college-age populations: multinational studies suggest that almost 20% of students have symptoms that meet past 12-month diagnostic criteria for major depressive disorder, and 16.7% have symptoms that meet criteria for generalized anxiety disorder; females have two to three times greater vulnerability to mood disorders than their male counterparts (Duffy et al. 2019; Essau et al. 2018). Indeed, college cohorts report higher levels of low mood, anxiety, and overall psychological distress than any other group in the general population, a concern that is exacerbated by the gap between the need for and the seeking of mental health services (Duffy et al. 2019; Stallman and Shocket 2009). In one large survey of university populations, in which students were asked about their overall sense of emotional well-being or distress in the preceding year, about 30% of the respondents endorsed finding intimate or family relationships "very difficult to handle," 21% reported overwhelming anxiety, just under 20% described feeling so depressed that it was difficult to function, and around 9% acknowledged considering suicide (American College Health Association 2019). In particular, the initial adjustment to the first semester at college marks a period of sharp decline in mental health (Bayram and Bilgel 2008).

A recent surge in rates of depression among university students, coinciding with the onset of the SARS-CoV-2 disease (COVID-19) pandemic, is hypothesized to reflect the following: loss of routines and social opportunities, the sense of having missed major precollege life transitional events (e.g., high school graduations, proms), and the additional stress of being laid off from one's job or of working under COVID-19 conditions among those with both student and essential worker status (Halliburton et al. 2021). LGBTQ+ students reported uniquely elevated levels of depression, anxiety, and general distress during the pandemic; some of these emerging adults were forced back into living situations with unsupportive families and cut off from their usual sources of companionship, such as campus-based friends and organizations (Halliburton et al. 2021).

Rates of depression begin a linear ascent during adolescence and continue to rise during the early years of emerging adulthood (Conway et al. 2017; Prenoveau et al. 2011; Villarroel and Terlizzi 2020). Certain anxiety disorders (separation anxiety, specific phobia) have an earlier onset, often making a first appearance during childhood (Essau et al. 2018). Although substantial research identifies the genetic variables, familial conditions, and early experiences that contribute to later mood and anxiety problems, less is known about the proximal factors that increase risk during emerging adulthood (Gutman and Sameroff 2004). Chronic interpersonal stress, childhood adversity, and both recent and more enduring negative life events are significant predictors of major depressive episodes; these factors may include a wide range of relational and environmental conditions, such as early trauma and adversity, ongoing parent-child conflict, overall lack of family support, social isolation, upheavals in personal circumstances, and recent relational losses and conflicts (Vacek and Whisman 2021; Vrshek-Schallhorn et al. 2015). Social interactions that involve perceived rejection or humiliation may be uniquely impactful in precipitating a depressive reaction (Vrshek-Schallhorn et al. 2015).

The high rate of both concurrent and sequential comorbidity of anxiety and depression is widely documented and is thought to reflect commonalities in both underlying biological mechanisms and symptom patterns; some studies suggest that as many as half of the patients with major depression also have symptoms that meet criteria for an anxiety disorder (Kessler et al. 2003). The prevalence of co-occurrence is especially concerning because having more than one condition increases an individual's risk for impaired functioning and self-harm. Both depression and anxiety pose significant, overlapping threats of interference in daily life from negative and disturbing thoughts, painful affects, changes in behaviors, and a range of physiological symptoms. However, mood and anxiety disorders represent distinct entities in certain ways: for example, whereas anxiety typically includes uncomfortable physiological arousal, along with preoccupation and anticipatory worry about what is to come, central features of depression are low levels of positive affect, a general loss of pleasure and motivation, and ruminations about perceived personal shortcomings and failures in the past (Heller et al. 2019).

Even relatively mild levels of depression and anxiety can significantly impede the emerging adult's ability to navigate social, academic, and work-related challenges: lowered mood, negative thoughts and feelings about the self, and worries and anxious ruminations create serious obstacles to autonomous functioning. Anhedonia, a foundational criterion of major depressive disorder, represents a qualitative change in motivation and enjoyment and a loss of the optimism and energy that are required to pursue novel interests and engage in social exploration. The phase-salient tasks of emerging adulthood—creating new friendships, mentorships, and romantic ties; independently managing demands and expectations at work and school; and engaging in self-discovery within multiple identity domains—require tolerance for uncertainty, sustained effort, and self-regulation, as well as at least a modicum of positive belief in the self and one's future potential. Ultimately, mood and anxiety symptoms and manifestations contribute to isolation, withdrawal, and avoidance and raise the risk of additional psychosocial problems, such as the use of substances (Gutman and Sameroff 2004). Derailments during this crucial developmental period disrupt the identity process and deprive the emerging adult of needed experience and competencies, potentially contributing to long-standing problems that extend into later established adulthood (Schulenberg et al. 2004). Moreover, rates of recurrence for depression and anxiety are high: although first adolescent major depressive episodes generally remit within 1–2 years, the rate of relapse within 5 years is almost 50% (Melvin et al. 2013); similarly, the presence of an anxiety disorder during adolescence marks a two- to threefold greater risk for anxiety during the emerging adulthood years (Essau et al. 2018).

Suicidality and Nonsuicidal Self-Injury

Suicide is the second leading cause of death for those in the 15- to 24-year age group; in a disturbing trend, rates of suicide within this cohort rose by more than 30% between the years 2000 and 2017 (Curtin and Heron 2019). Self-reports from college students indicate that almost a quarter endorse having experienced some form of suicidal feeling, and about 6%–9% assert that they have made a specific plan to end their lives (American College Health Association 2019; Mortier et al. 2018). Although the prevalence of ideation and attempts appears to peak in middle adolescence, the rate of suicide mortality rises in the early emerging adulthood phase, which suggests that the transition out of the teen years marks a time of particular vulnerability (Geoffroy et al. 2021).

Broad definitions of suicidal thinking and behavior include a range from more passive thoughts and feelings to actions designed to bring about harm: they encompass ruminations about death in general or about one's own demise in specific; the presence of suicidal thoughts, feelings, and actions; vague wishes to disappear; more specific plans for bringing about one's death; the stopping of treatments that are crucial for one's physical and mental health; and engagement in behaviors known to carry high levels of risk. A history of attempts and hospitalizations forms a particularly concerning backdrop to these various manifestations. Although suicidal thinking is typically conceptualized as verbal planning and ruminating, visual imagery about self-harm may represent an even more dangerous form of ideation (Lawrence et al. 2021). An extensive body of research has attempted to elucidate these factors, assess their correlates with other psychological conditions and variables in young people's lives, and ultimately address the pressing issue of identifying those at greatest risk. The following serves as a summary of current findings most relevant to the emerging adulthood phase.

Suicidality overlaps with some psychiatric conditions that are known to arise or intensify during the late teens and 20s. A diagnosis of major depressive disorder marks a potent risk factor; one study estimates that 5%–10% of adolescents who experience a first major episode are likely to die from suicide within 15 years (Weissman et al. 1999). Bipolar disorder (discussed further in the section "Schizophrenia and Bipolar Disorders" later in this chapter) is associated with a seriously increased level of risk, particularly during depressive episodes that occur early in the onset of the illness (Miller and Black 2020). Comorbid alcohol abuse substantially raises the likelihood of both ideation and attempts; the well-established link between alcohol use and suicidal behavior in college populations is hypothesized to reflect the following tendencies: the use of drinking as a coping mechanism for managing depression and negative affects, an underlying avoidant style of coping with distress, impulsivity, and poor problem-solving skills that increase the effect of complex social situations and stressors (Gonzalez 2019).

However, those who die from suicide are just as likely not to have symptoms that meet criteria for a diagnosable mental health condition, which has led researchers to elucidate a further range of stressful circumstances and psychological, familial, and historical correlates. Some of the known proximal factors that contribute to a young individual's risk include being hopeless about the future; experiencing the self as a burden to others; feeling a lack of belonging and loneliness; and feeling overwhelmed, defeated, or trapped vis-à-vis circumstances that are perceived as stressful and humiliating (O'Connor and Nock 2014; Rohde et al. 2013). Other variables include early childhood trauma and adversity, a history of exposure to someone else's suicide, a chronic tendency toward personal perfectionism and harsh self-criticism, and the presence of bodily illness (O'Connor and Nock 2014; Rohde et al. 2013). Although approximately 30% of young people who show suicidal thinking and nonsuicidal self-harm progress to making serious suicide attempts, preidentifying the individuals who make up this third is extremely difficult (Mars et al. 2019a). One major study suggested that although the presence of depression and other psychiatric disorders, along with a tendency toward impulsivity, is associated with the development of suicidal thoughts and with acts of nonsuicidal self-harm, it is not necessarily predictive of the transition to serious attempts; these researchers propose that the transition to serious attempts is correlated with a history of nonsuicidal self-harm, the use of cannabis and other drugs (perhaps via a pathway of lowered inhibitions, via impairments to judgment, or as a reflection of a maladaptive coping style), and exposure to suicide in friends or family (Mars et al. 2019a, 2019b).

A meta-review of adolescent and emerging adult suicidality found stark distinctions by gender. Although females are almost twice as likely to attempt suicide, males have a nearly threefold higher risk of death; hypotheses about these differences include the notion that females may be more likely to make use of help and verbal outlets for emotional pain (via friends, family, or professionals), whereas their male counterparts tend to attach stigma and shame to help-seeking behaviors (Miranda-Mendizabal et al. 2019). A systematic review of available research identified the major risk factors for suicide attempts, for both genders, as comprising the following: previous suicide attempts, a history of major depression or an anxiety disorder, childhood maltreatment, the experience of having been bullied, mental illness or substance abuse within the family, and a family history of suicidal behavior (Miranda-Mendizabal et al. 2019).

Emerging adults who are negotiating minority identities have even higher than usual vulnerability to suicidality. Research on transgender and other gender-diverse youths has reported rates of suicidal thinking and behavior as high as triple those of their age-mates; moreover, retrospective studies have reported a lifetime prevalence of suicidal thoughts as high as 50% and a lifetime prevalence of suicidal behaviors of 30% (Perez-Brumer et al. 2017; Vaughan 2018). Within ethnically diverse samples of emerging adults ages 18–25 years, discrimination and acculturation stresses are found to be predictive of suicide attempts; acculturation-related pressures may include perceived demands for assimilation in the social environment as well as the need to manage family expectations for maintaining values, customs, and practices that differ from one's own evolving desires and beliefs (Gomez et al. 2011; Polanco-Roman and Miranda 2013). Evidence indicates that strong ethnic identifications may protect against suicidality (e.g., Polanco-Roman and Miranda 2013), perhaps by providing the young individual with a sense of meaning and belonging and mitigating feelings of hopelessness. Cross (1995) suggested that discrete experiences of discrimination and racism may actually trigger and strengthen racial identity, because they lead the young individual to erect strong defenses and adaptive reactions to societal pressures.

Despite the extensive research on topics associated with suicidality, the ability to make predictions about who within the emerging adult cohort is at greatest danger remains elusive. Many writers propose that the risk for suicide is highest when a combination of risk factors intersects with the young person's here-and-now capability and the physical means to commit serious self-harm; when an individual is subject to recent disturbing events that increase tolerance for pain and death, suicide may feel more possible, especially in the face of a plan that can be actualized (Mars et al. 2019b; Stewart et al. 2017). An interpersonal theory of suicide that uses a desire-capability framework posits perceived burdensomeness and low belongingness as potent risk factors that create suicidal desire but suggests that the capability to act out lethal self-harm is acquired over time, in response to a cascade of painful events (Van Orden et al. 2010). A motivational-volitional framework emphasizes the role of immediate access to lethal methodologies in the completion of suicide (O'Connor 2011).

Nonsuicidal self-harm represents a distinct but related set of behaviors. Although these intentional acts of aggression (cutting, scratching, burning) against the body are generally distinguished by their lack of suicidal intent, self-harming behavior is associated with higher rates of suicidal ideation and suicide attempts; these correlations are particularly concerning because among postsecondary school students, the prevalence of nonsuicidal self-injury is as high as 20% (Boyne and Hamza 2022; Mars et al. 2019a, 2019b). Psychological predisposition to self-harm includes intense and poorly mitigated levels of shame, a tendency toward self-criticism, and intolerance of one's mistakes and failures; these represent especially problematic vulnerabilities during the inevitable trials, experimentations, and novel situations of the emerging adulthood period, when confronting personal missteps and flaws and discovering relative strengths and weaknesses mark an ongoing, universal experience (Mahtani et al. 2017). More proximal precipitants of self-injury often involve incidents of interpersonal stress, such as conflicts or rejections, that lead to escalating emotional dysregulation (Boyne and Hamza 2022). Several studies have suggested that young people recruit self-harming behaviors to act as a form of self-punishment that is perceived as deserved and to relieve and modulate powerful inner tensions and affects; during times of internal pressure, there may be repetitive, intrusive thoughts and intense urges to engage in self-injury (Boyne and Hamza 2022; Mahtani et al. 2017).

Alcohol and Substance Use

Rates of drug and alcohol use are marked by clear age-related patterns: prevalence begins to rise during adolescence, peaks in emerging adulthood, and starts to decline during the late 20s (Haller et al. 2010; Lynne-Landsman et al. 2010; Schulenberg et al. 2021). The normative trend toward decreasing use, beginning in the latter years of emerging adulthood, is sometimes referred to as the *maturing out* of substance-related behaviors and has been linked to improvements in self-regulation, increases in the stability of lifestyle, and incremental changes toward more intimate and committed relationships (Edgerton and Read 2018).

The typically high rates of both drinking and drug use during emerging adulthood can mask more pathological substance-related patterns and make it difficult to differentiate between those on a normative and those on a more problematic trajectory. Differentiating between typical use and disorder hinges on the extent to which an individual's overall functioning in major realms of life (social relationships, academic performance, occupational settings) is impaired, coupled with an inability to modify drug and alcohol behavior in the face of damaging consequences. Loss of friendships or romantic connections, deterioration in school performance, or getting fired from jobs can represent clear outward signs of interference from fre-

quent hangovers that impede next-day productivity, inappropriate and dis-
inhibited interpersonal behavior, and failure to complete tasks and fulfill
responsibilities. Such distinctions, however, are more straightforward in
the adult population, in which roles and responsibilities are more visible
and clear-cut; the ubiquity of alcohol and substance use among groups of
emerging adults, such as those in college who are frequently seen as just
partying, can lead to confusion around diagnosing the presence of an actual
disorder.

Overall drug use among emerging adults appears to have spiked during
the COVID-19 pandemic: in 2020, as many as 42% reported the use of marijuana within the past 12 months, with around 10% endorsing daily use; 19%
acknowledged past 12-month illicit drug use, with 4.5% for methylenedioxymethamphetamine (MDMA; ecstasy; Molly), 7.6% for hallucinogens,
and 6.8% for cocaine (Schulenberg et al. 2021). Frequent use of illicit stimulants is highly correlated with heavy episodic drinking, the use of additional
drugs, depression, and sleep problems; rates of use of these substances, as well
as diversion of prescribed stimulants, represent a serious problem among
emerging adults, both on and off college campuses (Tzilos et al. 2016). Although non-college-attending youths use illegal substances at slightly higher
rates than college students, more incidents of drinking occur on campus: approximately two-thirds of students report drinking alcohol during their current semester, and about half report heavy episodic drinking, a pattern of use
that is known to impede school performance and retention (Liguori and
Lonbaken 2015). Elevated drinking habits are not limited to undergraduates: a national survey of medical students found that almost one-third of
respondents had symptoms that met criteria for alcohol use or dependence;
a feeling of burnout, depression, and perceived poor psychological health
are highly correlated with elevated drinking (Jackson et al. 2016).

The role of the college environment in facilitating alcohol use is well
illustrated by the apparent decline in alcohol use among this population
during the COVID-19 pandemic, when many students were forced off
campus (Schulenberg et al. 2021). High rates of binge drinking—the consumption of enough alcohol within a 2-hour period to achieve a blood
alcohol concentration of 0.08 g/dL, which is typically achieved after five
drinks for men and four for women—among college populations are particularly problematic because this behavior correlates not only with academic
problems (e.g., missed classes and assignments) but also with increased
rates of physical injury, unplanned sex, sexual assault, and drunk driving
(National Institute on Alcohol Abuse and Alcoholism 2013; Stone et al.
2012). In one study, fully one-third of surveyed college students reported
having five or more drinks in a row within the past 2 weeks (Hamilton et
al. 2020).

Hypotheses about the environmental and social factors that increase drinking on campuses include the following: the transitional experience of reduced adult supervision and regulation, easy access to alcohol, the presence of peers who are drinking and the associated social pressures, and the stresses of student life and college academics; internal and developmental factors include the overlap of drinking habits with the pressures of emerging adulthood, the novel demands of identity exploration and increased autonomy, and the desire to experiment and test one's limits in the sphere of alcohol and other substances (Skidmore et al. 2016). Many college students take a casual view of their own and their peers' level of drinking and consider alcohol consumption an inherent component of the university experience; drinking, as well as sex, is often perceived as representative of normative postadolescent status (Goodman et al. 2016). Fellow students' drinking habits and drinking norms on campus are often overestimated; these perceptions, along with the positive motivations for drinking—sociability, relaxation, companionship, escape from worries and pressures—increase the likelihood of a young person using alcohol and tend to mitigate realistic appraisals of the negative effect on academic, emotional, and social functioning (Fournier et al. 2013). Even distinctly negative personal experiences, such as blacking out after binge drinking, are often rationalized and minimized (Wombacher et al. 2019).

The serious personal and societal costs of substance abuse and dependency—which are highly correlated with risks to one's own and others' physical and psychological health, functional impairments in academic and professional settings, and disruptions to relationships and families—have led to a substantial literature that seeks to delineate pathways toward disorder and predict individuals at high risk. A complex array of biological, developmental, familial, and other environmental variables, with cascading effects that influence one another both concurrently and longitudinally, have been identified as correlates of vulnerability to alcohol and substance use in the emerging adulthood phase; genetic vulnerability, a history of early trauma and stressful events, parental psychopathology (including the use of alcohol and substances), and high levels of family conflict have all been identified as risk factors (Handley et al. 2017; Stone et al. 2012). Adolescent antecedents include established patterns of drug and alcohol use, primary associations with peers who are using, and poor academic performance (Haller et al. 2010). Young men are at significantly greater risk than young women for more frequent drinking and steeper inclines in rates of alcohol use during emerging adulthood (Edgerton and Keough 2021). Transgender individuals are known to use substances at higher rates than their cisgender counterparts, a fact likely connected to the need to cope with exceedingly high levels of stress and depression (Watson et al. 2019).

Emerging adults who fail to modify levels of drinking and drug use by their late 20s are at greater risk for long-term alcohol and substance use disorders and for concomitant struggles in their subsequent occupational and interpersonal lives. In the United States, about 7% of the population have symptoms that meet criteria for either alcohol or substance use disorder, and deaths from drug overdoses have increased substantially in recent years; worldwide, around 5% of the global burden of disease and injury is linked to the use of alcohol (Center for Behavioral Health Statistics and Quality 2016; World Health Organization 2011). Enduring social and emotional issues include poor overall interpersonal skills, difficulties maintaining committed relationships, low self-esteem, antisocial behaviors, and ongoing affiliations with antisocial peers (Allen et al. 2021; Hussong et al. 2004).

Behavioral Addictions

In recent years, a growing body of research has addressed the increase in behavioral addictions within the emerging adult population. Many of these addictions involve a lack of control over the use of digital media; excessive time spent engaging on social platforms, playing video games, participating in internet gambling, and viewing media-based pornography represent common forms (Estévez et al. 2017). Rates of comorbidity for multiple problematic behaviors are high, and there is considerable overlap between alcohol or substance abuse and poor regulation of internet use (Estévez et al. 2017).

The following criteria are generally considered when evaluating pathological behavioral patterns: salience (i.e., devoting huge amounts of time to engaging in, thinking about, and planning the behavior); compulsive pursuit of the activity; tension and discomfort, including an uptick in depression and anxiety, when the behavior is not pursued; and continuation of the behavior despite negative repercussions in health, social, academic, and/or professional arenas of life (Guillot et al. 2016; Savolainen et al. 2018). Risk factors for the development of addictive behaviors overlap with those for drug and alcohol abuse: they include poor interpersonal skills, social isolation, weak emotional self-regulation and impulse control, low self-esteem, perceived lack of positive family support, and a paucity of healthy leisure outlets (Estévez et al. 2017; Stockdale and Coyne 2018). The detrimental effect of behavioral addictions extends beyond the immediate effects on emerging adulthood—poorer physical and mental health, problematic eating and sleeping routines, a decline in the quality of face-to-face social interactions, reduced academic and job performance, and increased levels of stress—and includes an increased risk for continued maladaptive patterns in the subsequent years of adult life (Guillot et al. 2016; Savolainen et al. 2018; Stockdale and Coyne 2018).

As emerging adults' access to digital media has proliferated, online gambling and pornography have emerged as growing concerns, especially for male users; primarily solitary in nature, these activities offer none of the potential interpersonal components of online video-gaming or social media use. Compulsive use of the internet to access explicit sexual content is associated with depression and a decline in the quality of real relationships; young individuals may perceive online sexual depictions and scenarios as reflecting reality, which can interfere with their motivation to pursue and enjoy face-to-face connections (Tan et al. 2022). Playing video games generally represents a harmless and stress-reducing diversion as well as an opportunity to play with others; excessive gaming, however, is correlated with reduced physical and mental health, a decline in motivation for nonvirtual socialization, and poorer performance in academic and occupational environments (Stockdale and Coyne 2018).

Identity Distress and Disorder

As discussed in Chapter 5 ("Identity in Emerging Adulthood"), a stable and coherent identity marks a foundational component of healthy psychological functioning. Marcia (2006) suggested that identity represents a personality structure, much like the ego and superego, with an initial configuration during late adolescence that is subject to successive subsequent modifications. Within traditional psychoanalytic theory, identity cohesion is seen as a phase-salient task of late adolescence; it corresponds with the development of the ego ideal, a system of moral beliefs, values, and aspirations that helps ground the young individual by maintaining consistent self-representations, self-esteem, and mood, even during external upheavals (Blos 1965, 1968; Ritvo 1971). Personality theorists conceptualize identity as a multifaceted component of personality that encompasses a stable sense of self of integration and continuity across different settings and others as well as abiding feelings (Jørgensen 2010).

Contemporary developmental theories suggest that identity formation represents a lengthy process that is active throughout the emerging adulthood decade and that many domains of self-definition remain in a state of flux from the late teens to the late 20s. Extensive research describes an ongoing process during which the young individual tries on a range of roles, relationships, interests, and attitudes, devoting a good deal of time and mental energy to experimentation, the seeking of social validation, and then further reflection. The lengthy duration of the emerging adulthood period opens up the potential for a prolonged course of self-discovery as well as ongoing exposure to uncertainty and instability around identity domains that are under active exploration. This process is accompanied by normative levels of distress and worry as the young person gradually moves toward making commitments in at least some major life areas; transient forms of anxiety, lowered mood, and diminished feelings of self-efficacy and self-worth may accompany the pressures of engaging in experimentation, trying on novel roles, seeking feedback from others, and making commitments (Luyckx et al. 2013). Among college students, the domains that cause the greatest anxiety typically involve friendships and career-related decisions (Palmeroni et al. 2020). A sense of worry and transient preoccupations (concern about the reactions of peers or about making a wrong choice) are expected; however, excessive distress, self-doubt, and negative affect may exacerbate internalizing symptoms, adversely affect needed feelings of optimism and competence, and impede academic and work functioning. Overly ruminative approaches to identity exploration can hinder the process and make it difficult for individuals to explore freely, seek and incorporate feedback, and ultimately make decisions about a course of action (Luyckx et al. 2013).

Identity distress, a typically transient experience, is distinct from identity disorder; the latter, which is at the heart of much research and theory on borderline personality, involves far more severe and enduring impairments in key areas of social, emotional, and behavioral functioning. Identity diffusion is marked by a painful sense of incoherence, feelings of emptiness, distorted views and fantasies about the self and others, vague or overly rigid perspectives, and a turn toward action-oriented outlets (including risky and injurious behaviors) for managing intense feelings (Ammaniti et al. 2015; Carlson et al. 2009; Erikson 1956). Personality theorists conceptualize well-integrated, stable representations of the self and self-with-others as crucial building blocks for a sense of personal continuity that is maintained over time and within shifting contexts; identity coherence is essential for committing emotionally to certain roles and values, managing affects and impulses, modulating reactions during inevitable minor relational disruptions, achieving empathy and concern for others, and sustaining intimate relationships (Jørgensen 2010; Kernberg 1974). A lack of cohesive identity is marked by significant relational difficulty and by trouble integrating sexual desires with loving feelings for the other person. Often, others are used as recipients for the projection of nonintegrated aspects of the self in an effort to maintain a sense of personal wholeness; moreover, autobiographical narratives may appear disjointed and poorly integrated, with difficulty connecting past with here-and-now experience (Jørgensen 2010; Kernberg 1974).

Identity diffusion represents a sine qua non for borderline personality disorder. This disorder has a prevalence of only 1%–2% within the general population, but it accounts for an outsize level of psychiatric care and for as many as 20% of psychiatric hospitalizations; fundamental characteristics include disturbances in behavior and affect, increased rates of suicidality and self-harm, cognitive distortions, and disruptive interpersonal patterns (American Psychiatric Association 2013; Ammaniti et al. 2015; Carlson et al. 2009). The complex etiology of borderline personality disorder involves inter-actions among multiple factors, including genetics, environmental adversity, exposure to maltreatment and other traumas, disorganized patterns of attach-ment, and parental hostility; these factors contribute to the erosion of stable self-representations, mentalizing capacities, and self-regulating capacities, qualities that are known to promote flexibility and resilience in the face of stressful circumstances and to correlate with good developmental outcomes in young people who are subject to early caregiving failures (Carlson et al. 2009). Comorbidities with borderline personality disorder are common: reduced access to effective emotional strategies, coupled with frequent exposure to environmental challenges, creates vulnerabilities to depression and anxiety, self-harm, and substance use (Ammaniti et al. 2015; Carlson et al. 2009).

Although clinicians have some reluctance to diagnose major personality disorders in adolescence because of worries about labeling very young in-dividuals and also assumptions that personality may undergo significant subsequent change, many practitioners consider adolescence a time when such disorders first appear; this perspective is supported by research that suggests that severe problems in attention, behavior, and emotional func-tioning during the teen years correlate with later diagnoses of borderline personality disorder (Carlson et al. 2009; Ensink et al. 2015). Like many de-velopmentally oriented clinicians, however, we take a cautious approach to diagnosing personality disorders in both adolescent and emerging adult populations; many of the domains that make up identity (social roles, sex-uality, personal values), as well as capacities for intimacy and even funda-mental aspects of self-regulation, are very much in flux and in the process of maturing. Moreover, conflictual relationships with family and authority figures may reflect ongoing developmental struggles in the areas of separa-tion and autonomy rather than enduring interpersonal patterns.

Eating Disorders

Eating disorders have a peak onset during late adolescence and affect about 13% of females; they are marked by potentially devastating effects on the young individual's mental and physical well-being, including increased risk for future poor health and unhealthy weight, depression, suicidality, and mortality (Stice et al. 2017; Verschueren et al. 2020). Anorexia nervosa, with its concomitant severe weight loss and effect on physical health, has one of the highest mortality rates of any mental disorder (Striegel-Moore and Bu-lik 2007). The transition into emerging adulthood is a period of high risk for the development of a range of eating problems, from unhealthy weight control behaviors and food restrictions to full-blown disorders; the latter include the following: anorexia nervosa (characterized by severe weight loss, often to the point of amenorrhea, and frequently accompanied by increased physical activity and overall preoccupation with food), bulimia nervosa (self-induced vomiting after eating in order to avoid weight gain), and binge-eating disorder (American Psychiatric Association 2013; Stice et al. 2017; Walsh and Devlin 1998). Indeed, almost 90% of college women report that they worry about how their bodies look, and more than half acknowledge moderate to severe attempts at dieting (Delene and Brogowicz 1990; Ventura et al. 2018).

During emerging adulthood, the prevalence of eating disorders is significantly higher among women than among men; over time, however, a substantial number of women recover and the gender gap narrows (Brown et al. 2020). Identity pathology is a frequent comorbid condition, because disordered eating is correlated with poor emotional self-regulation, intense negative feelings, and a sense of the physical self as an unintegrated object to be subject to one's control. The body, food, and eating offer concrete points of fixation that may serve as substitutes for focusing on inner experience and therefore provide an escape from painful affects (Stice et al. 2017). Lack of a strong, stable sense of self increases vulnerability to preoccupations with superficial appearances as well as to the internalization of unrealistic standards of physical perfection; an ideal body may be experienced as a key part of one's personal identity, and a potential gain in weight is then experienced as a threat to selfhood (Verschueren et al. 2020). The gap between one's body ideal, with its perfectionistic benchmarks for weight and shape, and the perception of one's actual body causes not only dissatisfaction but also acute distress, however implausible the goals and despite the obvious effects of weight-controlling behaviors on one's health (Ventura et al. 2018).

Sociocultural models stress additional pathways toward eating disorders. These approaches emphasize young women's exposure to cultural ideals, via media and other venues, leading to harsh self-scrutiny and inevitable dissatisfaction when they compare their personal physiques with ubiquitous images of low-weight, seemingly perfect-looking females; Western culture's objectification of women's bodies and idealization of thin physiques are seen as predisposing contemporary youths to the internalization of unhealthy cultural norms and ideals (Munsch et al. 2021; Striegel-Moore and Bulik 2007).

Schizophrenia and Bipolar Disorders

Emerging adulthood marks a period of peak onset of schizophrenia and bipolar disorders, relatively rare but serious illnesses. Schizophrenia and psychotic mood disorders are the conditions most frequently associated with psychosis and may involve hallucinations, delusions, disorganized thinking, and behavioral disturbances. Both bipolar disorder and schizophrenia follow a course that can unfold slowly, sometimes taking months or even years to fully express itself. These lengthy prodromal periods, which precede full-blown illness, are often marked by symptoms such as low or elevated mood, changes in affective reaction and expression, an increase in goal-directed behaviors, problems with sleep, declines in self-regulation, and gradual withdrawal from one's usual activities; attenuated psychotic symptoms, declines in socialization, and increased anxiety and depression may be subtle, initially escaping the notice of family and friends but posing increasing challenges to the emerging adult's capacity for independent functioning (McClellan 2018; Van Meter et al. 2016; Walker et al. 2010).

Schizophrenia, which has a prevalence rate of around 1%, causes long-term functional impairments in social, academic, and occupational realms; contemporary research suggests a multifactorial etiology and identifies the following variables as adding to an individual's risk: genetic predisposition, pregnancy and birth complications, childhood trauma, social isolation, and extensive substance use (with some evidence citing heavy use of cannabis and psychostimulants; McCutcheon et al. 2020; Stilo and Murray 2017). Bipolar disorders, which have a mean age at onset of 21–22 years, also interfere significantly with daily functioning and contribute to an increased risk for suicide (Berk et al. 2007). Prevalence within the 18- to 24-year age group is measured at 5% or 6%; although bipolar illness is widely viewed as a chronic condition, with a chance of relapse throughout the life span, some studies indicate that by the later years of emerging adulthood (ages 25–29), rates of illness decline to around 3% (Cicero et al. 2009). This notable age gradient may represent the complex array of factors that affect young individuals with underlying vulnerability, such as the developmental stressors of the emerging adulthood phase, exposure to psychoactive substances with neurodevelopmental effects, and the maturation of the prefrontal cortex that takes place during the third decade of life (Alloy et al. 2006). An onset of bipolar illness before emerging adulthood is associated with a worse prognosis, partly because of interference with ongoing developmental processes; in younger adolescents and children, this condition is often hard to distinguish from attentional and behavioral problems as well as from depression and severe states of anxiety (Alloy et al. 2006; Van Meter et al. 2016).

Conclusion

Emerging adulthood represents a period of great potential for psychological growth. At the same time, this phase coincides with the inception of new or the intensification of existing mental health vulnerabilities. Indeed, rates of anxiety, depression, eating disorders, overall psychological distress, and drug or alcohol use are higher than for any other time of life. Personality disorders are first diagnosed during this phase, and relatively rare but serious mental illnesses (schizophrenia, bipolar disorders) have their peak rate of onset. There is a notable gap between the psychiatric needs of this age group and their low rates of seeking professional help.

We use a developmental psychopathology lens to understand the complex factors that contribute to emerging adults' high rates of psychopathology and overall psychological distress; multiple biological, familial, developmental, and environmental variables interact with one another both longitudinally and concurrently to create patterns of risk and protection. The developmental tasks of emerging adult life—managing novel levels of autonomy; navigating the stresses and uncertainties of the identity process; and handling pressures that come from academic, work, and social sources—offer many young people new opportunities for self-expression, self-discovery, and solutions to prior conflicts. At the same time, these tasks and novel stresses may dovetail with individual vulnerabilities, contributing to a range of mental health risks.

KEY POINTS

- Rates of anxiety, depression, and overall psychological stress are extremely high among college-age cohorts; comorbidity of depressive and anxiety disorders is very common, and the recurrence of major depressive episodes and anxiety is also prevalent. These conditions have the potential to impede the emerging adult's need to immerse the self in novel experience and the capacity to summon sufficient energy, motivation, and confidence to forge new ties and experience.

- Rates of suicidality have risen in recent years, and suicide is the second most common cause of death in the emerging adult population. Risk factors include a history of suicide attempts, early childhood exposure to adversity, family psychiatric variables, the presence of psychiatric conditions, the person's sense of belonging and social connection, recent stressful events, and access to methods of self-harm.

- Substance and alcohol use peaks during emerging adulthood; failure to regulate such behaviors can contribute to serious relational, occupational, and academic problems during these years as well as during subsequent adulthood.

- Identity diffusion is distinct from normative identity distress. The latter marks typical levels of worry and preoccupation that often accompany the process of identity exploration; the former represents a state of inner confusion and a lack of personal cohesion that is characterized by poor emotional regulation, distortions in self- and other representations, and serious trouble sustaining close relationships.

- Eating disorders have a peak onset during early emerging adulthood, particularly among women. These disorders encompass a range of factors that include food restrictions, excessive attempts to reduce weight, and distorted body perceptions.

- Relatively rare but very serious psychiatric conditions, such as bipolar disorders and schizophrenia, typically first appear during emerging adulthood and may develop after lengthy prodromal periods.

References

Adams SH, Knopf DK, Park MJ: Prevalence and treatment of mental health and substance use problems in the early emerging adult years in the United States: findings from the 2010 National Survey on Drug Use and Health. Emerg Adulthood 2(3):163–172, 2014

Allen JP, Loeb EL, Narr RK, et al: Different factors predict adolescent substance use versus adult substance abuse: lessons from a social-developmental approach. Dev Psychopathol 33(3):792–802, 2021 32638695

Alloy LB, Abramson LY, Walshaw PD, et al: A cognitive vulnerability-stress perspective on bipolar spectrum disorders in a normative adolescent brain, cognitive, and emotional development context. Dev Psychopathol 18(4):1055–1103, 2006 17064429

American College Health Association: American College Health Association-National College Health Assessment II: undergraduate student reference group data report spring 2019. Silver Spring, MD, American College Health Association, 2019

American Psychiatric Association: Diagnostic and Statistical Manual of Mental Disorders, 5th Edition. Arlington, VA, American Psychiatric Association, 2013

Ammaniti M, Fontana A, Nicolais G: Borderline personality disorder in adolescence through the lens of the Interview of Personality Organization Processes in Adolescence (IPOP-A): clinical uses and implications. J Infant Child Adolesc Psychother 14(1):82–97, 2015

Arnett JJ: Emerging adulthood: a theory of development from the late teens through the twenties. Am Psychol 55(5):469–480, 2000 1084426

Arnett JJ, Žukauskienė R, Sugimura K: The new life stage of emerging adulthood at ages 18–29 years: implications for mental health. Lancet Psychiatry 1(7):569–576, 2014 26361316

Bayram N, Bilgel N: The prevalence and socio-demographic correlations of depression, anxiety and stress among a group of university students. Soc Psychiatry Psychiatr Epidemiol 43(8):667–672, 2008 18398558

Berk M, Dodd S, Callaly P, et al: History of illness prior to a diagnosis of bipolar disorder or schizoaffective disorder. J Affect Disord 103(1–3):181–186, 2007 17324469

Blos P: The initial stage of male adolescence. Psychoanal Study Child 20:145–164, 1965 5835539

Blos P: Character formation in adolescence. Psychoanal Study Child 23:245–263, 1968 5759022

Borelli JL, Snavely JE, Compare A, et al: Reflective functioning moderates the associations between perceptions of parental neglect and attachment in adolescence. Psychoanal Psychol 32(1):23–35, 2015

Borgogna NC, McDermott RC, Aita SL, et al: Anxiety and depression across gender and sexual minorities: implications for transgender, gender non-conforming, pansexual, demisexual, asexual, queer and questioning individuals. Psychology of Sexual Orientation and Gender 6(1):54–63, 2019

Boyne H, Hamza CA: Depressive symptoms, perceived stress, self-compassion and nonsuicidal self-injury among emerging adults: an examination of the between and within-person associations over time. Emerg Adulthood 10(5):1269–1285, 2022

Brown TA, Forney KJ, Klein KM, et al: A 30-year longitudinal study of body weight, dieting, and eating pathology across women and men from late adolescence to later midlife. J Abnorm Psychol 129(4):376–386, 2020 32309984

Burt KB, Paysnick AA: Resilience in the transition to adulthood. Dev Psychopathol 24(2):493–505, 2012 22559126

Carlson EA, Egeland B, Sroufe LA: A prospective investigation of the development of borderline personality symptoms. Dev Psychopathol 21(4):1311–1334, 2009 19825270

Center for Behavioral Health Statistics and Quality: Key Substance Use and Mental Health Indicators in the United States: Results From the 2015 National Survey on Drug Use and Health. Rockville, MD, Substance Abuse and Mental Health Services Administration, 2016

Cicchetti D, Rogosch FA: A developmental psychopathology perspective on adolescence. J Consult Clin Psychol 70(1):6–20, 2002

Cicero DC, Epler AJ, Sher KJ: Are there developmentally limited forms of bipolar disorder? J Abnorm Psychol 118(3):431–447, 2009 19685942

Conley CS, Kirsch AC, Dickson DA, et al: Negotiating the transition to college: developmental trajectories and gender differences in psychological functioning, cognitive-affective strategies and social well-being. Emerg Adulthood 2(3):195–210, 2014

Conway CC, Zinbarg RE, Mineka S, et al: Core dimensions of anxiety and depression change independently during adolescence. J Abnorm Psychol 126(2):160–172, 2017 28192011

Cross WE Jr: The psychology of nigrescence: revising the Cross model, in Handbook of Multicultural Counseling. Edited by Ponterotto JG, Casas JM, Suzuki LA, et al. Thousand Oaks, CA, Sage, 1995, pp 93–122

Curtin SC, Heron M: Death rates due to suicide and homicide among persons aged 10–24: United States, 2000–2017. NCHS Data Brief (352):1–8, 2019 31751202

Delene LM, Brogowicz AA: Student healthcare needs, attitudes, and behavior: marketing implications for college health centers. J Am Coll Health 38(4):157–164, 1990 2299049

Duffy ME, Twenge JM, Joiner TE: Trends in mood and anxiety symptoms and suicide-related outcomes among U.S. undergraduates, 2007–2018: evidence from two national surveys. J Adolesc Health 65(5):590–598, 2019 31279724

Edgerton JD, Keough MT: Identifying and predicting multiple trajectories of alcohol dependence symptoms in a Canadian sample of emerging adults. Emerg Adulthood 9(2):104–116, 2021

Edgerton JD, Read JP: Relationship role transitions and problem alcohol use in emerging adulthood. Emerg Adulthood 7(4):291–303, 2018

Eichler RJ: The university as a (potentially) facilitating environment. Contemp Psychoanal 47(3):289–317, 2011

Ensink K, Biberdzic M, Normandin L, et al: A developmental psychopathology and neurobiological model of borderline personality disorder in adolescence. J Infant Child Adolesc Psychother 14(1):46–69, 2015

Erikson EH: The problem of ego identity. J Am Psychoanal Assoc 4(1):56–121, 1956 13286157

Essau CA, Lewinsohn PM, Lim JX, et al: Incidence, recurrence and comorbidity of anxiety disorders in four major developmental stages. J Affect Disord 228:248–253, 2018 29304469

Estévez A, Jáuregui P, Sánchez-Marcos I, et al: Attachment and emotion regulation in substance addictions and behavioral addictions. J Behav Addict 6(4):534–544, 2017 29280395

Fournier AK, Hall E, Ricke P, et al: Alcohol and the social network: online social networking sites and college students' perceived drinking norms. Psychology of Popular Media Culture 2(2):86–95, 2013

Geoffroy MC, Orri M, Girard A, et al: Trajectories of suicide attempts from early adolescence to emerging adulthood: prospective 11-year follow-up of a Canadian cohort. Psychol Med 51(11):1933–1943, 2021 32290876

Gilmore KJ, Meersand P: Normal Child and Adolescent Development: A Psychodynamic Primer. Washington, DC, American Psychiatric Publishing, 2014

Gomez J, Miranda R, Polanco L: Acculturative stress, perceived discrimination, and vulnerability to suicide attempts among emerging adults. J Youth Adolesc 40(11):1465–1476, 2011 21717234

Gonzalez VM: Factors linking suicidal ideation with drinking to cope and alcohol problems in emerging adult college drinkers. Exp Clin Psychopharmacol 27(2):166–177, 2019 30556729

Goodman I, Henderson J, Peterson-Badali M, et al: Youth perspectives on the transition to adulthood: exploring the impact of problematic substance use and treatment seeking. Emerg Adulthood 4(2):92–103, 2016

Guillot CR, Bello MS, Tsai JY, et al: Longitudinal associations between anhedonia and internet-related addictive behaviors in emerging adults. Comput Human Behav 62:475–479, 2016 27182108

Gutman LM, Sameroff AJ: Continuities in depression from adolescence to young adulthood: contrasting ecological influences. Dev Psychopathol 16(4):967–984, 2004 15704823

Haller M, Handley E, Chassin L, et al: Developmental cascades: linking adolescent substance use, affiliation with substance use promoting peers, and academic achievement to adult substance use disorders. Dev Psychopathol 22(4):899–916, 2010 20883589

Halliburton AE, Hill MB, Dawson BL, et al: Increased stress, declining mental health: emerging adults' experiences in college during Covid-19. Emerg Adulthood 9(5):433–448, 2021

Hamilton HR, Armeli S, Tennen H: Drink (socially) and be merry: predicting enjoyment and self-perceptions from alcohol consumption among college students. Emerg Adulthood 9(4):415–421, 2020

Handley ED, Rogosch FA, Cicchetti D: From child maltreatment to emerging adult problem drinking: identification of a multilevel internalizing pathway among African American youth. Dev Psychopathol 29(5):1807–1821, 2017 29162188

Hastings PD, Serbin LA, Bukowski W, et al: Predicting psychosis-spectrum diagnoses in adulthood from social behaviors and neighborhood contexts in childhood. Dev Psychopathol 32(2):465–479, 2020 31014409

Heller AS, Fox AS, Davidson RJ: Parsing affective dynamics to identify risk for mood and anxiety disorders. Emotion 19(2):283–291, 2019 29863379

Hussong AM, Curran PJ, Moffitt TE, et al: Substance abuse hinders desistance in young adults' antisocial behavior. Dev Psychopathol 16(4):1029–1046, 2004 15704826

Jackson ER, Shanafelt TD, Hasan O, et al: Burnout and alcohol abuse/dependence among U.S. medical students. Acad Med 91(9):1251–1256, 2016 26934693

Jørgensen CR: Invited essay: identity and borderline personality disorder. J Pers Disord 24(3):344–364, 2010 20545499

Kernberg OF: Mature love: prerequisites and characteristics. J Am Psychoanal Assoc 22(4):743–768, 1974 4423688

Kessler RC, Berglund P, Demler O, et al: The epidemiology of major depressive disorder: results from the National Comorbidity Survey Replication (NCS-R). JAMA 289(23):3095–3105, 2003 12813115

Lawrence HR, Nesi J, Schwartz-Mette RA: Suicidal mental imagery: investigating a novel marker of suicide risk. Emerg Adulthood 10(5):1216–1221, 2021

Leebens PK, Williamson ED: Developmental psychopathology: risk and resilience in the transition to young adulthood. Child Adolesc Psychiatr Clin N Am 26(2):143–156, 2017 28314447

Liguori G, Lonbaken B: Alcohol consumption and academic retention in first-year college students. College Student Journal 49:69–77, 2015

Luyckx K, Klimstrat A, Duriez B, et al: Personal identity processes from adolescence through the late 20s: age trends, functionality, and depressive symptoms. Social Development 22:701–721, 2013

Lynne-Landsman SD, Bradshaw CP, Ialongo NS: Testing a developmental cascade model of adolescent substance use trajectories and young adult adjustment. Dev Psychopathol 22(4):933–948, 2010 20883591

Mahtani S, Melvin GA, Hasking P: Shame proneness, shame coping and functions of nonsuicidal self-injury (NSSI) among emerging adults: a developmental analysis. Emerg Adulthood 5(3):159–171, 2017

Malone JC, Piacentini E, Speranza M: Reclaiming the developmental lens for adolescent formulation and diagnosis: application of the PDM-2 to clinical cases. Psychoanal Psychol 35(3):339–345, 2018

Manago AM, Taylor T, Greenfield PM: Me and my 400 friends: the anatomy of college students' Facebook networks, their communication patterns, and well-being. Dev Psychol 48(2):369–380, 2012 22288367

Marcia JE: Ego identity and personality disorders. J Pers Disord 20(6):577–596, 2006 17192139

Marenco S, Weinberger DR: The neurodevelopmental hypothesis of schizophrenia: following a trail of evidence from cradle to grave. Dev Psychopathol 12(3):501–527, 2000 11014750

Mars B, Heron J, Klonsky ED, et al: Predictors of future suicide attempt among adolescents with suicidal thoughts or non-suicidal self-harm: a population-based birth cohort study. Lancet Psychiatry 6(4):327–337, 2019a 30879972

Mars B, Heron J, Klonsky ED, et al: What distinguishes adolescents with suicidal thoughts from those who have attempted suicide? A population-based birth cohort study. J Child Psychol Psychiatry 60(1):91–99, 2019b 29492978

McClellan J: Psychosis in children and adolescents. J Am Acad Child Adolesc Psychiatry 57(5):308–312, 2018 29706159

McCutcheon RA, Reis Marques T, Howes OD: Schizophrenia: an overview. JAMA Psychiatry 77(2):201–210, 2020 31664453

Melvin GA, Dudley AL, Gordon MS, et al: What happens to depressed adolescents? A follow-up study into early adulthood. J Affect Disord 151(1):298–305, 2013 23829999

Meyer IH: Prejudice, social stress, and mental health in lesbian, gay, and bisexual populations: conceptual issues and research evidence. Psychol Bull 129(5):674–697, 2003 12956539

Miller JN, Black DW: Bipolar disorder and suicide: a review. Curr Psychiatry Rep 22(2):6, 2020 31955273

Miranda-Mendizabal A, Castellví P, Parés-Badell O, et al: Gender differences in suicidal behavior in adolescents and young adults: systematic review and meta-analysis of longitudinal studies. Int J Public Health 64(2):265–283, 2019 30635683

Mortier P, Cuijpers P, Kiekens G, et al: The prevalence of suicidal thoughts and behaviours among college students: a meta-analysis. Psychol Med 48(4):554–565, 2018 28805169

Munsch S, Messerli-Bürgy N, Meyer AH, et al: Consequences of exposure to the thin ideal in mass media depend on moderators in young women: an experimental study. J Abnorm Psychol 130(5):498–511, 2021

National Institute on Alcohol Abuse and Alcoholism: Overview of alcohol consumption: moderate and binge drinking. 2013. Available at: https://www.niaaa.nih.gov/alcohol-health/overview-alcohol-consumption/moderate-binge-drinking. Accessed December 7, 2022.

Negriff S: Childhood adversities and mental health outcomes: does the perception or age of the event matter? Dev Psychopathol 33(3):778–791, 2021 32366345

O'Connor RC: Towards an integrated motivational–volitional model of suicidal behaviour, in International Handbook of Suicide Prevention: Research, Policy and Practice. Edited by O'Connor RC, Platt S, Gordon J. Chichester, UK, Wiley, 2011, pp 181–198

O'Connor RC, Nock MK: The psychology of suicidal behaviour. Lancet Psychiatry 1(1):73–85, 2014 26360404

Palmeroni N, Claes L, Verschueren M, et al: Identity distress throughout adolescence and emerging adulthood: age trends and associations with exploration and commitment processes. Emerg Adulthood 8(5):333–343, 2020

Perez-Brumer A, Day JK, Russell ST, et al: Prevalence and correlates of suicidal ideation among transgender youth in California: findings from a representative, population-based sample of high school students. J Am Acad Child Adolesc Psychiatry 56(9):739–746, 2017 28838578

Polanco-Roman L, Miranda R: Culturally related stress, hopelessness, and vulnerability to depressive symptoms and suicidal ideation in emerging adulthood. Behav Ther 44(1):75–87, 2013 23312428

Powers A, Casey BJ: The adolescent brain and the emergence and peak of psychopathology. J Infant Child Adolesc Psychother 14(1):3–15, 2015

Prenoveau JM, Craske MG, Zinbarg RE, et al: Are anxiety and depression just as stable as personality during late adolescence? Results from a three-year longitudinal latent variable study. J Abnorm Psychol 120(4):832–843, 2011 21604827

Reed-Fitzke K, Withers M, Ferraro AJ, et al: A growth curve analysis of self-esteem and depression throughout emerging adulthood: the role of the family. Emerg Adulthood 9(2):91–103, 2021

Ritvo S: Late adolescence: developmental and clinical considerations. Psychoanal Study Child 26:241–263, 1971 5163228

Rohde P, Lewinsohn PM, Klein DN, et al: Key characteristics of major depressive disorder occurring in childhood, adolescence, emerging adulthood, and adulthood. Clin Psychol Sci 1(1):41–53, 2013 24273703

Savolainen I, Kaakinen M, Sirola A, et al: Addictive behaviors and psychological distress among adolescents and emerging adults: a mediating role of peer group identification. Addict Behav Rep 7:75–81, 2018 29892700

Schulenberg JE, Zarrett NR: Mental health during emerging adulthood: continuity and discontinuity in courses, causes, and functions, in Emerging Adults in America: Coming of Age in the 21st Century. Edited by Arnett JJ, Tanner JL. Washington, DC, American Psychological Association, 2006, pp 135–172

Schulenberg JE, Sameroff AJ, Cicchetti D: The transition to adulthood as a critical juncture in the course of psychopathology and mental health. Dev Psychopathol 16(4):799–806, 2004 15704815

Schulenberg JE, Patrick ME, Johnston LD, et al: Monitoring the Future national survey results on drug use, 1975–2020: volume II, college students and adults ages 19–60. Monitoring the Future, 2021. Available at: https://monitoringthefuture.org/wp-content/uploads/2022/08/mtf-vol2_2020.pdf. Accessed December 7, 2022.

Skidmore CR, Kaufman EA, Crowell SE: Substance use among college students. Child Adolesc Psychiatr Clin N Am 25(4):735–753, 2016 27613349

Smith KM, Cobb KF, Reed-Fitzke K, et al: Connections between parental reciprocity and emerging adult depressive symptoms and loneliness: the role of peer social support. Can J Behav Sci 54(1):52–61, 2022

Stallman HM, Shocket I: Prevalence of mental health problems in Australian university health services. Aust Psychol 44(2):122–127, 2009

Stewart SM, Eaddy M, Horton SE, et al: The validity of the interpersonal theory of suicide in adolescence: a review. J Clin Child Adolesc Psychol 46(3):437–449, 2017 25864500

Stice E, Gau JM, Rohde P, et al: Risk factors that predict future onset of each DSM-5 eating disorder: predictive specificity in high-risk adolescent females. J Abnorm Psychol 126(1):38–51, 2017 27709979

Stilo SA, Murray RM: Non-genetic factors in schizophrenia. Curr Psychiatry Rep 21(10):100, 2017 31522306

Stockdale L, Coyne SM: Video game addiction in emerging adulthood: cross-sectional evidence of pathology in video game addicts as compared to matched healthy controls. J Affect Disord 225:265–272, 2018 28841491

Stone AL, Becker LG, Huber AM, et al: Review of risk and protective factors of substance use and problem use in emerging adulthood. Addict Behav 37(7):747–775, 2012 22445418

Striegel-Moore RH, Bulik CM: Risk factors for eating disorders. Am Psychol 62(3):181–198, 2007 17469897

Tan SA, Ng SHL, Hoo JJY, et al: The pornography use and its addiction among emerging adults in Malaysia: perceived realism as a mediator. PloS One 17(5):e0268724, 2022 35594283

Tzilos GK, Caviness CM, Anderson BJ, et al: Stimulant use and associated health risks among student and non-student emerging adults. Emerg Adulthood 4(4):298–302, 2016

Vacek S, Whisman MA: Traumatic events and adolescent psychopathology in a United States national probability sample. Psychol Trauma 13(3):277–283, 2021

Van Meter AR, Burke C, Youngstrom EA, et al: The bipolar prodrome: meta-analysis of symptom prevalence prior to initial or recurrent mood episodes. J Am Acad Child Adolesc Psychiatry 55(7):543–555, 2016 27343882

Van Orden KA, Witte TK, Cukrowicz KC, et al: The interpersonal theory of suicide. Psychol Rev 117(2):575–600, 2010 20438238

Vaughan SC: Suicidality in LGBTQ+ youth. Psychoanal Study Child 71(1):40–54, 2018

Ventura LM, Randall ET, Shapiro JB, et al: Looking good and making it seem easy: a prospective study of effortless perfectionism, body image, and BMI in unhealthy weight control behaviors among female adolescents and young adults. Emerg Adulthood 6(5):327–335, 2018

Verschueren M, Claes L, Gandhi A, et al: Identity and psychopathology: bridging developmental and clinical research. Emerg Adulthood 8(5):319–332, 2020

Villarroel MA, Terlizzi EP: Symptoms of depression among adults: United States, 2019. NCHS Data Brief, No 379. Hyattsville, MD, National Center for Health Statistics, 2020. Available at: https://www.cdc.gov/nchs/data/databriefs/db379-H.pdf. Accessed December 7, 2022.

Vrshek-Schallhorn S, Stroud CB, Mineka S, et al: Chronic and episodic interpersonal stress as statistically unique predictors of depression in two samples of emerging adults. J Abnorm Psychol 124(4):918–932, 2015 26301973

Walker E, Shapiro D, Esterberg M, et al: Neurodevelopment and schizophrenia: broadening the focus. Curr Dir Psychol Sci 19(4):204–208, 2010

Walsh BT, Devlin MJ: Eating disorders: progress and problems. Science 280(5368):1387–1390, 1998 9603723

Watson RJ, Veale JF, Gordon AR, et al: Risk and protective factors for transgender youths' substance use. Prev Med Rep 15:100905, 2019 31193847

Weissman MM, Wolk S, Goldstein RB, et al: Depressed adolescents grown up. JAMA 281(18):1707–1713, 1999 10328070

Werner KB, Cunningham-Williams RM, Ahuja M, et al: Patterns of gambling and substance use initiation in African American and white adolescents and young adults. Psychol Addict Behav 34(2):382–391, 2020 31750700

Wombacher K, Matig JJ, Sheff SE, et al: "It just kind of happens": college students' rationalizations for blackout drinking. Health Commun 34(1):1–10, 2019

World Health Organization: Global status report on noncommunicable diseases 2010. 2011. Available at: https://apps.who.int/iris/handle/10665/44579. Accessed December 7, 2022.

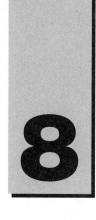

Therapeutic Modalities in the Treatment of Emerging Adults

In this chapter, we describe the range of mental health interventions available to emerging adults with the typical disorders of this age group and then focus our attention on psychoanalytically oriented treatment approaches, their indications, and their demonstrable benefits, with illustrative case material. As we have noted throughout this book, the full age range of emerging adulthood (the first part and the second part) typically includes considerable circumstantial and developmental change, with shifting locations and contexts; changing relationships with family, peers, teachers, and bosses; new configurations of identity and identity components; and ideally, an evolving sense of one's own capacities, values, purpose, and plan. Moreover, visible physical changes may extend into the 20s, and brain development and presumably cognitive development continues until at least age 25. These new findings have led contributors to the contemporary pediatric literature to favor the extension of late adolescence to age 24 (see Arain et al. 2013; Ledford 2018; Sawyer et al. 2018). During this time, aspects of mental life are in a period of active growth, synthesis, and deepening, historically referred to as a process of *consolidation* (Blos 1968; Blum 1985; Emde 1985). This term is, from our viewpoint, outdated in the twenty-first century because it evokes an identity formation that is solidified and inflexible.

Today, rapid social change, ongoing maturation, and evolving attitudes toward personhood demand constant revisions of identity and sense of self. These transformations—intrapsychic, environmental, and developmental—require that treatments for emerging adults be shaped to address their peculiar challenges. Throughout this developmental period, but especially in early emerging adulthood, instability, fragile achievement of autonomy, and vulnerability to the persuasive power of the peer group contribute to this population's susceptibility to its signature disorders, including substance use disorders, depression and suicidality, and risky behavior and accidental deaths, and to the difficulty in treating them.

For example, treatment modalities must have the flexibility to grapple with the idiosyncratic circumstances of this cohort in contemporary society, because instability in geographic location, employment, and relationships is typical (Arnett 2000; Escoll 1987; Lanz and Serido 2020). The authority of the traditional medical establishment has eroded: young people consult the internet for medical and mental health information, and word of mouth popularizes new developments in technology and psychopharmacology; emerging adults often arrive at the consultant's office with a preferred treatment plan based on these sources. Digital communication, including participation in social media, is a prominent feature of everyday experience and a notorious fount of misinformation. Moreover, the speed and globalization of information and communication (Turkle 2004) make the work of psychotherapy seem slow and arduous; for many, it can appear dated and inefficient.

Most forms of therapy, even preceding the exigencies of the SARS-CoV-2 disease (COVID-19) pandemic, struggle to bridge geographic moves and changes in daily schedule. Shifts in circumstances, such as moving from one institution to another (e.g., from college to a corporate job or from one start-up to another), can alter financial or contractual arrangements and make the continuation of a given treatment format impossible. In addition to diagnostic assessment, such issues ideally figure into treatment recommendations.

Some treatment approaches have been developed from the outset to adapt to these myriad circumstances. Notwithstanding the fact that emerging adulthood as a developmental entity has gained recognition only in the past two decades (Gilmore 2019; Gilmore and Meersand 2014; Knight and Miller 2017; Schechter et al. 2018), new forms of treatment have rapidly evolved to meet the specific needs of emerging adults, especially in the digital arena. Mental health apps designed for this age group are available to track moods and feelings, intercept impulses (e.g., to self-injure or use substances), measure physical activity, chart sobriety and substance use, document job searches, monitor focus, assess social behavior, and so on. In some instances, time-tested treatment modalities must be revamped to succeed with these transitional-age youths, and clinical services require expansion to deal with the contemporary circumstances of the opioid epidemic and peak alcohol consumption.

In what follows, we discuss problems associated with emerging adults' use of mental health services. We then briefly survey a range of programs and their successes and failures in addressing the significant treatment gap that has been identified in this most at-risk population. We then focus on psychodynamic interventions, their fundamental principles, their indications, and their vicissitudes.

Treatment Gap

The concept of a *treatment gap* refers to the absolute difference between the true prevalence of a disorder and the proportion of individuals affected by the disorder who receive treatment (Kohn et al. 2004). The treatment gap among emerging adults is of great concern in terms of both its immediate implications and its contribution to long-term disability. As noted in Chapter 7 ("Psychopathology and Emerging Adulthood"), emerging adulthood is a critical period for the onset of serious and lifelong mental health problems. It is considered one of the most vulnerable periods for the first appearance of psychiatric illnesses (Kessler et al. 2005); 75% of mental health and substance use disorders emerge before age 24 (Hunt and Eisenberg 2010) or age 25 (Rosenberg 2016). Of these mental health disorders, 40% involve a dual diagnosis with substance abuse; only one-tenth of the patients with a dual diagnosis who need help receive treatment (Hunt and Eisenberg 2010; Rosenberg 2016). Because this period also marks the transition to self-determined medical care, with treatment ideally and medicolegally initiated by the patients themselves, the treatment gap would seem to reflect a failure to reach and engage this population.

What are the impediments to engaging emerging adults? Pathways to treatment may differ by cohort or disorder (e.g., college students vs. young people in the workforce or alcohol use vs. drug use); according to the National Epidemiologic Survey on Alcohol and Related Conditions from 2008 (Blanco et al. 2008), prevalence varies only slightly in terms of the distribution of disorders in different socioeconomic strata, but the bottom line is that fewer than 25% of both working and college youths made use of available treatment in the year before the survey. In a more recent survey conducted by the World Health Organization as part of the International College Student Initiative (Ebert et al. 2019), fewer than one-quarter of college students in a range of countries reported a willingness to seek help. The most significant barriers were attitudinal: students' wish to handle the problem by themselves, their wish to talk to friends and relatives instead, and embarrassment associated with seeking professional help (Ebert et al. 2019,

p. 9). Other research, including a literature review by Gulliver et al. (2010) and a few studies by Cheng and colleagues (2013, 2015, 2018), found that mental health literacy among young people was an important foundation for willingness to use resources; the failure to recognize one's own suffering as a manifestation of mental disorder and/or illness arrested the process of getting the right kind of help at the threshold.

The emotion of *embarrassment* has a complex relationship with self-stigma and culture-based stigma; embarrassment and the more purely negative *shame* are affects elicited by the presence or mental representation of disapproving, rejecting, or disgusted significant others (peers, parents, community) leading to secrecy, hiding, or lying. The related self-stigma refers to the internalization of cultural or subcultural stereotypes and prejudices that are then applied to the self. These stereotypes arise from both the larger culture and the local community and can vary widely. Conceptualizations of mental illness depend on many factors, including racial/ethnic, religious, social status, age-based, and gender-based attitudes that permeate the cultural surround. Some prejudices are differentially associated with some mental illnesses and not others. For example, in many subcultural groups, drug addiction is subject to the moral condemnation that it is a deliberate choice; acknowledging its presence and seeking treatment are discouraged by the widespread belief that it is willfully chosen by the addicted person and therefore should be self-corrected. Some research on this topic has distinguished stigma around mental illness from stigma around *seeking help* for mental illness (Tucker et al. 2013); consenting to the role of help-seeker or patient is an additional threat to self-esteem and may be the more important impediment (Tucker et al. 2013, p. 528). Indeed, individuals with a history of severe mental illness and especially hospitalization retain lifelong self-stigma and shame (Mathison 2019).

As noted previously, both the illness and its treatment contribute stigmatizing identity components that intersect with racial/ethnic and gender identities. In a study that examined differences in help-seeking between ethnic groups within a college setting (DeFreitas et al. 2018), the problem of stigma was most pronounced among African American students, which the authors attributed to home-community attitudes and convictions about the nature of mental illness and its visible signs. However, prior research produced contradictory findings (Gonzalez et al. 2005; Shim et al. 2009) in that African Americans had more positive attitudes toward help-seeking than other groups did despite low rates of use. Asian Americans have been observed to have negative attitudes toward self-disclosure and help-seeking, presumably based on cultural beliefs. Among Latinx American and African American students alike, anxiety about treatment requiring interaction with someone different from themselves, such as someone racially or ethnically different, heightens reluctance to seek treatment.

Efforts to Engage Emerging Adult Patients

College Programs

Efforts to increase the use of mental health services have had to grapple with the fact that many programs are based on an adult model that is not attuned to the specific developmental needs of emerging adults (Osuch et al. 2016; Walker 2015). Given that emerging adulthood encompasses the period when potential lifelong disorders typically emerge, and that the treatment gap for these disorders is more than 50%, program developers focus on how best to engage this age group with sensitivity to their developmental needs (Kohn et al. 2004). Colleges have begun to vigorously address the mental health crisis among students at the point of orientation, with instructional videos; humorous skits about the travails of first-year life and how to get help; information about warning signs in oneself and others; and, in some cases, a greater presence of academic advisers, deans, and resident advisers, who may hold open office hours and check in with students of concern. The National Alliance on Mental Illness (NAMI) has developed NAMI on Campus clubs, offering start-up kits and other resources to facilitate the development of programs, guest speakers, and solidarity marches. A page on their website specifically directed at college students (www.NAMI.org/Get-involved/NAMI-on-campus) is a rich source of ideas and guidance. An important marker of the success of campus programs is the prevention of attempted and completed suicides among students. Unfortunately, suicide rates continue to rise for all age groups (Suicide Prevention Resource Center 2021), and suicide is the second leading cause of death among 17- to 24-year-olds regardless of college attendance (Kella 2021). It continues to occupy this position until the mid-40s, when it drops to the fourth leading cause of death.

On-campus programmatic efforts to discern mental health distress and to provide timely and needed help are not without cost to the colleges themselves. In an opinion piece in *Inside Higher Ed* (Dziech 2019), a professor who was deeply involved with a student who died from suicide delineated her concerns about the complexity of identifying those in critical danger and the complications for the institution: anxiety and depression are ubiquitous in this age group, the demand on college services is regularly increasing, and the cost of these services is high. Moreover, promising to provide services to students in need may be too ambitious for schools with limited resources and no systematized monitoring; students inevitably fall through the cracks.

Beyond College

The number of programs targeted especially for emerging adults has multiplied in response to the recognition of the latter as a developmental entity. Such programs include residential or wilderness programs and outpatient centers in addition to programs specifically geared to the identified problems of this generation.

A study of an outpatient treatment program called First Episode Mood and Anxiety Program (Osuch et al. 2019) showed that self-referral was a good predictor of sustained treatment results. Programmatic flexibility and a focus on "patients' needs and expressed wishes" (Osuch et al. 2019, p. 217) yield greater engagement and improvement. Self-referral and wraparound services provided at one site and tailored to the personal requirements of the individual patient—including individual, family, and addiction therapies—showed sustained participation and promising results.

However, such programs, with their communal feeling, freedom of choice about treatments, and focus on self-determination, work only for emerging adults whose striving for autonomy does not preclude the wish for professional guidance; they do not address some of the attitudes leading to the avoidance of help-seeking. A minimal level of mental health literacy is necessary to achieve the important first step of recognizing illness. Lack of literacy is both a product of and a contributor to the problems of stigma and self-stigma described in the previous section, "Treatment Gap."

Improving Literacy

Mental health literacy is the rate-limiting step in obtaining care. One approach to addressing the problem of literacy, Mental Health First Aid training programs, begun in 2001 in Australia by Kitchener and Jorm (2002), have spread across the globe. These programs are based on the idea that instruction in recognizing mental health problems and guides to intervention are as important as training in CPR. This initiative was first studied and found to be effective in rural Australia, where soccer coaches were trained to identify early signals or warning signs of mental illness and taught how to reach out to affected youths. With the additional mental health strain of COVID-19, such training became available online. The expectation is that widespread training of influential community members such as coaches, teachers, community leaders, and medical professionals will propagate enlightened views and provide helpful role models for young people and the community at large. Programs outside of academic centers must contend with the challenge of reaching numbers in incohesive and unstandardized environments.

It is important to note that the normative process of identity formation brings a degree of stress and anxiety, especially for those young people who feel stigmatized or "other" because they diverge from the "cultural master narrative," that is, those "ubiquitous, powerful cultural stories with which individuals negotiate in constructing personal identity" (McLean et al. 2017, p. 93). This conflict can trigger more serious disturbance if not addressed by either environmental measures or personal support. In the past, young people struggling with an outsider status due to race, sexual preferences, gender identification, immigration, or disability or, alternatively, due to the private realization of divergence from the master narrative were typically left to their own devices to define themselves, defend themselves, and find others like themselves. Programs and resources intended to stimulate discussion of religious, racial, gender, and other key components of identity are listed in the Child Welfare Information Gateway (www.childwelfare.gov); many grassroots organizations, discussion groups, and resource centers are available online.

Treatment for the New Disorders of Emerging Adulthood

Programs designed to treat common disorders of this age group, such as substance misuse and abuse, eating disorders, and borderline personality disorder, predate the designation of emerging adulthood as a developmental entity. More recently, there has been a wave of new programs that focus their outreach efforts specifically on emerging adults and the life problems that have become part of common parlance when speaking of this group. The yes-and-no status of emerging adults as autonomous, emancipated adults has been popularized by monikers such as *failure to launch*, *yo-yo* or *boomerangers*, *kidults*, and *go-nowhere* (Tuttle 2014). Efforts to address these related difficulties have shaped several programs aimed at facilitating the progression of faltering emerging adults. Although a return to the parental home is not the only way in which such faltering is signaled, it is an event that is widely recognized as a manifestation of developmental interruption or delay.

Inclusion of Parents

A recent Pew Research Center report noted that more than half of 18- to 29-year-olds live with one or both parents (Fry et al. 2020). This spike (up to 52% in 2020 compared with a still noteworthy 47% in 2019) was due primarily to early emerging adults (ages 19–24) living with parents as a result of the pandemic and its economic impact on this age group. The subjective experience of feeling in-between is matched by complicated responses from parents struggling with their 18- to 29-year-olds' difficult transition from dependency to full adult autonomy (and back again). Given that many emerging adults rely on parental support in the form of money or room and board, their relationship with their parents has a present-day impact, potentially reducing their confidence, decision-making ability, and sense of competence and augmenting anxiety and depression (Livesey and Rostain 2017). A combined treatment approach that involves periodic parental assessment and the inclusion of parents in the therapy allows the clinician to address the family system, including its cultural, generational, and idiosyncratic views of emancipation; psychiatric illness; addiction; and sexuality. The improved outcome of treatment for a range of disorders, such as psychosis, bipolar disorder, and drug addiction, has been demonstrable, which suggests that this modality should be included in training (Livesey and Rostain 2017).

Other programs have full-service facilities that offer a wide range of therapies focused on the specific needs of emerging adults. For example, the Columbia University Clinic for Anxiety and Related Disorders has the Launching Emerging Adults Program (LEAP), and McLean Hospital in Massachusetts has the Young Adult Mental Health Treatment Programs. These and many others provide a range of services, including cognitive-behavioral therapy (CBT), dialectical behavior therapy (DBT), day treatment, parent therapies, college preparation programs, and career guidance. Specialized programs for substance abuse and eating disorders similarly provide many services and family engagement programs.

Peer Involvement

Other modifications of established psychotherapies address the stated preferences and predilections of emerging adults to exclude parents; for example, the use of peers as "concerned significant others" instead of the more established use of family members has been shown to be promising in the treatment of substance use disorder (Smith et al. 2013) and in the treatment of serious mental illness (Aschbrenner and Brunette 2018). Such arrangements echo the positive experience of peer sponsorship in self-help organizations such as Alcoholics Anonymous and seem especially suited to the peer orientation of emerging adults.

Digital Enhancements

Given the time they spend on electronic devices (emerging adults spend 50% of their time connected to the internet) and their widespread ownership of smartphones (96% of 18- to 29-year-olds own smartphones) (Perrin 2021), emerging adults would seem the ideal population for using mental health apps. Indeed, there has been an explosion in mental health apps, but like many start-up internet phenomena, these programs have no oversight or regulation. A review of stand-alone apps with a specific focus on their use by adolescents and young adults (Leech et al. 2021) highlighted just how complicated it is to make a comparative analysis, given the diversity and idiosyncrasy of their approaches to disorders, inconsistency in age ranges in studies, frequency and overall duration of interventions, criteria for assessing distress, and variability of outcome measures. Most apps are based on "evidence based psychological principles and techniques, particularly cognitive behavior therapy and 'mindfulness'" (Leech et al. 2021, p. 4). Pooled data indicate improvement in depression and, importantly, no reported deterioration. Of note is that there is no Health Insurance Portability and Accountability Act (HIPAA) oversight, and privacy is frequently not maintained, which is a potential long-term complication. The reviewers concluded that the methodological problems involved in comparing apps in terms of their formats, their approaches, their underlying theory of illness (if any), and their assessments of improvement are staggering; further research is required. Evidence suggests that the presence of complex mental health conditions or comorbidities may benefit more from blended interventions, such as combined face-to-face and app-based support (Erbe et al. 2017), although randomized trials are still lacking. Although mental health apps are still a relatively new use of technology, they have nonetheless flooded the market (there at least 10,000 existing apps for mental health [Torous et al. 2018], and hundreds more appear daily). As noted, the apps are difficult to study, and therefore their efficacy is difficult to establish, but certain types of disorders, such as substance abuse and depression, appear to benefit from some of these programs.

But how does the clinician choose? Some professional organizations have developed evaluation methods to assess apps, to better guide practitioners on how to select from among them, to tailor them to supplement face-to-face treatment, or to make recommendations to patients who prefer that approach (Temkin et al. 2020). The American Psychiatric Association has one such model, a four-stage process assessing risk or privacy and safety, benefit and efficacy, engagement, and data sharing; the website dedicated to this project (www.psychiatry.org/psychiatrists/practice/mental-health-apps/app-evaluation-model) allows clinicians to post their assessments to aid others in the selection process, which essentially results in the creation of a curated library (Torous et al. 2018).

In addition to this proliferation of general mental health apps, other apps have been developed to aid in a particular treatment approach, presumably coordinated with the needs of mental health programs targeted at specific diagnoses, such as OCD, eating disorders, or substance abuse; some of these require clinician introduction and oversight. Some services focused on the treatment of a particular disorder, like a specified anxiety disorder, provide curated lists themselves (Temkin et al. 2020). They promote their value to patients and clinicians alike by monitoring symptoms, gathering behavioral data, and providing follow-up. These have seemed especially useful during the pandemic and in areas where access to services is severely limited. Pocket Skills, a mobile app designed to support DBT skills, comes with a conversational eMarsha (to represent the founder of DBT, Marsha Linehan) and has shown efficacy in helping participants maintain and improve skills (Schroeder et al. 2018). Similarly, a promising brief intervention for disadvantaged emerging adults recruited while visiting an emergency department used motivational interviewing to curb substance use and unsafe sex, with the embellishment of "mobile boosters" (i.e., daily messaging). A pilot study documented considerable user satisfaction, especially if the follow-up messaging was playful and not relentlessly drug related (Bonar et al. 2021). In general, digital apps are increasingly designed to supplement well-established evidence-based therapies by promoting skill practice and implementation with user-friendly notifications.

Evidence-Based Therapies Using Specific Strategies

Evidence-based psychotherapies, which arise from certain traditions in psychology and psychiatry, share many features despite having radically different theoretical underpinnings. For example, functional analytic psychotherapy was derived from Skinner's ideas; in contrast, DBT, which is an outgrowth of CBT, and transference-focused psychotherapy (TFP) arose as variations on psychoanalytic thinking. All these approaches include attention to distorted cognitions and to the repercussions of the latter in behavior. They use methods that document the automatic thinking patterns that are part of many disorders, identifying associated recurrent avoidance strategies that are often self-destructive or self-undermining. Each uses techniques ultimately intended to facilitate the patient's own recognition of disturbed thinking. These efforts may be supported by psychoeducation, meditation, practiced self-reflection, or mindfulness; all these approaches rely on the therapeutic relationship to highlight and address the deleterious effect of pathological patterns of thinking and behaving on expectations and communications in the here-and-now therapeutic relationship.

All these different methods include the enumeration of specific tasks that establish the agenda and parameters of the therapy. There is often a contractual arrangement arising from an extended consultation that seeks to establish an atmosphere of safety for both the therapist and the patient; intense emotions and reactions are welcome into discussion but must be verbalized rather than enacted. Because characteristic defensive behaviors resulting in isolation, avoidance, and passivity perpetuate paralysis, an important part of the guidelines is that constructive actions must be *initiated* to address the problems that arise in real time.

Some of these therapies can be combined with other interventions, including interactive mental health apps, psychodynamic therapies, and selected techniques from other behavioral therapies. Many evidence-based therapies began as treatments for a specific disorder but subsequently were found useful for treating others that share features, such as repetitive self-destructive behaviors, impulsivity, and susceptibility to panicky feelings. Current practice shows that the specific indications for given therapies have expanded, that diagnoses can be addressed by a range of approaches, and that combining techniques is effective (Reyes-Ortega et al. 2020).

Cognitive-Behavioral Therapy

CBT was first developed by Beck (1963, 1964) as a treatment for depression. It is based on the idea that many psychic states, such as depression and anxiety, are accompanied and perpetuated by problematic *information processing*. The tendency of depressed people to view events as evidence of personal flaws or failures traps them in a negative spiral of hopelessness and defeat. CBT does not offer hypotheses about the *origins* of the depressive mood, which is implicitly acknowledged to be the result of genetics, neurobiology, and other causes. The purview of CBT concerns the depressive cognitions that maintain depressive states (Wright et al. 2014). The depressed person consistently interprets events as negative, as reflections of inadequacy or moral turpitude, or as proof of personality defects. Many of these cognitions are *automatic* and not subject to logic or rational thinking. These include catastrophic thinking, arbitrary inferences, personalization, and selective abstraction that isolates single elements of an experience to draw a negative conclusion; all of these pathological cognitions serve to confirm the patient's worldview. The cognitive structures that take over are called *schemas*; they are established early in life and are relatively inaccessible to conscious thought but determine the way information is screened and processed; some of these schemas are relatively quiescent until triggered by an event or experience. Some examples pertinent to this population are "If I don't know what I want to do in life, then I am a loser" and "If I tell my parents that I am gay, then they will abandon me." Teaching the patient to monitor mental states and cognitions promotes self-awareness and a collaborative partnership between patient and therapist. The therapy follows a general plan in which the overall therapeutic agenda is determined at commencement, subject to regular modifications at the beginning of each session as more immediate agendas arise; psychoeducation is prominent.

The patient-clinician relationship is viewed as "collaborative empiricism," in which the therapist and patient work as an "investigative team" to identify these distorted cognitions and schemas (Wright et al. 2014, p. 1127).

In addition to addressing and correcting pathological cognitions in depression, CBT focuses on the behavioral component; behaviors and behavioral inhibitions associated with erroneous thinking are uncovered and countermanded by directives to resume formerly rewarding experiences that have been abandoned because of loss of motivation, pleasure, or aspiration. Often the process requires breaking down the activity into smaller pieces to provide the patient with a sense of accomplishment and positivity. This "behavioral activation"—the directed reengagement with activities of life—has intrinsic mood-elevating effects (Macrodimitris et al. 2010).

Within the category of CBT, exposure therapy is a demonstrably effective approach to treating phobias, OCD, and other fear-based disorders. According to proponents, this technique is underused because it elicits "exposophobia" (Schare and Wyatt 2013, p. 252, also quoted by Springer and Tolin 2020, p. 10) in clinicians—that is, clinicians fear making their patients worse. Practice in easing patients into addressing their phobic anxiety in slow increments can reduce therapists' reluctance, although follow-up refreshers are often required. In emerging adults, such a technique is used in programs intended to address the typical presenting complaint of feeling stuck; by parsing this state into a combination of social anxiety disorder, fear of failure, and other depressive cognitions, exposure therapy combined with standard CBT cognitive modifications has proved helpful. Even exposure therapy in which the feared object or behavior is complex, such as applying for a job or going to a campus event, has resulted in useful behavioral activation.

CBT's target population has now come to include anxiety disorders such as phobias, OCD and obsessive-compulsive traits, PTSD, suicidality, substance abuse, eating disorders, personality disorders, bipolar disorder, and psychosis. CBT is often conceptualized as adjunctive to other treatments, such as hospitalization, medication, and psychodynamic psychotherapies. Many of these disorders appear or mushroom in emerging adulthood. A supplemental course of CBT can provide momentum for psychoanalysis or a psychodynamic treatment when a symptom, such as paralyzing perfectionism or social anxiety disorder, results in widespread avoidance and isolation, thereby arresting forward movement.

Emotional Dysregulation Therapies

Personality disorders are conceptualized on a spectrum of severity in terms of mental organization and symptomatology. Recommendations emerge from careful assessment of anxiety level and affect tolerance, impulse control, identity cohesion, attachment anxiety, self-destructiveness (including sui-cidality), the capacity to form relationships, and the ability to self-reflect. Because late adolescence and emerging adulthood are times of peak suicide risk (Suicide Prevention Resource Center 2021), and because borderline personality disorder is often floridly expressed beginning in adolescence, treatments like DBT and TFP have special relevance to the emerging adult period.

Dialectical Behavior Therapy

DBT was created by Marsha Linehan in the context of her own misdiagno-sis with schizophrenia in adolescence and her inpatient experience. It is derived from cognitive-behavioral principles to treat parasuicidality (in-cluding any intentional self-injurious behavior, from cutting to suicide) and emotional dysregulation.

Linehan described DBT as principle based rather than solely manual-ized. Even in the most unexpected or extreme situations, the therapist can rely on one of three paradigms for interventions: the acceptance paradigm, the change paradigm, or the dialectical paradigm, wherein the tension be-tween acceptance and change is negotiated. These paradigms highlight the challenge of maintaining an accepting posture toward patients, however pessimistic and hostile, while continuing to develop strategies for change. Because work with borderline patients can easily lead to clinician burnout, when the therapist feels defeated by patients' resistance, their emotional lability, and their resorting to familiar maladaptive patterns, contractual agreements are central. In what is called "pretreatment," a careful assess-ment of the patient is followed by a series of steps that importantly include a psychoeducational component describing the therapy and what is expected of the patient and clinician in the process. The pretreatment sessions ideally result in the patient committing to the terms and agreeing to a treatment plan that identifies behavioral targets. One proponent, Swenson (2016), de-scribed this early conversation as a clarification of what makes "life worth living" (p. 7) in order to establish a shared agenda.

The classical structure of DBT includes skills training in a group set-ting, individual psychotherapy, telephone consultation, and therapist con-sultation team meetings (May et al. 2016). Skills training involves capacities that derive from Eastern meditation principles and work synergistically: these are core mindfulness, distress tolerance, interpersonal effectiveness, and emotional regulation. The telephone consultation component provides a resource for patients who are contemplating self-injurious behavior; the contractual agreement is that they must call their therapist before any ac-tion is taken. The consultation team meeting is a regularly planned discussion by all treatment providers of a given patient. Because of the value of DBT for treating suicidal patients, training modules are proliferating among psychiatric residency programs (Brodsky et al. 2017).

Transference-Focused Psychotherapy

Severe identity diffusion is considered an indication for a special type of therapy: TFP. This modality is derived from psychoanalytic theory and uses some of the same tools as psychoanalytic psychotherapy.

TFP aims to improve affect regulation, reduce impulsive behavior, and enhance interpersonal stability in individuals with borderline personality disorder. Achieving greater integration and cohesion of identity constitutes a major goal, because these patients typically demonstrate highly distorted, rigid, and inconsistent internal representations of the self (Jørgensen 2010; Yeomans et al. 2017). Within this treatment model, the therapeutic relationship serves as the main vehicle for effecting change: patient-clinician interactions, as they unfold in the here and now, are explicated to help make connections between behavior and internal states; promote self-observation and reflection; and elucidate deeply held (often unconscious) beliefs, expectations, and fantasies about the self and others (Normandin et al. 2015; Yeomans et al. 2017).

In the past few years, the TFP approach has been modified to serve adolescent patients, the cohort in which borderline psychopathology is often first diagnosed (for our discussion of personality disorders in this age group, see Chapter 7). Indeed, relatively early intervention—during the teens or early 20s when symptoms, behaviors, and relational difficulties begin to cohere into a recognizable pattern of personality disorder—is considered foundational to a good adult outcome because of this condition's potential disruption to wide swaths of personal and professional life (Normandin et al. 2015). TFP for adolescents takes into account the young person's ongoing brain maturation and ego development and their interface with the pressures of age-salient developmental tasks; separation from family, increased responsibility for the self, deepening capacities for intimate relationships, and the establishment of personal identity are considered major achievements that are made more difficult to negotiate by the borderline adolescent's impulsivity, fragile self-esteem, poor emotional self-control, and difficulty sustaining stable interpersonal bonds (Ammaniti et al. 2015; Ensink et al. 2015; Normandin et al. 2015). In our view, the latter two tasks—developing deepening relationships and establishing identity coherence—are best conceptualized as ongoing processes that usually begin during the late teens and early 20s, as the emerging adult explores multiple aspects of self and identity, including gender, sexuality, and social roles. Our approach to diagnosing identity and relational impairments in these co-horts is cautious, as described in Chapter 5 ("Identity in Emerging Adult-hood") and Chapter 7, because clinical presentations are heavily influenced by the young person's normative immersion in experimentation and flux, which often leads to inconsistent and even chaotic-seeming behaviors.

Clinicians who use TFP for adolescents conduct structural diagnostic interviews to determine the young patient's level of personality organiza-tion; a close evaluation of identity (i.e., an adaptable but coherent sense of self vs. identity diffusion), reliance on primitive defenses (such as splitting and denial), and capacity for reality testing are seen as foundational for the diagnosis of borderline pathology. The borderline emerging adult often lacks coherent strategies for emotional self-control and tends toward po-tentially destructive behavioral outlets (drug use, self-harm) in order to ob-tain affective relief in the short term (Normandin et al. 2015). Etiologies and antecedents of borderline pathology are complex, involving an inter-play among biologically based temperamental factors, environmental chal-lenges, trauma, and deficits in the areas of attention-based control and mentalization; these vulnerabilities create obstacles not only for the young person's ability to meet age expectations but also for the treatment itself. The clinician may set limits, including creating specific contracts for safety, to help manage impulsivity, suicidality, or other forms of risk behaviors (Normandin et al. 2015).

Psychoanalytically Informed Treatments

The Mind According to Psychoanalytic Theory

Psychoanalysis and its various psychotherapeutic offshoots are informed by a basic orientation toward the mind and by a set of conceptualizations and principles that guide clinical work. There are significant disagreements among the many schools of psychoanalysis extant in North America and across the globe in terms of the way the mind develops and the relative im-portance of intrapsychic components and the interpersonal world, but these schools are united by foundational ideas (for an in-depth exploration of these ideas, see Auchincloss 2015). Most psychoanalytic theories include some version of the following ideas:

1. Mental life is both *conscious* and *unconscious*. Although there are several types of unconscious, such as in procedural memories like the capacity to ride a bicycle, the unconscious mind of interest to psychoanalysis is the *dynamic unconscious*. This unconscious is the repository of forbidden wishes, drives, and aspects of the self held out of awareness by *defenses*, including *repres-*

sion, splitting, and dissociation. Elements of unconscious content can be glimpsed in dream content, slips of the tongue, parapraxes, and "forgetting" (e.g., forgetting an important event like an anniversary).

2. *Signs and symptoms* reflect the dynamic conflict among drives, impulses, and wishes; the superego, which regulates self-esteem and guilt; and the ego, which defends against outward expression. Elucidating a patient's defenses provides important information for the clinician; defensive organization is directly linked to diagnosis and assessment of personality structure. Although diagnostic considerations are an important part of assessment, medication recommendations, and management, the psychoanalytically informed clinician looks beyond diagnosis and views signs, symptoms, and the associated defenses as meaningful representations of ego organization and ego strength, clues to central organizing unconscious fantasy, and guideposts to core conflicts and trauma. The exploration of the content of conflicts that elicit defenses and, from a different angle, the effect of the defenses on thinking (Busch 2013) are both part of the work of psychotherapy. And because consultation can immediately elicit defensiveness because of the fantasied threat it poses, defenses are often the first indication of how a given patient's mind works.

3. Signs, symptoms, and personality organization are also shaped by *constitutional endowment, interpersonal experience, trauma,* and myriad other factors that impinge on individual ontogenesis. Many of these interfacing systems may come under scrutiny in psychodynamic treatment, which alleviates some of their deleterious impact. However, some aspects of endowment and trauma may ultimately be understood as irreducible factors that must be grappled with but cannot be fully dissolved.

4. The relationship that develops between patient and clinician is a fundamental tool of treatment because it becomes the premier source of knowledge not only about the patient's interpersonal world but also about unconscious fantasy. Most contemporary thinkers carefully consider the patient's and the therapist's subjectivities as they emerge in the relationship, because they provide invaluable information about the patient's mental life. The ever-changing and evolving constellation of *transference and countertransference* is viewed as the here-and-now context in which many characteristic and long-standing drives, defenses, attitudes, and fantasies emerge with an immediacy that makes them especially accessible to interpretive work and self-understanding. Both patients and therapists must collaborate to address conflicts or feelings that arise, mistakes that occur, and, importantly, pressures to enact these in the actual relationship.

5. *Enactments* are powerful re-creations of interpersonal conflicts that draw in both patient and therapist and their unconscious fantasies and feelings; these fantasies and feelings are then *enacted* in the relationship. Because of

the "evocative coercive power" of the transference-countertransference relationship, both parties feel like they are responding to the actions of the other (McLaughlin 1991, p. 598). Interpersonal theorists argue that enactments are the fundamental raw material of the analytic work, in which patient and therapist participate, and these enactments provide clues to the "unthought known" (Bollas 1987) in both parties. The clinician's capacity to see and reflect on these cocreations and to help the patient understand them is often crucial to the success of the treatment. Historically, psychoanalytically oriented treatments were said to rely on verbalization to achieve insight (Grand 1995), but enactments have achieved important therapeutic status as the nonverbal illuminations of conflicts in and between analyst and patient that can then be understood with words.

6. In addition, *insightfulness*, a term introduced by Sugarman (2006, p. 98), is an acquired suite of mental processes that includes the capacity to self-reflect, mentalize (i.e., apply theory of mind), and develop intersubjective awareness. Sugarman describes insightfulness as the stable ability to mentalize and reflect on one's own mental functions, which develops in early childhood and can be cultivated in treatment; it is essential to analytic work with all age groups. This idea brings together the artificially separated roles of interpretation and the patient-analyst relationship in achieving change.

7. Psychoanalytic approaches benefit from a *developmental perspective* that recognizes that personality evolution begins to emerge at birth, with the first exchange with the caregiver, and that ego capacities and the resulting defenses emerge in a sequence that depends on biological maturation as well as environmental nurturance and stimulation. A culturally dictated, uniform set of expected milestones and progressions in ego capacities, established by the environment and mediated by caregivers, work in concert with biological maturation to lead the infant through childhood and the myriad requirements, demands, and constraints of socioeconomic, environmental, cultural, and familial conditions. As developmental psychoanalysts, we are always interested in the interplay of developmental processes, mental conflict, environmental provision, and the culture at large; we are prepared to modify our methodology to facilitate the optimal therapeutic conditions for the exploration of the mind of the person before us. This developmental orientation is an important lens for viewing emerging adults, because they are in a period of active development.

It is *usually* true that the population actively seeking individual psychodynamic treatment, especially in a climate in which there are many structured, time-limited approaches, is self-selected and usually more familiar with the benefits of talk therapy from their families, experience, or reading. Some of this group, once they begin psychodynamic therapy, develop a growing appreciation for the greater self-reflective capacity and insight they develop through this modality and for their ability to see conflicts in others and their own interpersonal foibles; because of their newly achieved self-reflection and insightfulness, they are often the go-to person for friends in distress and thereby serve as an unofficial mental health first aid counselor.

Given the aforementioned principles as backdrop, we now describe basic features of the clinical orientation that grew from this model and then delineate the principles of the technique and the specific challenges posed by treating this age group. Importantly, our view is informed by the recognition that development and psychological conflict remain entwined throughout this period, in contrast to the view that developmental issues have diminished in the 20s in concert with the waning biological driver (Gilmore 2019). The gains achieved through psychoanalysis and psychodynamic psychotherapy not only maximize the efficacy of auxiliary therapies such as medication and specific focused interventions such as TFP, CBT, or DBT (Plakun 2012) but also improve adaptation and resilience in adulthood. This is because such treatments result in the enhancement of enduring mental capacities such as self-awareness, theory of mind, introspection informed by gradual recognition of defensive operations and warded-off affects, and the capacity for self-regulation.

The Therapist's Orientation

A Way of Looking

Psychoanalysis is, as Erikson (1950, 1995) simply stated, "a way of looking at things." This way is informed by the idea that feelings and behavior have meaning and can be gradually understood through the process of self-reflection. It does not insist that every behavior or feeling has an etiology traceable to or entirely determined by psychological causes. It does not attempt to offer a simple answer as to *why* a person has this or that problem or trait but rather *how* that person came to be that way. This reflects a nonlinear systems view of development and mental life: we identify contributions, not singular causes. It also reflects the principle of *multiple function*—any one trait or symptom can simultaneously serve as a solution or way of managing a range of internal conflicts; over the course of development, solutions are repurposed and elaborated to serve current needs.

The guiding principle is that the mind makes meanings and psychological content by recruiting elements of biological endowment (including physical features, talents, drive, cognitive potential, and other givens), the provisions afforded by the interpersonal world, and personal history and experience for purposes of managing conflicts, securing attachments, and experiencing pleasure (Abrams 1990). Early experience plays an outsize role in shaping object relations and fundamental attitudes toward others; this does not preclude the powerful effect of subsequent experience and trauma, nor does it minimize the information and therapeutic power of the here and now.

A Way of Listening

Psychoanalysis and related psychotherapies are also informed by a particular way of listening (Arlow 1995), because these treatments are, in large part, verbal discourse—the analyst listens for hidden meanings, feelings, narratives, connections, and omissions in the patient's verbal production. In the early stages of assessment, listening is more comprehensive than the search for meanings, because it may include history-taking and diagnostic assessment. An important part of the psychoanalytically oriented assessment is evaluating the patient's potential to do the work of treatment—that is, ego strength, reality testing, self-reflectiveness, rigidity of defenses, interest in the mind, and recognition that therapy may lead to confrontation with unwanted parts of the self. Most of these capacities are in nascent form or exist as potentials because they are developed or augmented in the course of treatment. The therapist listens to determine the severity of illness; to assess character pathology; to note the intrusion of conflict; to see defenses in operation; to assess ego capacities; to observe relationships (both by description and by the early emergence in the transference of ways of being with and experiencing the other); and to explore theories of why and for what help is needed, how it came to be this way, what has led to the decision to take action at this moment in time, and what hopes for improvement are brought into the consulting room.

In order to propose psychodynamic treatment to a patient, the therapist may have to clarify its open-ended structure and preferred modality of *free association*. Suggesting that the patient say whatever comes to mind derives from the idea that how a person approaches the process, the way and the order in which leading conflicts and worries emerge, and the degree to which interferences arise in the patient's thinking and narrative are crucial clues about the personality and the course of treatment. As treatment gets underway, this other, more open-ended way of listening enters into the relationship. This way of listening is attuned to the discovery of hidden themes, meaningful connections, and observations of defenses in action.

Early in the development of psychoanalytic technique, the fundamental rules of *abstinence*, *neutrality*, and *anonymity* were presented as the achievable and desirable analytic attitudes in listening, but contemporary theorists recognize that these are impossible and even distracting standards. No therapist or psychoanalyst can completely suspend their own biases or opinions, reveal nothing about themselves, or abstain from all action. Therapists bring their subjectivity and values to every treatment they participate in; what is essential is that therapists know themselves, can self-reflect, and recognize their subjectivity operating in every clinical interaction. Coordinated self- and patient observation is essential and provides yet another level of understanding. Some adolescent theorists suggest that maintaining these standards simply as ideals alerts the therapist to the particular challenges that emerging adults bring to the relationship (Chused 1990).

Assessment and Induction of Psychodynamic Treatment With Emerging Adults

What are the specific considerations in recommending psychodynamic treatment to emerging adults? It is rare in our contemporary society for a young patient to consult with a psychodynamic psychotherapist with a clear intention of pursuing psychoanalysis. Most patients, especially those with no previous treatment, are unfamiliar with the demands and duration of this form of therapy and unclear why and how it works. They present their complaints and symptoms with little awareness of their meaning, how they fit into the narrative arc in their life story, or their current use as compromise formations that have maintained stability until now. The psychoanalytic therapist must be discriminating and assess the patient carefully for this type of treatment. The therapist also needs to engage the patient in work that may seem meandering and peripheral to the presenting complaint.

Suitability

When assessing a patient, the clinician keeps in mind a series of questions about the severity of the patient's disorder; the nature of preferred defenses; and the presence of certain ego capacities, including the potential for self-reflection, theory of mind, attachment, and the willingness to commit to a lengthy treatment. In regard to diagnostic issues, the presence of florid psychosis is, almost without exception, a contraindication for intensive exploratory treatment without lengthy stabilization. Severe and acute illnesses usually require ego support or ego bolstering and may need pragmatic interventions. They often benefit from medication, which does not, in itself, preclude intensive treatment in nonpsychotic disorders. Patients with moderately severe mood disorders may be treatable analytically, optimally when euthymic. In patients with a dual diagnosis, the substance use component may prohibit psychodynamic treatment when it is the preeminent focus of the patient, dwarfing other conflicts and anxieties. Beyond these major contraindications, others may rule out this type of treatment or require that it be a collaborative endeavor with other specialties. For example, patients with eating disorders, trichotillomania, OCD, and similar disorders may benefit from a course of CBT simultaneously or in series with psychodynamic treatment.

As noted earlier in the subsection "A Way of Looking," psychoanalysis is a way of looking at things and a way of seeing them (Erikson 1950, 1995) that searches for meaning and motives in the patient's struggles, seeks to uncover and integrate unacceptable parts of the self, and seeks to facilitate the patient's self-reflection. The therapist listens (Arlow 1995) for underlying conflicts, themes, and meanings of which the patient is not fully aware. To introduce patients to this way of seeing and listening to things, the clinician may determine that with certain patients, perhaps especially emerging adult patients, some form of psychoeducation may be necessary. The lack of familiarity with dynamic thinking and treatments may render the recommendation for frequent sessions frightening, as if it implies severe mental illness. The central importance of work in the transference may be similarly experienced as threatening. It is often helpful to point out that the patient's feelings toward the psychotherapist provide important clues for understanding the patient's interpersonal conflicts in relationships in general. Similarly, tentative interpretations or links can be offered to spark a patient's interest in the presence of unconscious motives, meanings, and conflicts; the narrative arc of such meanings over the patient's personal history; and the operation of characteristic defenses that hamper their awareness. There may be the barest glimmers of readiness to grapple with this way of thinking; whether patients gather momentum is the critical question.

Thus, in the course of assessing suitability, therapists inevitably make comments that amount to trial interpretations; they offer observations of links among thoughts, emotions, actions, experience, and relationships that are intended both to show the value of their nascent understanding of the patient's life story and to determine whether the patient can reflect on such links, clarify or correct them, and make some use of them. The patient who summarily dismisses these forays into interpretive work may benefit from another attempt at engagement, embedded in a clarification about the importance of making links that give meaning and coherence to the patient's story. This then provides a further opportunity to assess receptivity to the psychoanalytic orientation and readiness to make use of this way of seeing and hearing things.

The following vignette shows the degree to which the first and sometimes even the second impression of a patient's accessibility may be misleading; in this case, the patient's openness and enthusiasm while setting the first appointment led his potential therapist to be optimistic about his receptiveness to psychoanalytically oriented psychotherapy or psychoanalysis. A few other positive indications were identified in this first phone call: Diego, age 28, was a graduate student in neuroscience from a family full of psychoanalysts, psychiatrists, and psychologists; he had had a positive experience in a brief dynamic treatment in college; and he described his desire to pursue treatment now in terms of unresolved issues in his career and his love life. Diego enthusiastically announced his desire to do "talk therapy"; he noted that the referral source had assured him that Dr. D was an excellent choice for this type of treatment. This introduction did not prepare Dr. D for their first meeting.

Case Vignette: Diego

Diego arrived early for the scheduled appointment. When Dr. D opened the door to the waiting room to greet him, he was surprised to see Diego, casually dressed in jeans and lugging a backpack, looking disgruntled and unfriendly. Diego did not make eye contact, did not accept Dr. D's outstretched hand to shake, and momentarily hesitated when entering the office. Without any familiarity with this patient to guide him, Dr. D was puzzled and unable to orient himself. He mentally scrolled through the little he knew about Diego and juxtaposed that with the typical reaction the office and waiting room elicited, especially in young people. Dr. D rented the space from a revered senior colleague whose elegance and affluence were legendary in the psychoanalytic community. He guessed, rightly as it became clear, that Diego was responding adversely to the well-appointed office and the prestigious location. Dr. D also wondered what Diego might have discovered by googling him (an action almost inevitable in this population), because a book of essays about training that Dr. D had edited had been recently published to considerable acclaim even in the lay press. Dr. D felt that he had to address Diego's demeanor to clear the air and hopefully arrest what already looked like a negative transference reaction. He observed aloud his impression that Diego was uncomfortable; he wondered if there was something on his mind that had caused his initial enthusiasm to transform so abruptly. Diego responded with a barrage of critiques of the neighborhood and the office, of Dr. D's accomplishments, and of his curriculum vitae. Although Dr. D understood this as defensive reaction, it was sufficiently cutting and derisive that he was taken aback; he feared that, given both his and Diego's state of mind, anything approaching an interpretation of Diego's defensiveness would likely exacerbate it.

Dr. D tried to listen to Diego's diatribe uninterrupted for a while, doing his best to be open to details to see what he could learn about Diego from his reaction. There were many references to Dr. D's apparent investment in the superficial trappings of success and money and his apparent acceptance of the established hierarchy and traditional values, as further shown by the "lightweight" book that he had edited. Dr. D was aware that he was himself feeling irritated, even insulted. His own defensiveness mirrored Diego's state of mind. He chose the first opening to say that he got the feeling that

Diego was disappointed and that he must have been expecting something very different. Diego nodded but continued unabated. As the session wore on, Dr. D ventured to suggest that Diego seemed annoyed, even scornful, of things he viewed as showy displays of elite status and affirmation of the status quo. Diego was equally scornful of this "obvious" inference. Before the session ended, Dr. D entertained the idea of referring Diego elsewhere, but he waited to see if Diego requested another visit, which he did.

Dr. D thought that this first appointment with Diego was distinctly unpromising. He felt worn out by absorbing insults and was discouraged by Diego's unwillingness to reflect on his apparently reflexive stance of hostile defensiveness. Dr. D reminded himself that this was the very first encounter, that he knew very little about Diego's personal experience or conflicts. He thought it was worth pursuing the assessment further, in part persuaded by Diego's spontaneous request for a second meeting: perhaps this was a glimmer of recognition that his reaction was problematic.

In the second appointment, Diego said that he had thought a lot about his scorn; it reminded him of the atmosphere between him and his father in high school when the latter expected him to "shape up," apply himself, and earn A's. Dr. D also learned that Diego's parents had split up at the end of his junior year in high school when infidelity on the father's part came to light. The family's socioeconomic status suffered when the father departed, because he was "shockingly stingy" in the financial arrangements, even though he was a very wealthy man.

Because the atmosphere in the session was less hostile, Dr. D decided he might gently suggest that Diego had given him a taste of what it was like to feel belittled and vaguely threatened with rejection—both of these reactions seemed related to Diego's own adolescent experience. Diego's apparent willingness to hear Dr. D's reaction was especially encouraging. Indeed, over the course of the next several months, Diego said that he thought a lot about what Dr. D said about Diego's "rant." He spontaneously connected it to problems with his boyfriend and with his boss; he observed that in both relationships, the urge to disparage was irresistible when he felt even mildly criticized or outdone.

This vignette highlights how any aspect of the treatment situation—the office, the neighborhood, the appearance of the therapist, and sometimes undisclosed online research—can influence the patient's feelings about the clinician sight unseen and set the stage for transference reactions in the very first meeting. These can be based on any number of factors, including object representations established in childhood or the patient's sociopolitical viewpoint about the establishment or conventional values. Such preconceptions can coalesce into transference configurations well before the patient enters the office, when the therapist is likely entirely unfamiliar with the patient's story. In this case, Dr. D took a chance in disclosing how Diego's behavior made him (the therapist) feel. Depending on their level of object relatedness, some patients experience such a response as a shift of focus, a narcissistic attack, or defeated acknowledgment of the correctness of the critique. Instead, Diego became thoughtful and made connections—a promising indication of his openness to psychoanalytic thinking.

This vignette also highlights an important feature of this age group: they respond best to a frank conversation rather than one in which the therapist relies on a professional stance. They want to see the person inhabiting the role and want the therapist to be a sincere participant.

Induction

Even when trial interpretations are well received and the therapist has gathered sufficient information to confidently suggest a psychodynamic treatment, some patients may desire a discussion of other modalities, such as CBT, to understand their potential as alternatives or supplements to the psychodynamic process. Laying out the advantages and disadvantages of the recommended therapy and explaining alternatives underscore the therapist's concern for the patient's well-being and freedom of choice. This is especially important for therapists with a training objective, such as residents and analytic candidates; often the educational and clinical goals can both be met, but the patient's needs and readiness may conflict with the educational opportunity for the trainee. A review of the rationales for each, reasonable expectations of change, and what is required of the patient in terms of participation in a range of therapies is usually helpful.

The Course of Treatment With Emerging Adults: Does the List of Five Features Help?

The emerging adult population presents with specific challenges for treatment. Although Arnett's five features—role or identity exploration, instability, feeling in-between, self-focus, and wide-open possibilities—do not fully capture the developmental experience, they do serve as useful descriptors of emerging adults' behavior, preoccupations, and circumstances. They can also alert the clinician to common disruptions in the therapy of this cohort.

Feeling in-between refers to emerging adults' experience of being neither adolescent nor adult. The subjective uncertainty of status often heightens the insistence on autonomy from parental influence. When that position generalizes to other adults, it may interfere with establishing and sustaining a treatment relationship; intensive therapy invokes childhood feelings, including dependency, passivity, and the range of attachment styles. Moreover, it may require further reliance on parents because of the need for financial support. Even in colleges and universities where mental health services may be free and available, individual therapy is usually limited to a certain number of sessions. Individuals who require further psychotherapy are typically referred elsewhere, requiring out-of-pocket or insurance payment, both of which are usually dependent on parents. Although some parents are knowledgeable and respectful of the privacy of the therapeutic relationship, others intrude—through entitled demands for regular phone contact or meetings. Managing these intrusions challenges the clinician to maintain therapist-patient confidentiality, thereby setting limits on information sharing without alienating parents and without alarming the patient. If the emerging adult patient becomes suspicious of parent-therapist collusion, wariness and secrecy may contaminate the treatment.

The state of feeling in-between teenager and adult can make some emerging adults sensitive to adults telling them what to do or treating them like kids. They may chafe when a therapist tries too hard to be cool or even when the therapist maintains a nonjudgmental, neutral position that can be construed as lofty and condescending. Some typical enactments of this age group involve attempts to provoke the therapist. In Diego's case, his immediate stance of hostile disparagement was an attempt to engage Dr. D in his version of father-son conflict. Other examples include reports of flagrant defiance of rules in order to elicit authoritarian disapproval (Chused 1990), which paradoxically reasserts the parent-child dynamic. For example, the patient may describe a violation of institutional rules, including drug use on campus, cheating, stealing, destroying property, or violations of guidelines governing COVID-19 precautions and testing. Whether patients offer these "confessions" sheepishly or gleefully, they reveal their ambivalence about autonomy and responsibility, baiting the therapist to become the authority who reprimands or controls. Work in the transference-countertransference relationship can clarify the adolescent provocation in the behavior, which unconsciously places the onus for responsible decision-making on the grownups. Gradually the patient may be able to observe this dynamic as it unfolds and forgo the urge to force that response (Strenger 2004), instead working with the therapist on internal conflict around becoming an adult.

In instances like these, the concept of neutrality serves as a beacon to orient the clinician, who is inevitably drawn into enactments. This is equally true of enactments that are not explicitly about rule violations but tap into therapists' parental feelings or personal regrets about their own adolescent violations. In the following vignette, the therapist, Dr. T, lost her inquiring stance and struggled to regain neutrality when her late adolescent patient was increasingly impulsive and potentially self-damaging in the public space of a university chat room.

Case Vignette: Jessica

Jessica had been about to start college when the COVID-19 crisis struck; she elected to do a gap year at home rather than begin her much anticipated college experience off campus and online. At age 19, she had finally arrived in person to start her "real" campus life. She and her boyfriend of 3 years, Alan, had talked during their shared gap year about how they would handle the upcoming separation when they went to their separate colleges: they considered trying long distance (requiring a 4-hour car trip) or breaking up "by decree." They agreed to stay together, although in retrospect, Jessica acknowledged her growing awareness that Alan was ambivalent. Within 3 weeks of starting college, Alan texted to say that he wanted to end their relationship. Jessica was surprised and hurt by the announcement; after it sank in, she became enraged by Alan's poor timing and need to rush something that, she insisted, they both knew would have occurred "naturally" without drama. Most hurtful was the fact that Alan refused to participate in further discussion; he said that he just wanted to make a clean break.

Jessica had already been in twice-weekly therapy with Dr. T for several years, months before the relationship with Alan had begun. Treatment was initiated by her parents because they thought that she seemed less mature at age 14—less interested in parties, romance, makeup, and fashion—than her peers. In early middle school, she had been an all-around popular kid— a good athlete, good student, and nice person. However, her mother observed that, as she approached high school, Jess was increasingly left out of some "important" insider gossip and parties. Some of Jessica's former friends were beginning to hang out with the boys, wear makeup, and dress "sexy." Although her mother greatly preferred Jessica's sporty and modest demeanor, she was concerned that Jess was getting a reputation as a "dork" and was being seen by her classmates as immature. Jessica herself claimed not to care; she was dedicated to sports and to doing well at school; she happily spent her weekends with her family.

Dr. T, a psychiatrist and psychoanalyst in her late 30s, remembered well her own social awkwardness in middle school, high school, and college, something she finally overcame when she started therapy during medical school. She recognized that she approached Jessica's case as if she already understood her new patient via her own experience and knew that she had to be careful about overidentifying with her. When Dr. T met Jessica, this identification was immediately modulated by Jessica's lack of introspection; Dr. T was surprised to discover how little access Jessica had to her thoughts and feelings. Dr. T hypothesized that this obliviousness was another manifestation of Jessica's naivete and innocence. Jessica became somewhat more open in the consultation period and took up a few ideas Dr. T offered; she began to recognize instances of her denial of emotion and her defensive deployment of smiles and laughter to cover distress or anger. This insight, however small, suggested to Dr. T that Jessica had promise as a psychotherapy patient: she seemed eager to talk about the events in her life; she was always offering her dreams for discussion; and her pleasure in learning of all kinds was genuine, despite the excessive focus on grades. Jessica's sexuality was initially impossible to assess, because she acknowledged no interest in either gender, no flirtations, and remarkably little fantasy.

However, a "bonding" trip at the end of ninth grade abruptly changed that picture. Jessica reported that, on this 3-day trip, she immediately started spending time with Alan, who had just entered their school at the beginning of high school. She said that she "had seen him around" and knew his reputation because he was also an athlete and a good student. But now there was an upsurge of interest and excitement; she said it was "love at first sight." Their relationship blossomed and became serious in a matter of months. Jessica rapidly transformed into a young woman with a sex life who was impatient with her uptight parents; she was determined to get birth control pills without consulting her mother and was willing to lie to get private time with Alan. Alan was only slightly more experienced but was very motivated to advance their intimacy; luckily his affection for Jessica matched his sexual desire. He even declared his wish to marry her someday. Jessica's confiding and open relationship with her mother suddenly went silent, to the dismay of both parents. Their former relaxed attitude about her social life shifted to outright prohibition of private time with Alan; they were convinced that it was Alan who wanted to move fast sexually and that he was pressuring Jessica. With growing evidence of Alan's devotion over the course of the next months plus numerous shouting matches with Jessica about her right to have a private life, her parents accepted the reality that the young couple was as deeply attached as they were sexual.

As the work progressed into her COVID-19 gap year, Dr. T saw the multiple arenas in which Jessica's prior innocence was still evident; despite her sexual awakening, she was naively gullible and seemed to lack the street smarts typical of a city girl. There were numerous examples of Jessica's childlike trust of older men who approached her in the park suggesting that they "be running buddies" or meet after dark to play night Frisbee. Awkward moments regularly ensued when Jessica eventually recognized the come-on and resorted to avoidance and hiding to discourage unwanted advances. Dr. T better understood from these examples how her parents might have concluded that Alan pressured and Jessica gave in; the pattern of submission to a "nice" approach with a not-so-subtle sexual motive was ongoing. Dr. T also became aware of other facets of Jessica's "sneaky side." For example, in her weekly job as babysitter, Jessica was intent on getting around what she saw as parents' unfair rules in order to gratify her young charges with forbidden toys, bubblegum, and chocolate.

A new manifestation of these conflicting tendencies emerged in Jessica's gap year when she got an internship at a financial institution. During orientation, she was oblivious to flirtations and sexual interest from her fellow trainees; lacking caution in regard to these approaches made it difficult for her to reassert her boundaries. At the same time, her intolerance of her investment bank's infamous "toxic masculinity" led to some "talking back" to her superiors that bordered on unprofessional and hot-headed. Dr. T worked hard to engage Jessica's reflections around these complexities. When Dr. T pointed something out, Jessica often used giddy excitement to deny that anything serious or meaningful was being enacted. Dr. T's efforts to move her toward introspection met with increasing resistance, because by Jessica's description, Dr. T was "beginning to sound just like my mother."

Nonetheless, Jessica had asked to keep meeting with Dr. T remotely; this was an immediate source of comfort when the relationship with Alan ended. After his breakup text message, Alan blocked her on all social media "in order to make a clean break." Jessica's reaction revealed the kaleidoscope of emotions familiar to Dr. T; she rapidly cycled through hurt and grief, rage and retaliatory fantasies, giddy laughter, and an urgent need to replace Alan. Dr. T noted with some concern that Jessica seemed driven to engage in casual hookups with anyone showing interest. This concern was heightened when Jessica described her plan to get even with Alan by asking a mutual friend at his college to denounce him in the school's "anonymous" chat room, accusing him of pressuring girls sexually in high school and then abruptly dropping them. Dr. T heard this plan with some alarm; she was not only uneasy about Jessica's plan to wreak vengeance on Alan but also worried that Jess might be easily identified as the jilted and vindictive lover who lacked self-control. Jessica's status in her new college peer group and her chance to have a fresh start might be derailed by the indiscriminate hookups and/or the revenge tactics, labeling her as out of control and aggressive. Dr. T departed from her stance as a listening and inquiring presence; she told Jessica that she was managing the pain of loss though vengeful action and not giving herself the chance to mourn. These comments had the distressing effect of rendering Jessica silent, after which she announced, "I know you are right, but I am still going to do it."

Dr. T took a step back and did some reflection of her own. She realized that she was feeling too concerned about Jessica making a misstep that, in Dr. T's mind, could color her whole college experience and maybe even get her into serious trouble; Dr. T was not familiar with the technology of this anonymous chat room, which she suspected was, at the very least, closely monitored by the college. Dr. T further reflected that she did not fully understand the complexity of her own response to Jessica and had passed up the opportunity to explore Jessica's revenge fantasy. Dr. T talked over her countertransference reaction in her own supervision and came away with a better understanding of how she both identified with and was angry at Jessica's juvenile behavior. She saw "saving her" as a means of redeeming the treatment and undoing some of her own missteps and mistakes during her college years. Dr. T also became aware that she was now fully identified with Jessica's parents' attempts to rein her in. These observations allowed Dr. T to restore a reasonable degree of neutrality, sufficient to appreciate the intense distress that was covered over by Jessica's false sense of omnipotence and her gleeful affect around her revenge plan. She was relieved when Jessica announced at the beginning of their next session that she had not followed through on her impulse; although still struggling with it, she was more open to exploring it.

This vignette illustrates that neutrality is an ideal that is impossible to sustain in pure form in practice, especially with the younger emerging adult population. Because these late adolescents feel and act in-between, many of their defenses are at least initially not verbalized but rather enacted—for example, in partying and defying adults. Provocation is often part of the enactment, requiring the therapist to think carefully about departures from neutrality as intense feelings and reactions get stirred up by the patient. Exploring her own participation in the enactment unfolding in the transference and countertransference ultimately allowed Dr. T to analyze the process with the patient.

The vignette also shows that the term *feeling in-between* does not do justice to the complicated state that it so names. For the early emerging adult, mastering the challenge of forgoing the role of provocateur or passive adolescent and moving toward the consistent self-determination of imminent adulthood is not a smooth or steady process. This vacillation is one type of *instability*, a feature that characterizes emerging adults in many arenas—intrapsychic, interpersonal, and geographic. Identity and sense of self are in flux, plans are unformulated or subject to frequent change, and geographic moves can be sudden and impulsive. (Both moving from and returning to family homes were widespread among many age groups during the COVID-19 pandemic—see Chapter 4, "What Is Distinct About the Second Part of Emerging Adulthood?") Instability is associated with many typical behavioral phenomena, such as boomeranging, dropping in and out of college, changing jobs frequently, and postponing relationship commitments. In this climate, flexibility on the part of the clinician may be essential to sustaining a treatment, even though continuity is foundational to this modality and in-person sessions are especially beneficial. Indeed, in the context of instability in so many facets of life, regular sessions, if achievable, can serve to anchor the young person and provide consistency; nonetheless, insistence on a traditional format can devolve into a power struggle when the emerging adult's current circumstances (or need to assert autonomy) make it too difficult. These realities must figure into recommendations for treatment (Jacobs and Chused 1987). For example, in consultation with a highly suitable emerging adult who may be moving across the country, the clinician can recommend psychodynamic treatment of the appropriate frequency as the ideal treatment choice, acknowledging that treatment may have to wait until the patient relocates (or decides to stay put). Given that instability may persist over a decade, it is sometimes advisable to offer an alternative format; engaging the patient in a modified psychodynamic therapy may boost the interest and commitment necessary for intensive treatment at a later date. A clinician's flexibility and patience can gradually facilitate the desired format, even if it happens elsewhere.

In addition to adolescent and adult fluctuations, other forms of developmental instability may figure into treatment recommendations. Narcissistic self-preoccupation, a typical component of late adolescent development, is now designated as another typical feature of emerging adults, termed *self-focus*. This may temporarily interfere with sustaining an intensive treatment (Adatto 1966; Blos 1962), because a workable transference does not readily develop. Can self-focus be distinguished from the more ominous form of narcissism characteristic of borderline personality disorder? We believe that the type of self-focus common in emerging adults constitutes a different, developmental type of narcissism, in which self-focus reflects the degree to which the task of forming an identity and establishing a workable sense of self consumes mental life. This distinction has been challenged by other observers, such as Jean Twenge, who debated Jeffrey Arnett in the first issue of the journal *Emerging Adulthood* (Arnett 2013): Twenge argued that *self-focus* is simply a euphemism for *narcissism* and that narcissistic pathology and its deleterious consequences have increased dramatically in this age group. Arnett argued that self-focus is a developmental phenomenon, more in line with psychoanalytic thinking that recognizes the prolonged preoccupation of emerging adults with their identities and the psychosocial moratorium society provides for identity exploration. Furthermore, to the extent that grandiosity is evident, it is often harnessed to serve a noble purpose (Bronk 2012) and to propel young people to action (e.g., Greta Thunberg as an environmental activist or Emma Gonzalez as a survivor of the Parkland, Florida, shooting and an impassioned advocate for gun control).

There are other arguments with Arnett's perspective, including the view that many features of emerging adulthood are typical adolescent behaviors or, as suggested previously, manifestations of borderline psychopathology (see Chapter 7). The midcentury psychoanalytic commentators (Adatto 1966; Blos 1962) suggested that a narcissistic self-focus in late adolescence is essential to the developmental process, even if it is an impediment to full engagement in analytic treatment. These writers argued that dedicating energy to identity formation, personality integration, the quest for meaning, and the search for objects outside the family makes younger emerging adults too self-absorbed to engage in analyzing the transference until some of their developmental tasks have progressed. The presumably positive experience of another of Arnett's features, *wide-open possibilities*, may serve as a similar kind of resistance, because emerging adults can be so preoccupied with their real-life options, which may come with concrete changes in schedule, location, politics, and attitudes, that they do not have the attention span for a lengthy and laborious treatment process.

Finally, but most important, the developmental task of *role (or identity) exploration* would appear to be eminently compatible with psychoanalytic treatment; historically, the far briefer identity crisis first described by Erikson was seen to benefit from intensive treatment, even when stalled in a state of prolonged adolescence (see Chapter 3, "Late Adolescence"). The importance of the idea of emerging adulthood, however, is that it is not psychopathology or arrested development per se but a widespread generational phenomenon that appeared in the context of broad cultural shifts—changing economies; the disintegration of traditional institutions, pathways, and value systems; prolonged life expectancy; delayed childbearing; and many other factors. It is not the result of individual disturbance but rather a part of the contemporary normative developmental sequence. The role exploration that extends over a decade encompasses not only the various components of identity but also the meaning of adulthood in contemporary society, especially in the context of formerly discrete categories such as race, environment, truth, democracy, and gender. The current situation underscores the importance of the psychoanalytic capacities of seeing and listening and of being receptive to the realities of contemporary life. As the norms and pathways of prior generations vanish, the resulting prolongation of identity exploration is a societal phenomenon that does not invariably reflect a borderline diagnosis.

Arnett's (2004) original list of five distinguishing features of emerging adulthood (i.e., role exploration, instability, feeling in-between, self-focus, and wide-open possibilities) is helpful but does not fully inform the clinician about special dilemmas of emerging adulthood and the challenges arising from the interface of individual psychology, development, new cultural demands, and new ways of being in a changed world. The developmental agenda of emerging adulthood unfolds within the powerful and continuous transformations of techno-culture, the ubiquity of social media, and global society. The presence of this new phase is related to a radically altered culture that is alien to the parents' and sometimes the therapist's generation (although this is already changing as the first generation of emerging adults become parents and psychiatrists). The degree to which the culture is unfamiliar may lead to overpathologizing of normative behaviors and developmental challenges.

The Role of Transference and Countertransference in Emerging Adult Treatment

As suggested in this examination of psychoanalytically oriented treatments of emerging adults, the importance of the therapeutic relationship, originating in psychoanalytic theorizing, is an element in most forms of treatment, especially the one-on-one therapies described in this chapter. The vignettes about Diego and Jessica highlight the importance of the therapist's self-reflection and insights into the inevitable enactments that are the most visible indications that the relationship is now the "playing field" (Winnicott 1968, 1971). It is in the therapeutic space that the relationships, conflicts, and emotions of the patient are revealed through enactments, attitudes, dreams, and fantasies with the therapist-participant.

This does not mean that attention should not be paid to the important input and opportunities of the outside world. Emerging adults are eagerly acting in the world—leaving home; engaging in romantic and sexual relationships; experimenting with sexual preferences, gender identifications, and roles; exploring interests introduced by school, jobs, or peers; and participating in one type or another of youth culture. They are also acting on the world, driving technology, and seeking solutions to problems left by past generations.

Conclusion

We have highlighted the growing array of mental health services available to the vulnerable emerging adult population, from traditional talk therapy to apps, DBT groups, and more. Each of these has its usefulness and indications. Among these, we believe that psychoanalytic principles and insights provide a guide for therapists to understand and think about their patients, even if another treatment modality is used.

What makes a psychoanalytic clinical approach recognizable, specific, and preferable, whether it be psychoanalysis itself or psychoanalytically informed psychotherapy? Contemporary psychoanalysis is by no means a unitary entity, but there are certain basic ideas that despite variations are recognizable in a range of approaches. Indeed, Freud himself noted that the recognition of transference and resistance (Freud 1913/1958) and unconscious mental processes (Freud 1923–1925/1961) defines the psychoanalytic approach to mental life, and these elements are part of every theoretical school. The legacy of psychoanalytic thinking is represented in approaches that are evidence based and manualized, such as CBT (Mares 2022). The specific indications for an actual psychoanalytic treatment include a personality within the neurotic range, the capacity to reflect, and the ability to engage in the relationship with the therapist. The patient must be invested in the exploration of meanings, relationships, and mental processes. In turn, the therapist must be mindful of the developmental vulnerabilities characteristic of emerging adulthood and their ready recruitment by mental conflict (Abrams et al. 1999).

KEY POINTS

- Emerging adults constitute a psychiatrically vulnerable population at a crucial developmental moment when the onus of procuring medical care falls on them. Parents are no longer expected to monitor their well-being, make regular doctor's appointments, and hover over their care.

- Treatment use by emerging adults is often impeded by a lack of mental health literacy, stigma, self-stigma, and difficulty accessing suitable programs that understand and respect their special needs.

- Available treatments and services are struggling to provide care given the significant surge in major psychiatric illnesses, including personality disorders, substance use, psychosis, and suicidality, in the emerging adult population. Among these treatments are cognitive-behavioral therapy, dialectical behavior therapy, and transference-focused psychotherapy, which have shown demonstrable benefits in their target patient groups.

- College-based suicide prevention programs (e.g., those developed by the National Alliance on Mental Illness) are increasingly widespread and active in education, recognition, and support for both suicidal patients and their peers. These have yet to make a significant dent in the high rate of suicide among college students.

- Outreach and special treatment programs and mental health literacy training have been designed to engage young people, get help to those in need, and sustain their treatment.

- Psychoanalytically informed treatments can be invaluable during this extended active formation of personality encompassed by emerging adulthood.

References

Abrams S: The psychoanalytic process: the developmental and the integrative. Psychoanal Q 59(4):650–677, 1990 2267274

Abrams S, Neubauer PB, Solnit AJ: Coordinating the developmental and psychoanalytic processes: three case reports. Introduction. Psychoanal Study Child 54:19–24, 1999 10748626

Adatto CP: On the metamorphosis from adolescence into adulthood. J Am Psychoanal Assoc 14(3):485–509, 1966 6007436

Ammaniti M, Fontana A, Nicolais G: Borderline personality disorder in adolescence through the lens of the Interview of Personality Organization Processes in Adolescence (IPOP-A): clinical uses and implications. J Infant Child Adolesc Psychother 14(1):82–97, 2015

Arain M, Haque M, Johal L, et al: Maturation of the adolescent brain. Neuropsychiatr Dis Treat 9:449–461, 2013 23579318

Arlow JA: Stilted listening: psychoanalysis as discourse. Psychoanal Q 64(2):215–233, 1995 7652100

Arnett JJ: Emerging adulthood: a theory of development from the late teens through the twenties. Am Psychol 55(5):469–480, 2000 1084426

Arnett JJ: Emerging Adulthood: The Winding Road From the Late Teens Through the Twenties. New York, Oxford University Press, 2004

Arnett JJ: The evidence for generation we and against generation me. Emerg Adulthood 1(1):5–10, 2013

Aschbrenner KA, Brunette MF: The role of peers in health interventions for serious mental illness. Psychiatr Serv 69(5):497, 2018 29712540

Auchincloss EL: The Psychoanalytic Model of the Mind. Arlington, VA, American Psychiatric Publishing, 2015

Beck AT: Thinking and depression, I: idiosyncratic content and cognitive distortions. Arch Gen Psychiatry 9:324–333, 1963 14045261

Beck AT: Thinking and depression, II: theory and therapy. Arch Gen Psychiatry 10:561–571, 1964 14159256

Blanco C, Okuda M, Wright C, et al: Mental health of college students and their non-college-attending peers: results from the National Epidemiologic Study on Alcohol and Related Conditions. Arch Gen Psychiatry 65(12):1429–1437, 2008 19047530

Blos P: Intensive psychotherapy in relation to the various phases of the adolescent period. Am J Orthopsychiatry 32:901–910, 1962 13971819

Blos P: Character formation in adolescence. Psychoanal Study Child 23:245–263, 1968 5759022

Blum HP: Superego formation, adolescent transformation, and the adult neurosis. J Am Psychoanal Assoc 33(4):887–909, 1985 3843604

Bollas C: The Shadow of the Object: Psychoanalysis of the Unthought Known. London, Free Association Books, 1987

Bonar EE, Cunningham RM, Sweezea EC, et al: Piloting a brief intervention plus mobile boosters for drug use among emerging adults receiving emergency department care. Drug Alcohol Depend 221:108625, 2021 33631541

Brodsky BS, Cabaniss DL, Arbuckle M, et al: Teaching dialectical behavior therapy to psychiatry residents: the Columbia Psychiatry Residency DBT curriculum. Acad Psychiatry 41(1):10–15, 2017 27481266

Bronk KC: A grounded theory of the development of noble youth purpose. J Adolesc Res 27(1):78–109, 2012

Busch F: Creating a Psychoanalytic Mind: A Psychoanalytic Method and Theory. London, Routledge, 2013

Cheng HL, Kwan KL, Sevig T: Racial and ethnic minority college students' stigma associated with seeking psychological help: examining psychocultural correlates. J Couns Psychol 60(1):98–111, 2013 23356468

Cheng HL, McDermott RC, Lopez FG: Mental health, self-stigma, and help-seeking intentions among emerging adults: an attachment perspective. Couns Psychol 43(3):463–487, 2015

Cheng HL, Wang C, McDermott RC, et al: Self-stigma, mental health literacy, and attitudes toward seeking psychological help. J Couns Dev 96(1):64–74, 2018

Chused JF: Neutrality in the analysis of action-prone adolescents. J Am Psychoanal Assoc 38(3):679–704, 1990 2229881

DeFreitas SC, Crone T, DeLeon M, et al: Perceived and personal mental health stigma in Latino and African American college students. Front Public Health 6:49, 2018 29536000

Dziech BW: The costs of overpromising. Inside Higher Ed, October 8, 2019. Available at: https://www.insidehighered.com/views/2019/10/08/colleges-have-oversimplified-mental-health-crisis-and-overpromised-when-it-comes. Accessed September 25, 2021.

Ebert DD, Mortier P, Kaehlke F, et al: Barriers of mental health treatment utilization among first-year college students: first cross-national results from the WHO World Mental Health International College Student Initiative. Int J Methods Psychiatr Res 28(2):e1782, 2019 31069905

Emde RN: From adolescence to midlife: remodeling the structure of adult development. J Am Psychoanal Assoc 33:59–112, 1985

Ensink K, Biberdzic M, Normandin L, et al: A developmental psychopathology and neurobiological model of borderline personality disorder in adolescence. J Infant Child Adolesc Psychother 14(1):46–69, 2015

Erbe D, Eichert HC, Riper H, et al: Blending face-to-face and internet-based interventions for the treatment of mental disorders in adults: systematic review. J Med Internet Res 19(9):e306, 2017 28916506

Erikson EH: Childhood and Society. New York, WW Norton, 1950

Erikson EH: A Way of Looking at Things – Selected Papers From 1930 to 1980. Edited by Schlein S. New York, WW Norton, 1995

Escoll PJ: Psychoanalysis of young adults: an overview. Psychoanal Inq 7(1):5–30, 1987

Freud S: On beginning the treatment (further recommendations on the technique of psycho-analysis I) (1913), in The Standard Edition of the Complete Psychological Works of Sigmund Freud, Vol 12. Translated and edited by Strachey J. London, Hogarth Press, 1958, pp 121–144

Freud S: The resistances to psycho-analysis (1923–1925), in The Standard Edition of the Complete Psychological Works of Sigmund Freud, Vol 19. Translated and edited by Strachey J. London, Hogarth Press, 1961, pp 211–224

Fry R, Passel JS, Cohn D: A majority of young adults in the U.S. live with their parents for the first time since the Great Depression. Pew Research Center, September 4, 2020. Available at: https://www.pewresearch.org/fact-tank/2020/09/04/a-majority-of-young-adults-in-the-u-s-live-with-their-parents-for-the-first-time-since-the-great-depression. Accessed August 20, 2021.

Gilmore K: Is emerging adulthood a new developmental phase? J Am Psychoanal Assoc 67(4):625–653, 2019 31604388

Gilmore KJ, Meersand P: Normal Child and Adolescent Development: A Psychodynamic Primer. Washington, DC, American Psychiatric Publishing, 2014

Gonzalez JM, Alegria M, Prihoda TJ: How do attitudes toward mental health treatment vary by age, gender, and ethnicity/race in young adults? J Community Psychol 33(1):611–629, 2005 19921079

Grand S: A classic revisited: clinical and theoretical reflections on Stone's Widening scope of indications for psychoanalysis. J Am Psychoanal Assoc 43(3):741–764, 1995 8568153

Gulliver A, Griffiths KM, Christensen H: Perceived barriers and facilitators to mental health help-seeking in young people: a systematic review. BMC Psychiatry 10:113, 2010 21192795

Hunt J, Eisenberg D: Mental health problems and help-seeking behavior among college students. J Adolesc Health 46(1):3–10, 2010 20123251

Jacobs TJ, Chused JF: Psychoanalysis of the young adult: theory and technique. Panel report. J Am Psychoanal Assoc 35(1):175–187, 1987 3584817

Jørgensen CR: Invited essay: identity and borderline personality disorder. J Pers Disord 24(3):344–364, 2010 20545499

Kella S: The imperfect storm: college students and suicide. Harvard Political Review, August 10, 2021. Available at: https://harvardpolitics.com/the-imperfect-storm. Accessed September 22, 2021.

Kessler RC, Berglund P, Demler O, et al: Lifetime prevalence and age-of-onset distributions of DSM-IV disorders in the National Comorbidity Survey Replication. Arch Gen Psychiatry 62(6):593–602, 2005 15939837

Kitchener BA, Jorm AF: Mental health first aid training for the public: evaluation of effects on knowledge, attitudes and helping behavior. BMC Psychiatry 2:10, 2002 12359045

Knight R, Miller JM: Emerging adulthood: a developmental phase: an introduction to the section. Psychoanal Study Child 70(1):5–7, 2017

Kohn R, Saxena S, Levav I, et al: The treatment gap in mental health care. Bull World Health Organ 82(11):858–866, 2004 15640922

Lanz M, Serido J: Introduction to special issue financial and life instability: obstacles to and opportunities for emerging adult development and future well-being. Emerg Adulthood 8(6):439–442, 2020

Ledford H: Who exactly counts as an adolescent? Nature 554(7693):429–432, 2018 29469127

Leech T, Dorstyn D, Taylor A, et al: Mental health apps for adolescents and young adults: a systematic review of randomised controlled trials. Child Youth Serv Rev 127:106073, 2021

Livesey CM, Rostain AL: Involving parents/family in treatment during the transition from late adolescence to young adulthood: rationale, strategies, ethics, and legal issues. Child Adolesc Psychiatr Clin N Am 26(2):199–216, 2017 28314451

Macrodimitris SD, Hamilton KE, Backs-Dermott BJ, et al: CBT basics: a group approach to teaching fundamental cognitive-behavioral skills. J Cogn Psychother 24(2):132–146, 2010

Mares L: Unconscious processes in psychoanalysis, CBT, and schema therapy. J Psychother Integr 32(4):443–452, 2022

Mathison LA: Internalized stigma of mental illness: more than a scale. Stigma Health 4(2):165–169, 2019

May JM, Richardi TM, Barth KS: Dialectical behavior therapy as treatment for borderline personality disorder. Ment Health Clin 6(2):62–67, 2016 29955449

McLaughlin JT: Clinical and theoretical aspects of enactment. J Am Psychoanal Assoc 39(3):595–614, 1991 1939990

McLean KC, Shucard H, Syed M: Applying the master narrative framework to gender identity development in emerging adulthood. Emerg Adulthood 5:93–105, 2017

National Alliance on Mental Illness: NAMI on campus: because mental health matters. Available at: https://www.nami.org/get-involved/nami-on-campus. Accessed December 8, 2022.

Normandin L, Ensink K, Kernberg OF: Transference-focused psychotherapy for borderline adolescents: a neurobiologically informed psychodynamic psychotherapy. J Infant Child Adolesc Psychother 14(1):98–110, 2015

Osuch EA, Vingilis E, Fisman S, et al: Early intervention in mood and anxiety disorders: the first episode mood and anxiety program (FEMAP). Healthc Q 18:42–49, 2016

Osuch E, Vingilis E, Summerhurst C, et al: Process evaluation of a treatment program for mood and anxiety disorders among emerging adults: preentry factors, engagement, and outcomes. Psychiatr Serv 70(3):211–218, 2019 30821209

Perrin A: Mobile technology and home broadband 2021. Pew Research Center, June 3, 2021. Available at: https://www.pewresearch.org/internet/2021/06/03/mobile-technology-and-home-broadband-2021. Accessed August 15, 2021.

Plakun E: Treatment resistance and psychodynamic psychiatry: concepts psychiatry needs from psychoanalysis. Psychodyn Psychiatry 40(2):183–209, 2012 23006116

Reyes-Ortega MA, Miranda EM, Fresán A, et al: Clinical efficacy of a combined acceptance and commitment therapy, dialectical behavioural therapy, and functional analytic psychotherapy intervention in patients with borderline personality disorder. Psychol Psychother 93(3):474–489, 2020 31246370

Rosenberg L: Bridging the gap between adolescence and adulthood: the challenges of emerging adults. J Behav Health Serv Res 43(4):518–520, 2016 27678111

Sawyer SM, Azzopardi PS, Wickremarathne D, et al: The age of adolescence. Lancet Child Adolesc Health 2(3):223–228, 2018 30169257

Schare ML, Wyatt KP: On the evolving nature of exposure therapy. Behav Modif 37:243–256, 2013

Schechter M, Herbstman B, Ronningstam E, et al: Emerging adults, identity development, and suicidality: implications for psychoanalytic psychotherapy. Psychoanal Study Child 71(1):20–39, 2018

Schroeder J, Wilkes C, Rowan K, et al: Pocket skills: a conversational mobile web app to support dialectical behavioral therapy, in Proceedings of the 2018 CHI Conference on Human Factors in Computing Systems, Montreal, QC, Canada, April 21–26, 2018. Paper No 398. New York, Association for Computing Machinery, 2018, pp 1–15

Shim RS, Compton MT, Rust G, et al: Race-ethnicity as a predictor of attitudes toward mental health treatment seeking. Psychiatr Serv 60(10):1336–1341, 2009 19797373

Smith DC, Cleeland L, Middleton A, et al: Willingness and appropriateness of peers participating in emerging adults' substance misuse treatment. J Subst Abuse Treat 45(1):148–154, 2013 23462152

Springer KS, Tolin DF: The Big Book of Exposures: Innovative, Creative and Effective CBT-Based Exposures for Treating Anxiety-Related Disorders. Oakland, CA, New Harbinger Publications, 2020

Strenger C: The Designed Self: Psychoanalysis and Contemporary Identities. New York, Routledge, 2004

Sugarman A: Mentalization, insightfulness, and therapeutic action: the importance of mental organization. Int J Psychoanal 87(Pt 4):965–987, 2006 16877247

Suicide Prevention Resource Center: Scope of the problem: suicide by age. 2021. Available at: https://sprc.org/about-suicide/scope-of-the-problem/suicide-by-age. Accessed October 10, 2021.

Swenson CR: DBT Principles in Action: Acceptance, Change, and Dialectics. New York, Guilford, 2016

Temkin AB, Schild J, Falk A, et al: Mobile apps for youth anxiety disorders: a review of the evidence and forecast of future innovations. Prof Psychol Res Pr 51(4):400–413, 2020

Torous J, Nicholas J, Larsen ME, et al: Clinical review of user engagement with mental health smartphone apps: evidence, theory and improvements. Evid Based Ment Health 21(3):116–119, 2018 29871870

Tucker JR, Hammer JH, Vogel DL, et al: Disentangling self-stigma: are mental illness and help-seeking self-stigmas different? J Couns Psychol 60(4):520–531, 2013 23815629

Turkle S: Whither psychoanalysis in computer culture? Psychoanal Psychol 21(1):16–30, 2004

Tuttle B: Here's how many students could save $50,000 on college—but aren't. Time Magazine, April 7, 2014. Available at: https://www.time.com/52020/heres-how-many-students-could-save-50000-on-college-but-arent. Accessed December 7, 2022.

Twenge JM: Overwhelming evidence for generation me: a reply to Arnett. Emerg Adulthood 1(1):21–26, 2013

Walker JS: A theory of change for positive developmental approaches to improving outcomes among emerging adults with serious mental health conditions. J Behav Health Serv Res 42(2):131–149, 2015 25694066

Winnicott DW: Playing: its theoretical status in the clinical situation. Int J Psychoanal 49(4):591–599, 1968 4180041

Winnicott DW: Playing and Reality. Harmondsworth, UK, Pelican Books, 1971

Wright JH, Thase ME, Beck AT: Cognitive-behavior therapy, in The American Psychiatric Publishing Textbook of Psychiatry, 6th Edition. Edited by Hales RE, Yudofsky SC, Roberts LW. Arlington, VA, American Psychiatric Publishing, 2014, pp 1119–1160

Yeomans FE, Delaney JC, Levy KN: Behavioral activation in TFP: the role of the treatment contract in transference-focused psychotherapy. Psychotherapy (Chic) 54(3):260–266, 2017 28922005

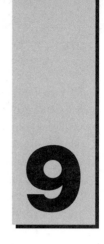

Conclusion

Standing too close to the great changes that have already taken
place or are beginning to, and without a glimmering of the
future that is being shaped, we ourselves are at a loss as to the
significance of the impressions which press upon us and as to
the value of the judgments which we form.

Freud (1915/1957, p. 275)

The concept of emerging adulthood is more than two decades
old and by now securely ensconced in contemporary thinking about young
adult development. Developmental science is indebted to Jeffrey Arnett for
his important insight into developmental progression during the passage
from ages 18 to 29 years in the twenty-first century. His astute observations
about shifts in society and fundamental changes in the way young people
think about themselves and their futures alerted the scientific community
to a phenomenon in need of study and explication. Despite the massive accumulation of new data, there have been controversies around its premises,
gaps in the research, and most importantly, orthodoxy in theory that has not
been modified since its inception. As psychoanalytic thinkers, we find ourselves returning to a few key questions and concerns about the theory, the
research, and the literature on emerging adulthood.

Why Do Away With Late Adolescence?

One of our objections to the formulation of Arnett's theory is that, in its original form, it amounted to rebranding a familiar phase, historically considered
late adolescence (from 18 to 23 or 24 years old), with a new name. As research

into the emerging adult phenomenon accumulated over the years, the range was extended, albeit inconsistently, to 18–29 years old, with little justification or discussion. Although we believe that this new range is in fact crucial to the concept, for reasons we discuss shortly, the unfortunate legacy of Arnett's original age range is that it focused the research on college student subjects and diminished efforts to study the less accessible 24- to 29-year-old cohort. From our point of view, this creates another inconsistency: late adolescent experience, as embodied by the college student, is now understood to characterize the entire 11–12 years of emerging adulthood, washing out all the consequential changes that take place between ages 18 and 30, perhaps especially 24–29.

Moreover, the choice to eliminate the term *late adolescence* and incorporate its time frame into the unitary stretch of emerging adulthood is increasingly challenged by new discoveries. Although taken for granted by today's emerging adulthood scholars, this assumption is at odds not only with the historical position of the "father of adolescence," G. Stanley Hall (1904), and psychoanalytic thinkers from the second half of the twentieth century (Blos 1962; Erikson 1968; E. Laufer 1986; M. Laufer 1986) onward but also with contemporary pediatric viewpoints. The latter have reformulated adolescent parameters based on new data indicating physical, including neuroanatomical, development until the mid- to late 20s, in addition to the similar extension of typical adolescent psychosocial features (such as the sustained salience of the peer group and risky behaviors). Such findings are used to support suggestions, for example in *The Lancet Child & Adolescent Health* (Sawyer et al. 2018), *Neuropsychiatric Disease and Treatment* (Arain et al. 2013), and *Nature* (Ledford 2018), that the end point of adolescent development should be extended to age 24. This aligns with our idea that late adolescence continues into the college years and that the inflection point Arnett used as the onset of emerging adulthood better serves as the onset of late adolescence.

From a different vantage point, Erikson's (1968) seminal work on identity formation in late adolescence highlighted the college experience as the sine qua non institutional psychosocial moratorium, a 4-year playground dedicated to identity explorations. Even though most late adolescents in the United States get only 1 or 2 years of that experience, college represents a unique interlude in which young people are halfway released from the role of the child and halfway granted autonomy and self-determination while still under the watchful eye of a distant authority. In the safety of college, young people learn, some for the first time, to monitor their daily functioning—to get up for class, to do their assignments, to negotiate a new social world, and to pursue their interests—and in many cases, to handle socioeconomic, class, sexual, and racial differences that require interpersonal finesse, all while being housed and fed by the institution. College life, however brief, creates a protected environment in which to connect with others sharing the moment, despite their vast differences. Late adolescents in this setting are free to choose their own crowd and their own academic and extracurricular agenda, and they are compelled to independently manage an array of interpersonal circumstances that require judgment, intuition, emotional awareness, and a new level of acceptance and interest in differences. The predictable foil created by the closely hovering presence of parents and teachers in mid-adolescence is attenuated in the college setting. Absent this easy adversary, late adolescents enlarge their perspectives, become more self-reflective, and often bring their teenage rebellion into social movements that address the larger culture.

Even without any college exposure, many high school graduates engage in some version of identity exploration and individuation, often by trial and error, moving from job to job, yo-yoing between their childhood home and independent or shared domiciles, and mingling with an expanded cast of characters. For many, youth culture offers a degree of exploration and experimentation within its purview while satisfying typical late adolescent predilections, like peer focus, risky activities, and resistance to the adult world. Despite the many commonalities in participants, differences in background and origins are usually sufficient to make youth cultural gatherings an opportunity to mingle with unfamiliar others. Like college, but far less structured and conventional, these groups allow intermediate steps in the journey toward complete autonomy.

Today's late adolescents are keenly aware that identity exploration will continue through the 20s. They anticipate an extended, open-ended period of exploration and experimentation without commitment as part of their foreseeable futures. For example, most college students graduate with no premeditated plan for life (McGraw Hill 2017); they often feel uncertain, unprepared, and undecided about steps that may lead to a viable career. Many are still unsure of significant identity components and their own moral convictions. Similarly, working youths do not necessarily identify with their first jobs or industry sectors and are reluctant to get stuck in a work trajectory that limits future potential. Both college students and working youths may require several years of trial and correction to discover a viable identity. Rockiness in work and social development in the mid- to late 20s among college graduates and working emerging adults alike often strikes the parent generation as misdirected, confused, and ill-fated. This group is still engaged in identity work at a time of life when it was already resolved in previous generations.

In our opinion, the continuation of identity exploration, instability, and self-focus into the late 20s is the real signature experience of emerging adulthood. Among the 24- to 30-year-olds, we see most clearly the new juxtaposition of personality development set loose from traditional pathways and traditional adult roles, now in lively and creative interaction with a new cultural surround. Continued identity work requires that the journey through late emerging adulthood be sustained by sufficient personality stability to permit flexibility and adaptability. Successful late emerging adults have the capacity to maintain a degree of fluidity, steadied by slowly evolving identity integration, growing superego reliability, a sense of purpose, and the capacity for self-reflection and perspective-taking throughout the 20s, not necessarily tied to any fixed adult outcome. This is the emerging adult adaptation to the radical changes and opportunities that constitute twenty-first-century Western culture.

Folding the late adolescent experience into a decade of emerging adulthood may inadvertently diminish the importance of its novel extension and homogenize the vast developmental transformations that occur between high school graduation and age 29 years. Arnett's original cohort of college students, mostly late adolescents, have mistakenly become the exemplars of a period in which the real differences from the past are present in nascent form but only flower in their futures. The tilt toward the first half of this period in the literature reinforces the idea of a unitary developmental period, thereby obscuring the complexity of the change processes that occur in it. Furthermore, it deflects attention from what is most new in the concept of emerging adulthood; the tasks of identity formation and the formulation of the adult plan (Arnett 2018) are not resolved in late adolescence but go on to occupy the mental lives of people throughout their 20s. (This extension has an effect on late adolescents because that age group is under no real pressure, at least by peer expectations, to get settled.) The societal factors contributing to this shift come from a variety of changes, including the ascendance of a knowledge economy that requires new levels of education and skills, the explosion of the digital world and the proliferation of new roles associated with it, the shift in women's position in the workplace and culture, advances in medical science and technology that allow the postponement of marriage and child-rearing, and the extension of life expectancy.

Is Emerging Adulthood Primarily a Time Frame or a Specific Set of Features That Highlight the Novel Way It Is Now Traversed?

If we put aside the question of late adolescence, another significant concern about the categorization of emerging adulthood as applied in the research arises from a fundamental lack of clarity: is the cohort simply defined by age or by characteristic features? If the subjects are deemed emerging adults solely because they fall within the age range of 18–29, then the specific idea about the new way of traversing the passage gets obscured; in contrast, if the category is determined by its features, then emerging adulthood is present only when individuals manifest at least some of the five features. To elucidate the boundaries of this new phase, Arnett (2016) stated, "Emerging adulthood can be considered to exist wherever there is a period of at least several years between the end of adolescence—meaning the attainment of physical and sexual maturity and the completion of secondary school—and the entry into stable adult roles in love and work" (p. 234). (As noted in Chapter 8, "Therapeutic Modalities in the Treatment of Emerging Adults," the current position among contributors to the pediatric literature is that development is not completed until the mid-20s.) Arnett's statement, which is intended to clarify parameters and draw attention to the time delay in adult roles, rests on two problematic assumptions we have alluded to already: that adolescence ends at age 18 in coordination with the national kindergarten–grade 12 educational mandate and that adulthood is signaled by entry into traditional adult roles. The end point in Arnett's formulation underscores that his criteria for the termination of emerging adulthood are unchanged from the centuries-old traditional markers of adulthood, even if they are considerably delayed by widespread demographic trends (e.g., later marriage) and the demands of a changed culture. Despite claims that Arnett's "established adulthood" (Mehta et al. 2020) is a distinct phase, it is mostly in regard to the delay of traditional achievements into the 30s that it departs from standard conceptualizations. However, as Arnett noted in the first introduction of the concept of emerging adulthood (Arnett 2000), the equation of traditional markers with the onset of adulthood is strongly contested by emerging adults themselves. The historical linking of those so-called adult markers with an actual conviction of adulthood needs updating: adulthood now requires a new concept.

Does the use of Arnett's five features provide a better guide for categorizing and characterizing emerging adults? The widespread use of the reified five features as the pillars of emerging adult experience has come under question by Arnett himself. In an article addressing the problem, Arnett (2016) insisted, "I never proposed that those five features would prove to be universal features of emerging adulthood. On the contrary, I emphasized that there would surely be variations in the paths that people would take through emerging adulthood, depending on cultural context and economic circumstances" (p. 228). The five features were further demoted in Arnett and Mitra's (2020) publication "Are the Features of Emerging Adulthood Developmentally Distinctive? A Comparison of Ages 18–60 in the United States." Using the familiar survey methodology, these authors confirm the incidence of the features in 18- to 29-year-olds but also document the statistically significant endorsement of all but one of the same features (with the exclusion of feeling in-between) in age groups up to 60. Such findings add a new level of uncertainty to the specificity of emerging adulthood: age range and characteristic features are apparently neither intrinsically linked nor unique to the cohort.

Does Emerging Adulthood Really Exist in the Forgotten Half?

The question of whether emerging adulthood really exists in the forgotten half, which has plagued the field from the beginning, is related to the confusion over time frame versus developmental experience. Arnett insisted that the theory of emerging adulthood does not exclusively apply to the privileged, white, affluent college student; it is applicable to other classes, racial/ethnic groups, and youths in other countries. His response to the frequent critique that his theory pertains to only one segment of the population is to say "one stage, many paths....There are many possible paths through any life stage, with variations not only by social class but also by gender, ethnicity, sexual orientation, and cultural context" (Arnett 2016, p. 234). Once again, we come to a somewhat elusive position. On the one hand, emerging adulthood is a rich developmental life stage occupying the lengthened interval between the end of schooling and the assumption of adult roles, in which role exploration is prominent and optimism is high. On the other hand, some populations pass through these years as emerging adults but follow paths devoid of experimentation and developmental opportunities. For example, do young people who must earn a living, support a family, and/or abandon dreams of graduate schooling because of finances have less of the developmental experience than more privileged cohorts? Arnett's rejoinder is that they may have a shorter interval than their affluent peers, but they still take longer to get jobs and get married than their equivalent cohort of half a century earlier, thereby ensuring that they have an emerging adulthood. But does the mere addition of a few years of struggle make this a true emerging adult experience? To us, the true experience must include the opportunity to experiment; to feel uncommitted; to try anything; or to be guided by predilections, consolidating interests, or whim— all in pace with the transformations of society.

How Does Emerging Adulthood End?

Another unsolved puzzle of emerging adulthood is how it comes to an end—intrapsychically, interpersonally, and in the eyes of society. To us, it diminishes the significance of Arnett's important insight to suggest that emerging adulthood ends with the same old "established adulthood" (Mehta et al. 2020), only later. In fact, we believe that adulthood is in a process of transformation and that it has already proved to be very different.

Throughout development, young people are socialized to develop fantasies and internalized representations of adulthood as reflected in their parents, families, and culture; such representations undergo their own developmental progression in the mind, evolving through the phases shaped by maturing socioemotional, cognitive, and physical capacities; intrapsychic conflicts; and experience. Today's young people, even as early as grade school, see a different kind of adulthood as represented by their heroes, not only teen idols, although these are plentiful, but more likely late emerging adults who have achieved recognition in their areas of interest and are already forging an adulthood different from the past model. The rising generation of young emerging adults see their open-ended pathway and understand its requirement that they create and follow their own vision. Although we understand that the use of the formulation "transition to adulthood" diminishes the legitimacy of the phase of emerging adulthood as one of "becoming" rather than a state of "being" (Arnett 2014), the transition terminology identifies a fundamental quality of development: all development is transitional and emerging. Emerging adults are preoccupied with their lives in the here and now, but every year that passes allows their own meanings of adulthood to mature and become clearer. Over the entire course of this lengthy period, they are, consciously and unconsciously, grappling with their notions of what lies ahead. But what adulthood are they seeing and imagining? According to cultural historian James Davison Hunter (2009), "Adulthood is undergoing just as significant a transformation as youth, and these are inextricably linked to each other."

Emerging adults themselves endorse certain attitudes and capacities that signify the new adulthood:

- The ability to make decisions on their own
- Financial independence
- The ability to control their emotions
- Consideration for others
- The establishment of an equal relationship with their parents (Wood et al. 2018)

In contrast to the old markers, these accomplishments are almost entirely socioemotional and personal, without reference to societal roles like job, domicile, spouse, and parent.

In Chapter 1, "A Brief Review of Developmental Theory," we reviewed developmental theories and their conceptualization of how development happens. What drives the process, and how does it work? How can young people traverse this prolonged interval, make good developmental use of it, and emerge on the other side with this list of capacities in place? This process is usually termed *maturation*, a word applied to the manner in which all entities, from trees to stars to humans, achieve the adult form. Traditionally, many theories of human development simply relied on adult roles as maturing agents, but the achievement of those roles is not necessarily a goal for the new version of adulthood, now delinked from traditional markers.

In developmental science, the concept of maturation has not achieved consensus (Rocque 2015), in part because, like most things developmental, it occurs in the context of culture and involves the ongoing evolution of many interfacing systems that may be uneven, idiosyncratic, and in some instances deficient. Consistent with the ascendant scientific paradigm, the leading contemporary approach to maturation is the *integrated maturation theory*, which defines maturation according to nonlinear systems as the interface of multiple domains, including the psychosocial arena, adult social roles, identity formation, civic responsibility, and neurocognitive development (McCuish and Gushue 2022). This multisystem model of maturation suggests that a confluence of factors—neurological, psychosocial, environmental, and others—contribute to a capacity for more measured self-regulation and socioemotional intelligence, including considering other perspectives, recognizing consequences, taking personal responsibility for decisions and actions, and maintaining temperance (McCuish and Gushue 2022).

A frequently cited component of the maturational process is the evolution of *executive function*, a capacity that appears in early childhood and evolves through the 20s. A comprehensive review of the literature on this topic (Bagetta and Alexander 2016) noted its widespread use but lack of crisp definitional clarity and consensus. These authors distilled various attempts to characterize executive function to the following: "1) it guides action and behaviors essential to aspects of learning and everyday human performance tasks; 2) it contributes to the monitoring or regulation of such tasks; and 3) it pertains not only to the cognitive domain, but also socioemotional and behavioral domains of human performance" (Bagetta and Alexander 2016, p. 22).

Executive capacities such as the ability to arrive at flexible and adaptive solutions, ready use of a preexisting knowledge base, and reflection on context and future consequences (Prencipe et al. 2011) require both a level of mental development and environmental circumstances that allow for relatively cool contemplation, in contrast to the emotionally fraught or stressful states that can derail executive function. Similarly, the development of executive function requires manageable levels of internal and environmental stimuli; it is neurodevelopmentally constructed according to its use, beginning early in childhood, and available for activation over the course of a lifetime (Rueda and Paz-Alonso 2013). Genetic correlates (including neuroanatomical development) dynamically interface with environmental factors, and their mutual interactions lead to a range of phenotypes with different potentials (Weil 1978; Zelazo 2013). In early life, executive function is manifested by essential capacities such as self-regulation, multitasking, and delay tolerance, all essential for success in school and family life. With development, executive function comes to serve many systems (Zelazo and Carlson 2012) in the full range of arenas—advanced schooling, interpersonal relationships, sustained competitive endeavors, and so on. The evolution of this multifaceted function in the late 20s allows the emerging adult to disengage from the characteristic auto-processing of adolescence: to reflectively reprocess (Zelazo 2015) information, conflicts, or problems and to rely increasingly on the mobilization of reliable thinking, problem-solving, and complexity management, even in settings with high emotional valence. In its fully developed form, it is harnessed to monitoring, regulating, and integrating human experience and performance in cognitive, socioemotional, and behavioral domains; these developments lend a quality of thoughtfulness and self-regulation that is observable as a reliable sign of a maturing individual.

In addition to these evolving ego capacities, the subjective conviction of adulthood, like most aspects of identity, relies on recognition by others (Blatterer 2007; Erikson 1968). In the absence of agreed-on markers and scripts that can be checked off like the historical to-do list, the quest for recognition by others may seem daunting. Late adolescents' attraction to their preferred youth culture shapes their immediate goals and provides reinforcement by the peer group. But over the course of emerging adulthood, they rely less on scaffolding by their peers; they instead seek signposts that link them to the adulthood they envision. As they contemplate their evolving representations of adulthood and juxtapose their particular assets, possibilities, achievements, potentialities, personality features, and realities (such as gender, race, financial resources, minority status, or privilege) with their idea of adulthood, they are able to have some control over the adulthood they intend to inhabit. The outcome of this process ideally is a bespoke adulthood, including meaningful indicators that the surrounding culture can honor, even if entirely novel. And although we agree that emerging adulthood cannot be reduced to a mere transition, it does form the crucial preamble in which maturation to a conscious and individualized version of adulthood occurs.

What does this look like in terms of psychodynamic conceptualizations of mental life? Maturation requires a stable and reliable superego, which plays an important role in the establishment of consistent self-regulation of impulses and mood and the capacity for measured action, for moral convictions, for the management of desires in the light of conscience, and for responsible and compassionate relationships. It requires a well-integrated ego, with the smooth operation of high-level defenses, anxiety tolerance, and relatedness accompanied by an acceptance of flaws and deficiencies in the self and others, a capacity to manage ambivalence, and an ability to maintain interpersonal boundaries. Maturation and evolving executive capacities allow emerging adults to take perspective, recognize their own subjectivity, and consider the perspectives of others, thereby applying a sophisticated version of theory of mind. These qualities also allow for the honest measure of one's dreams against one's real capacities and actual environmental provision, with necessary modification or renunciation of some of those dreams with equanimity. These capacities are not uniform in any one individual, but the possession of even a few can be enough to demonstrate adulthood to the outside world.

The implication is that the achievement of adulthood is now individualized and idiosyncratic. But the accumulation of individual testimonies suggests that there are a few consistent themes, some of which may seem like the old concrete markers but actually go beyond them: First are the capacities for flexibility and adaptability such that new circumstances are neither discouraging nor insurmountable. Then there are the familiar accomplishments, with added socioemotional features: making a living and feeling a commitment to contributing to the upkeep of self and family; doing work that requires dedication, expertise, and experience; shouldering responsibility in the workplace; having children with the conscious awareness of lifelong obligation—these are some of the moments that are accompanied by a keen consciousness of adulthood. In such moments, the internal balance of autonomy and relatedness (Luyten et al. 2019), the confidence in self-regulation and the conviction of one's worth to others, the readiness to adapt as required by circumstances (including natural and humanmade catastrophes and personal trauma), and the willingness to reflect while maintaining perspective provide a sense of agency and value. Such may be the requirements of the new adulthood, one that is self-contained, portable, subject to self-scrutiny, and ready to change as necessary. And while still just a glimmering, it will clearly be different from the twentieth-century stereotype.

KEY POINTS

- Emerging adulthood is a contemporary phenomenon referring to the extended interval between mandatory schooling and the achievement of adulthood.

- The developmental tasks of identity formation and role experimentation occupy this interval.

- This developmental modification has occurred in a new cultural era that is fully mediated and driven by an informational and technological economy.

- The achievement of adulthood rests on the maturation of executive function, emotional regulation, invested object relations, and a personal plan rather than on the traditional markers of adulthood: completion of education, entrance into the workforce, financial independence, marriage, and children.

References

Arain M, Haque M, Johal L, et al: Maturation of the adolescent brain. Neuropsychiatr Dis Treat 9:449–461, 2013 23579318

Arnett JJ: Emerging adulthood: a theory of development from the late teens through the twenties. Am Psychol 55(5):469–480, 2000 1084426

Arnett JJ: Emerging Adulthood: The Winding Road From the Late Teens Through the Twenties, 2nd Edition. New York, Oxford University Press, 2014

Arnett JJ: Does emerging adulthood theory apply across social classes? National data on a persistent question. Emerg Adulthood 4(4):227–235, 2016

Arnett JJ: Happily stressed: the complexity of well-being in midlife. J Adult Dev 25(4):270–278, 2018

Arnett JJ, Mitra D: Are the features of emerging adulthood developmentally distinctive? A comparison of ages 18–60 in the United States. Emerg Adulthood 8(5):412–419, 2020

Bagetta P, Alexander PA: Conceptualization and operationalization of executive function. Mind Brain Educ 10(1):10–33, 2016

Blatterer H: Adulthood: the contemporary redefinition of a social category. Sociological Research Online 12(4):1–11, 2007

Blos P: On Adolescence: A Psychoanalytic Interpretation. New York, Free Press of Glencoe, 1962

Erikson EH: Identity: Youth and Crisis. New York, WW Norton, 1968

Freud S: Thoughts for the times on war and death (1915), Chapter 1: The Disillusionment of War, in The Standard Edition of the Complete Psychological Works of Sigmund Freud, Vol 14. Translated and edited by Strachey J. London, Hogarth Press, 1957, pp 275–288

Hall GS: Adolescence in literature biography and history, in Adolescence: Its Psychology and Its Relationship to Physiology, Anthropology, Sociology, Sex, Crime, Religion and Education, Vol 1. New York, D Appleton and Company, 1904, pp 513–589

Hunter JD: Wither adulthood? The Hedgehog Review, Spring 2009. Available at: https://hedgehogreview.com/issues/youth-culture/articles/wither-adulthood. Accessed November 30, 2022.

Laufer E: Psychoanalytic psychotherapy as an intervention with university students. Psychoanal Psychother 2(2):111–119, 1986

Laufer M: Adolescence and psychosis. Int J Psychoanal 67(Pt 3):367–372, 1986 3744692

Ledford H: Who exactly counts as an adolescent? Nature 554(7693):429–432, 2018 29469127

Luyten P, Campbell C, Fonagy P: Reflections on the contributions of Sidney J. Blatt: the dialectical needs for autonomy, relatedness, and the emergence of epistemic trust. Psychoanalytic Psychology 36(4):328–334, 2019

McCuish EC, Gushue K: Maturation as a promoter of change in features of psychopathy between adolescence and emerging adulthood. Youth Violence Juv Justice 20(1):3–21, 2022

McGraw Hill: New survey: fewer than half of college seniors feel "very prepared" for a career. May 8, 2017. Available at: https://www.mheducation.com/news-media/press-releases/2017-future-workforce-survey.html. Accessed December 8, 2022.

Mehta CM, Arnett JJ, Palmer CG, et al: Established adulthood: a new conception of ages 30 to 45. Am Psychol 75(4):431–444, 2020 32378940

Prencipe A, Kesek A, Cohen J, et al: Development of hot and cool executive function during the transition to adolescence. J Exp Child Psychol 108(3):621–637, 2011 21044790

Rocque M: The lost concept: the (re) emerging link between maturation and desistance from crime. Criminology and Criminal Justice 15(3):340–360, 2015

Rueda MR, Paz-Alonso PM: Executive function and emotional development, in Encyclopedia on Early Childhood Development. Edited by Tremblay RE, Boivin M, Peters RDeV. Montreal, QC, Canada, CEECD, 2013, pp 17–21

Sawyer SM, Azzopardi PS, Wickremarathne D, et al: The age of adolescence. Lancet Child Adolesc Health 2(3):223–228, 2018 30169257

Weil AP: Maturational variations and genetic-dynamic issues. J Am Psychoanal Assoc 26(3):461–491, 1978 7017734

Wood D, Crapnell T, Lau L, et al: Emerging adulthood as a critical stage in the life course, in Handbook of Life Course Health Development. Edited by Halfon N, Forrest CB, Lerner RM, et al. New York, Springer, 2018, pp 123–143

Zelazo PD: Reflections on the development of executive function: commentary on Knapp and Morton, Munakata et al., Rueda and Paz-Alonso, Benson and Sabbagh, Hook et al., and Blair, in Encyclopedia on Early Childhood Development. Edited by Tremblay RE, Boivin M, Peters RDeV. Montreal, QC, Canada, CEECD, 2013, pp 42–46

Zelazo PD: Executive function: reflection, iterative reprocessing, complexity, and the developing brain. Dev Rev 38:55–68, 2015

Zelazo PD, Carlson SM: Hot and cool executive function in childhood and adolescence: development and plasticity. Child Dev Perspect 6(4):354–360, 2012

Index